Clinical Nursing Practices

For Churchill Livingstone:

Commissioning editor: Ellen Green
Project development editor: Mairi McCubbin
Project manager: Valerie Burgess
Project controller: Derek Robertson
Design direction: Judith Wright
Sales promotion executive: Hilary Brown

Clinical Nursing Practices

Elizabeth M Jamieson RGN ONC RCT RNT

Janice M McCall BA RGN RCNT

Rona Blythe SRN SCM RCT RNT

Lesley A Whyte BA MPhil RGN DN RNT

Lecturers, Department of Nursing and Community Health, Glasgow Caledonian University

THIRD EDITION

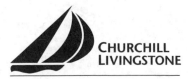

CHURCHILL
LIVINGSTONE

NEW YORK EDINBURGH LONDON MADRID MELBOURNE SAN FRANCISCO AND TOKYO 1997

CHURCHILL LIVINGSTONE
Medical Division of Pearson Professional Limited

Distributed in the United States of America by Churchill
Livingstone, 650 Avenue of the Americas, New York,
N.Y. 10011, and by associated companies, branches and
representatives throughout the world.

First edition 1988
Second edition 1992
Third edition 1997

ISBN 0 443 05290 5

British Library Cataloguing in Publication Data
A catalogue record for this book is available from the British
Library.

Library of Congress Cataloging in Publication Data
A catalog record for this book is available from the Library of
Congress.

Medical knowledge is constantly changing. As new
information becomes available, changes in treatment,
procedures, equipment and the use of drugs become necessary.
The editors/authors/contributors and the publishers have, as
far as it is possible, taken care to ensure that the information
given in this text is accurate and up to date. However, readers
are strongly advised to confirm that information, especially
with regard to drug usage, complies with the latest legislation
and standards of practice.

The
publisher's
policy is to use
**paper manufactured
from sustainable forests**

Produced through Longman Malaysia, PP

Contents

Preface to the third edition

Since the first edition of this book was published in 1988, there have been significant changes in the environment in which nursing intervention occurs – changes that are reflected in this new edition. The implementation of Project 2000 has resulted in greater emphasis on nurse education, and on preparing nurses of the future to work both in the community and in an institutional setting (DoH 1989[1]). In this third edition, we have, therefore, encouraged the reader to look at the practices in relation to caring for patients at home or in an institution, which may include a hospital, residential home, nursing home or hospice. For greater clarity, we have changed some of the headings and adapted others. A section on 'Patient education: key points' has been added to each practice, and is described in more detail on page *xiv* of the Introduction. Although the book has been considerably updated, the educational philosophy underpinning it remains unchanged.

We are grateful for the help of Winifred Logan, who acted as consultant for the first two editions of the book. Win has now retired, but we will always appreciate her professional expertise, her insistence on well-researched and referenced material, her wonderful command of the English language and her meticulous attention to detail. We enjoyed a very happy working relationship and will always value her friendship.

For this edition, we have asked our colleague Lesley Whyte to join us, and have benefited from her expertise on nursing in the community. Lesley has a joint appointment as a Lecturer in the Department of Nurisng and Community Health at Glasgow Caledonian University, and as a District Nursing Sister with the Central Scotland Health Care Trust.

We hope that the updated material, to reflect nursing trends, will ensure that this book will continue to be useful for registered nurses, as well as student nurses.

1997

E.M.J.
J.M.Mc.
R.B.
L.A.W.

1. Department of Health 1989 Caring for people. Community care agenda. HMSO, London

Introduction

Over a hundred years ago, Florence Nightingale argued that good nursing must contain a strong 'thinking' as well as a 'doing' component. 'Observation tells us the facts, reflection tells us the meaning of the fact . . . observation tells us how the patient is, reflection tells us what is to be done'.

Unfortunately, many people still think of nursing as a series of tasks. They do not realise that, as well as possessing manual skills, nurses need knowledge and the ability to think and reflect about a task if it is to be done effectively.

This book has been written to further the aim, alluded to by Nightingale, of integrating theory and practice in nursing. The focus of the book is nursing practices, by which is meant not simply the tasks themselves but also the thinking which surrounds them.

The purpose of this Introduction, which we hope all users of the book will read, is:

- to provide readers with a brief introduction to the theoretical background of the book and refer them to the more substantial texts on the subject for further study
- to explain the relationship between nursing models, in particular the Roper, Logan and Tierney model for nursing, and the content of this book
- to summarize briefly the main headings used for each practice and what each heading covers.

The theoretical background in nursing

This book is necessary because, unfortunately, not only the public think of nursing as a series of tasks. Despite Nightingale's emphasis on the need for a combination of cognitive skills and manual dexterity, the theme of 'functional orientation' has persisted in the nursing profession itself. Loomis (1974) defines 'functional orientation' as being busy doing procedures rather than thinking, reflecting and problem-solving, and maintains that this orientation originates from the early inclusion of nurse training programmes in hospital settings which socialised nurses into being intellectually subordinate. So, she argues, as a group they developed an attitude of task orientation, and nursing remained at a practical level only, rather than developing a theoretical level on which to base practice. Despite this indictment, there have been many nurses who did not consider that 'doing' and 'thinking' were mutually exclusive; who have struggled to emphasise the need to identify the theoretical base for practice, and who have eschewed blind obedience to ritual, routine and unquestioning tradition, seeing nursing as both art and a science (Conway 1994).

The development of nursing models

During the last three decades, a number of nurse writers and practitioners have published their attempts to identify the theoretical base of nursing. Some have undertaken research to corroborate their hypotheses. Of late there has been healthy debate about which comes first – do theories grow out of what nursing is and how nurses deliver care, or is a theoretical framework developed first, providing guidelines for the practice?

In pursuit of theory development, certain writers have attempted to clarify their thinking by using a model for nursing (the term 'conceptual framework' is sometimes used) as an intermediate step to theory development.

Fawett (1984), discussing models from a variety of disciplines, maintains that each evolved from the empirical observations and intuitive insights of scholars, and/or deductions that creatively combine ideas from several fields of enquiry. However, she continues, each model includes only those concepts which the model-builders considered a relevant representation of the real world, and an aid to understanding.

Using models has come to be part of the search for the knowledge base of nursing. Of course, models are useful in any disciplines as a visual representation of a theoretical framework. They indicate the main concepts, and just as importantly, show the relationship between the concepts – even when these relationships have not yet been rigorously tested by research. Each model is one person's individual interpretation of the discipline, offered as an aid to further thinking, and is a growing point, the basis of a reciprocal relationship (Fawcett 1992).

To concentrate on thinking to the exclusion of nursing practice, of course, is folly. Nursing is a practice discipline. However, Walsh (1994) has shown how the practical application of models in the clinical setting can enhance patient care.

The relationship of this book to nursing models

This book has been written with examples related to one particular model for nursing – the Roper, Logan and Tierney model – although the content can be used with any other model. The Roper, Logan and Tierney model was selected because for 12 years the authors of this book, all lecturers, have been using it sucessfully in the practice setting with students on a degree programme for nursing. These same students also learn to apply other models for nursing in the practice setting, but because the Roper, Logan and Tierney model is so readily understandable, it was selected for use here. This is important as, with the development of caring teams in community settings, the activities of living are readily understood by all the professions allied to medicine.

Roper, Logan and Tierney present their model in full in *The Elements of Nursing* (1996), which readers are urged to study carefully. The Roper, Logan and Tierney model has five main concepts:

- activities of living (ALs)
- lifespan
- dependence–independence continuum

- factors related to ALs:
  — physical
  — psychological
  — sociocultural (including spiritual/religious and ethical)
  — environmental
  — politicoeconomic (including legal)
- individuality and individualising nursing
  — assesing lifespan
  — planning
  — evaluating.

These five concepts and the relationships between them have to be considered when making a nursing plan, and therefore when carrying out a nursing practice which is part of that plan. The following three examples should illustrate this point.

Example 1

The important nursing action of explaining to the patient (and family when appropriate) what will occur during an intervention, and seeking consent and cooperation, relates to the AL of Communicating. At face value, this activity may seem to involve merely the physical action of listening and talking. But of course there are important psychological and sociocultural considerations, for example choosing language suited to the patient's age (stage of the lifespan), degree of dependence/independence, and sociocultural background. The related non-verbal communication is also important, and includes more than the simple physical manifestation of 'talking'. Sometimes communicating may mean helping the patient adjust to changes in his usual lifestyle, which may involve psychological, sociocultural, environmental and politicoeconomic factors.

Example 2

Isolation nursing also shows clearly that nursing practices are much more than merely physical tasks. Washing hands and safely disposing of used equipment are patently physical activities which relate to the AL of Maintaining a Safe Environment. However, psychological and social factors feature importantly in isolation nursing, for example, ensuring that the patient does not feel alone when 'reverse barrier nursing' is required or, in 'barrier nursing'. Avoiding the patient's feeling ostracised or stigmatised because his eating and sanitary utensils are kept separate from those of other patients, and his clothing and body discharges are handled by individuals with gloved hands. Nursing someone with HIV gives rise also to important ethical considerations, an aspect which has been well publicised recently in the professional literature and the mass media.

Example 3

In almost every nursing practice, the patient's privacy is mentioned: the need to protect the patient's privacy, to preserve dignity; to prevent embarrassment; to be sensitive to the patient's anxiety because of even a temporary change in body image such as the presence of a catheter or a stoma bag. Using bed screens and covering the patient as much as possible are physical activities, but there are also psychological and sociocultural considerations related, for example, to the AL of Expressing Sexuality, i.e. femininity, masculinity.

These three examples highlight the importance of the decision to relate nursing practices to a nursing model. It should ensure the following:

- that the patient's individuality is always uppermost in the nurse's mind
- that important aspects of nursing which relate to (but are not part of) the physical activity itself are not omitted.
- that the theoretical basis of all nursing practices is not forgotten — the base both in nursing theory and in other disciplines such as the physical and social sciences and the humanities.

Finally, there are two further ways in which the link between the nursing practices and the Roper, Logan and Tierney model has been made apparent:

- The nursing practices are discussed within the framework of the 12 ALs as used in the Roper, Logan and Tierney model for nursing.
- This use of the ALs is quite purposeful; it is hoped that it will reinforce in the nurse's mind the relationship of the nursing practices to the broader theoretical base.

The nursing practices: the main headings

Knowing that this book would be 'dipped into' rather than read from cover to cover we felt it was important to present the information for each practice in a consistent format. This should allow the reader to use the book easily and quickly, once he or she has become familiar with the way in which the material is presented and, in particular, what can be found under the main headings used for each practice. These are:

- Learning outcomes
- Background knowledge required
- Indications and rationale for . . .
- Outline of the procedure
- Equipment
- Guidelines and rationale for this nursing practice
- Relevance to the activities of living
- Patient education: key points
- References
- Further reading

A brief summary is given below of the material covered under each of these headings.

Learning outcomes

The material under this heading indicates what the nurse should know after reading and studying this practice, in combination with his or her existing personal knowledge and knowledge from other sources – the physical and social sciences, the humanities, and professional nursing literature.

It may be necessary, of course, for experienced nursing staff (teaching and clinical) to demonstrate the manual aspects of the practice.

Background knowledge required

Included here are suggested areas of physiology and anatomy which should be reviewed to promote safe manual practice. Knowledge of physical aspects is emphasised because the practices described in the book are physical tasks and must be performed safely. (The relationship of psychosocial theory to the physical practice, and the importance of combining the two, are dealt with more fully under the subsequent heading 'Relevance to the activities of living'.)

In addition, cross-references to related nursing practices are given here, and the nurse's attention is also drawn to the need to consult health authority policy if it is likely to have a particular bearing on this practice, both in a community and an institutional setting.

Indications and rationale for . . .

Under this heading a definition of the nursing practice is given where relevant, and common disease conditions, or other instances for which the practice might be undertaken, are mentioned. It was deliberately decided not to give a definition at the beginning of each practice, but rather to place it in its context – that is, alongside examples of circumstances which may give rise to the practice. Definitions given in isolation may lead to the mistaken view that the nursing practices are tasks with a beginning and an end, rather than part of a nursing plan which requires thought and reflection. The rationale will be given where applicable in continuous text, but highlighted in italics.

Outline of the procedure

This heading appears for those few procedures normally performed by a medical practitioner, where the nurse is present to nurse the patient and/or assist the medical staff (a part of nursing which is 'doctor-initiated'). A brief description of the sequence of events is given, so that the nursing student can follow the steps intelligently; information about the position of the patient during the procedure is usually included, some of the commonly used tests are described, and the role of the nurse is emphasised. 'Outline of the procedure' may also appear if a particular theory needs to be highlighted.

Equipment

The material under this heading is a list of the equipment commonly used for the particular nursing practice. As far as possible, general terms such as 'local anaesthetic' or 'water-based lotion for cleansing the skin' are used, and specific brand names are merely cited as examples. Where appropriate, some equipment is described: for example the different types of catheter used in urinary catheterisation; the types of packaging used for IV infusions and how they are connected to the infusion system; the various parts of the lumbar puncture needle.

In many instances, diagrams or drawings of actual pieces of equipment are provided to supplement the text.

Guidelines and rationale for this nursing practice

The general principles for the practice are outlined here and the rationale highlighted in italics. The following points should be noted:

- Near the beginning of the guidelines, the nurse is alerted to 'observe the patient throughout the nursing practice': some suggested observations are given under the subsequent heading 'Relevance to the activities of living'.
- At the end of the guidelines, there is a statement 'document the nursing practice appropriately, observe after-effects and report abnormal findings immediately'. The meaning attached to these three phrases is discussed below:
  - The wording '*document each nursing practice appropriately*' was chosen carefully: discussion of methods of documentation would merit a separate book, and therefore has not been attempted here. In each ward, clinic or community setting, a method of documentation will have been decided upon; indeed, in some authorities nursing data are recorded on computers.
  - '*Observe after-effects*' is really a follow-on to the earlier guideline 'observe the patient throughout the nursing practice': it is part of the process of evaluating outcome – an integral phase of the process of nursing (individualising nursing).
  - '*Report abnormal findings immediately*' alerts the student to the need not just to document the practice but to report abnormal findings immediately to the nurse in charge. Abnormal findings often require immediate action, for example altering the site of an IV infusion needle when there is evidence of fluid infiltrating the tissues around the site, discontinuing a drug because of the appearance of a rash, or investigating the cause of pain in the calf of the leg following surgery, which can be indicative of deep venous thrombosis.

Relevance to the activities of living

Observing is a crucial part of nursing, and Nightingale comments on its importance in the quotation given at the beginning of this Introduction. However, rather than giving a list of observations to be made before, during and after each nursing practice, the authors thought it would be much more helpful to present observations as and when they related – and only when they *directly* related – to the ALs suggested in the Roper, Logan and Tierney model for nursing. Usually the reference is to the patient's ALs, but when relevant, the nurse's responsibilities are also given by AL. For example, under Maintaining a

Safe Environment, there is reference to the nurse's responsibility to all patients, to him or herself and to other members of staff in observing the general principles for preventing cross-infection.

Moreover, whereas under the second heading 'Background information', material on the physical aspects of each practice is cited (because the content of the book is essentially concerned with observable physical procedures which must be carried out safely) this section *combines* physical science knowledge with the psychosocial and humanities knowledge which must be used before, during and after each nursing practice. It is this integrated thinking process which differentiates the performance of a routine physical task – even when performed dextrously – from a nursing practice. It demands assessment, planning and evaluation related to the specific practice within the context of the patient's total plan of care. Each nursing practice is an important part (but still only a part) of a total nursing plan.

Patient education: key points

Health promotion and health education are key components in the development of a healthy community. With earlier discharge from hospital and increased care in the community, the importance of educating the patient in relation to his own health and his own well-being cannot be over emphasised.

This section includes aspects of patient education which will help to give the patient increasing confidence in his own self care in relation to particular nursing practices.

References

This list includes books, articles and research reports relevant to each nursing practice referenced in the text. Where possible there have been selected from readily available material and most references provide suggestions for further reading around the topic. This guided search and self-search is intended to encouraged nurses to look at a variety of sources, to learn about research findings and to understand the reason behind specific practices in the context of a total care plan. Research articles and reports are used whenever possible. Clinical reviews discussing research have also been useful references. In some instances case studies have been used to reinforce the text.

Further reading

This list includes books and research reports which will be helpful to further understanding of the topic, making it a rewarding learning experience.

In addition, the authors assume that readers are using supplementary texts in related fields such as the sciences and humanities. Also, to gain full benefit from this book, the reader should be conversant with *The Elements of Nursing* (Roper, Logan and Tierney 1996).

In conclusion, we hope that this Introduction will provide a throught-provoking foundation for the nursing practices which follow. The practices are as succinct as possible for ease of reference and we are confident that readers who assimilate the principles outlined in the Introduction will be able to utilise the practices with individuality – while respecting the patient's special needs – and with the depth of thought which all nursing actions deserve and, indeed, should demand.

It is important to emphasise too that, apart from maintaining a legal record, well-charted practices and observations are essential in developing nursing theory. In fact, Benner (1984) goes further and maintains that the practices and expertise of good nurse clinicians contain a wealth of untapped knowledge, which will not expand unless nurses systematically record for themselves what they learn from their own practice experience.

References

Benner P 1984 From novice to expert: excellence and power in clinical nursing practice. Addison Wesley, Menlo Park, California

Conway J 1994 Reflections: the art and science of nursing and the theory – practice gap. British Journal of Nursing 3(3) February 10: 114–118

Fawcett J 1984 Analysis and evaluation of conceptual models of nursing. F A Davis, Philadelphia, p 4

Fawcett J 1992 Conceptual models in nursing practice; the reciprocal relationship. Journal of Advance Nursing 17: 224–226.

Loomis M 1974 Collegiate nursing education: an ambivalent professionalism. In: Meleis A (ed) 1985 Theoretical nursing: development and progress. Lippincott, Philadelphia, p 38

Roper N, Logan W, Tierney A 1996 The elements of nursing. 4th edn. Churchill Livingstone, Edinburgh

Walsh M 1991 Nursing models in clinical practice. The way forward. Ballière Tindall, London.

1 Administration of Medicines

There are seven parts to this section:

1 Principles of medicine administration
2 Routes of medicine administration
3 Immunisation
4 Syringe driver pumps
5 Anaphylaxis
6 Patient controlled analgesic devices
7 Patient compliance devices.

The concluding section 'Relevance to the activities of living' refers to all practices.

Learning outcomes

By the end of this section you should know how to:

- prepare the patient for this practice
- collect and prepare the equipment
- carry out administration of medicines
- educate the patient on follow-up care.

Background knowledge required

Review of:

- pharmacology of the medicine to be administered
- metric system of volume and weight used in a dose calculation of a medication
- HMSO 1985 Misuse of Drugs Act 1971 (reprinted 1985)
- United Kingdom Central Council for Nursing, Midwifery and Health Visiting (UKCC) 1992 *The Scope of Professional Practice*
- UKCC 1992 *Standards for the Administration of Medicines*
- HMSO 1992 *Medicinal Products: Prescription by Nurses Act*
- Department of Health 1992 *Immunisation against Infectious Disease* (new edition due 1996)
- health authority policy regarding the patient's medicine prescription and recording documents, administration of drugs, disposal of equipment, and management of anaphylactic shock.

Indications and rationale for administration of medicines

A medication can be administered by a variety of routes and for many different reasons:

- *to prevent disease*
- *to cure disease*

  - *to alleviate pain or other symptoms caused by disease, injury or surgery*
  - *to alleviate a manifestation of disease.*

Outline of the procedure

Administration of medicine encompasses many different procedures, depending on the needs of the patient. The UKCC (1992) lays great emphasis on issues of accountability for any nurse undertaking this practice. It is important that the following guidelines are used in conjunction with health authority policy as there may be policy or procedural differences (such as the grade and number of nurses required to undertake these practices).

Equipment

Patient's medicine prescription and recording documents

Trolley, tray or a suitable work surface for equipment

Medication to be administered

Equipment for use during medicine administration, e.g.:

— oral administration: medicine glass or spoon, glass of water

— injection: appropriately-sized sterile needles and syringe, disposable gloves, alcohol-impregnated cleansing swab, cotton wool, adhesive plaster

Sharpsbox

Receptacle for soiled material

Equipment/medication for the treatment of anaphylactic shock (as per health authority policy).

1   Principles of medicine administration

Guidelines and rationale for this nursing practice

All forms of medicine administration

  - discuss the procedure with the patient, asking whether he has any known allergy to the drug, and obtain his consent (this may not always be possible, for example when the patient is unconscious) *to inform the patient about the procedure, discuss any concerns or queries, identify any known allergies and ensure that the patient is aware of his rights as a patient*
  - wash hands *to reduce risk of cross-infection*
  - select a suitable clean surface and lay out equipment *to provide a suitable protected work surface*
  - observe the patient throughout this procedure *to identify any potential reactions to the medicine*
  - identify the medicine to be administered on the prescription document. The prescription should be complete and legible *to ensure that all details about the medicine can be clearly identified on the prescription documentation*
  - check that the medicine has not already been administered *to ensure that only one dose of the medicine is given*
  - select the appropriate medicine against the prescription documentation *to ensure that the correct medicine is administered*

- check the medicine name, dosage, timing and expiry date. If the medication has been dispensed to a specific patient then check that his name is on the container *to ensure that all the relevant details are listed on the medicine container*
- remove the prescribed dosage from the container *to ensure that the correct amount of medicine is removed from the container*
- check the prescription and dosage against the medicine container *to ensure that the medicine details match*
- identify the patient to whom the medicine is to be administered. In an institution this will normally be done by checking the details on the patient's identification bracelet. In a community setting verbal verification should be obtained from either the patient or the carer *to ensure that the medicine is administered to the correct patient*
- administer the medicine by the route prescribed
- dispose of contaminated equipment according to health authority policy *to prevent transmission of infection*
- ensure that patient is comfortable following the administration of the medicine *to identify any reaction to the medication*
- follow local policy regarding the time that a nurse must remain with a patient following the administration of certain medicines. This is particularly relevant where the medicine is being administered in the patient's own home or in a treatment room *to ensure prompt recognition and treatment of any reaction to the drug (see* Anaphylaxis, p. 12*)*
- record the medication details on the patient documentation, monitor any after-effects and report abnormal findings immediately *to ensure that there is a permanent record of the medicine administration and that any side-effects are reported to medical staff.*

Controlled medicines

Institutional setting The administration of a controlled medicine within an institutional setting must involve two nurses, one of whom is a registered nurse practitioner. A controlled drug register is kept on each ward or department giving details of the stock and administration of controlled drugs.

- as for All forms of medicine administration to the guideline 'check that the medicine has not already been administered'
- remove the appropriate medicine from the controlled drug store, check the stock number with the number detailed in the register with the other nurse *to ensure that the number of drugs in the container matches the number recorded in the register*
- check the date of the prescription *to ensure that the medicine is administered on the correct date*
- check the time of administration *to ensure that the medicine is given at the correct time*
- check the method of administration *to ensure the correct route of administration*
- remove the appropriate dose from the stock of controlled medicine, checking the name and dosage with the second nurse. Check and record the stock

number of the remaining controlled medicine *to ensure that the correct dose is withdrawn from the container and the remaining balance recorded*
- enter into the controlled medicine record sheet the appropriate details *to ensure a permanent record of the administration details (date, time, patient's name, drug dosage and initial of staff)*
- continue as for All forms of medicine administration.

Community setting The administration of a controlled medicine within the patient's own home may be carried out by the patient or carer (this would be the normal practice for medicines in tablet or liquid form).

When medicines are given by injection, suppository or via a syringe driver this is normally carried out by the community nurse(s). The number and grade of staff depend on health authority policy.

Controlled medicines belong to the patient and remain within his home. Advice should be given to the patient/carer on the safe storage of these medicines.

A controlled medicine record sheet giving details of any medicine administered by the nurse and a balance of stock should be placed in the patient's house along with a special prescription sheet for controlled medicines (completed and signed by the general practitioner).

- as for All forms of medicine administration to the guideline 'check that the medicine has not already been administered'
- check the stock number of medicines with the number detailed in the controlled drug record sheet *to ensure the number of medicines in the container matches the number recorded in the drug record*
- check the date of the prescription *to ensure that the medicine is administered on the correct date*
- check the time of administration *to ensure that the drug is given at the correct time*
- check the method of administration *to ensure the correct route of administration*
- remove the appropriate dose from the stock of controlled medicines, checking the name and dosage. Check and record the stock number of the remaining controlled medicines *to ensure that the correct dose is withdrawn from the container and the remaining balance recorded*
- enter into the controlled drug record sheet the appropriate details *to ensure a permanent record of the administration details (date, time, medicine dosage and signature of staff)*
- continue as for All forms of medicine administration.

2   Routes of medicine administration

Oral preparation

- as for All forms of medicine administration to the guideline which begins 'remove the prescribed dosage....'

- remove the required number of tablets, pills or cachets from the medicine container without contaminating the preparation. Place into the medicine glass or medicine spoon *to ensure that the correct drug dosage is dispensed*

or

- shake the liquid medicine preparation well. Pour into the appropriate container at eye level and on a solid flat surface *to ensure accurate drug dose measurement*
- check the medicine prescription and dosage against the container *to ensure that the correct medicine and dosage has been dispensed*`
- identify the patient *to ensure that the medicine is administered to the correct person*
- administer the medicine and offer the patient water (if allowed) *to aid swallowing of an oral preparation*. If the medicine is a powder which requires to be mixed with water then the instructions on the container should be followed *to ensure that the medicine moves efficiently down the oesophagus into the stomach*.
- continue as for All forms of medicine administration.

Injection preparations — intramuscular and subcutaneous routes

Equipment

Appropriate-sized needles (21 G, 23 G and 25 G) and syringes

Alcohol-impregnated swab

Drug ampoule or vial

Diluent if required

File

Disposable gloves

Gauze swab

Sterile adhesive plaster.

Guidelines and rationale for injections

- as for All forms of medicine administration, follow guideline which begins 'check the medicine name, dosage, timing and expiry date'
- put on gloves *to prevent contamination by medicine and to protect against blood-borne infection*.

Ampoule

- snap the neck of the ampoule using a gauze swab *to protect the nurse from laceration by glass splinters*
- if any glass enters the ampoule discard it and start the process with another ampoule *as glass particles may have contaminated the medicine*
- if the solution is already present in the ampoule draw up the required amount of medicine into the syringe

- if the medicine is in powder form draw up the required amount of diluent and inject it slowly into the powder within the ampoule *to enable the medicine to be dissolved in diluent*
- gently rotate the ampoule and inspect it for any visible particles of undissolved powder *to ensure that the powder is fully dissolved*
- withdraw the required amount of drug solution into the syringe *to ensure that the correct amount of medicine is dispensed*
- gently tap the side of the barrel with the finger *to move any air bubbles to the neck of the syringe to enable them to be expelled prior to injecting the solution.*

Vial

- remove the protective cap and cleanse the rubber top with an alcohol-impregnated swab *to cleanse the entry point*
- insert the first needle, ensuring that the tip is above the fluid level *to release the vacuum within the vial*
- draw air into the syringe attached to the second needle to equal the amount of solution to be withdrawn from the vial *to enable easier withdrawal of solution from the vial*
- insert the second needle attached to the syringe and expel air into the vial. Draw up the required amount of drug, expelling any air bubbles prior to removing the needle from the vial *to prevent spray of the drug solution into the atmosphere on withdrawal of the needle*
- if the medicine is in powder form draw up the required amount of diluent and inject it slowly into the powder within the vial *to enable the medicine to be dissolved in diluent*
- gently rotate the ampoule and inspect for any visible particles of undissolved powder *to ensure that the powder is fully dissolved*
- change the needle to the required size for the route of administration; *if an intramuscular injection is to be given a clean needle prevents irritation of the subcutaneous tissue as the needle is being inserted into the muscle* (Stilwell 1991)
- place the prepared syringe and the empty ampoule or vial on a foil tray *to retain the original drug container so that a final check can be made prior to administering the medicine*
- identify the patient to whom the medicine is to be administered and recheck the prescription details with the medicine, container, and dosage drawn up in the syringe *to ensure the correct medicine is administered to the correct patient*
- ensure the patient's privacy
- cleanse the skin surface (if required). The policy on skin cleansing prior to injection varies according to the health authority concerned (Lawrence et al 1994). Patients receiving insulin injections should not have the area cleansed with an alcohol-impregnated swab as this will toughen the skin over time
- expose the chosen site and inject the drug.

Intramuscular injection

Sites for intramuscular injection are shown in Figure 1.1. Using the non-

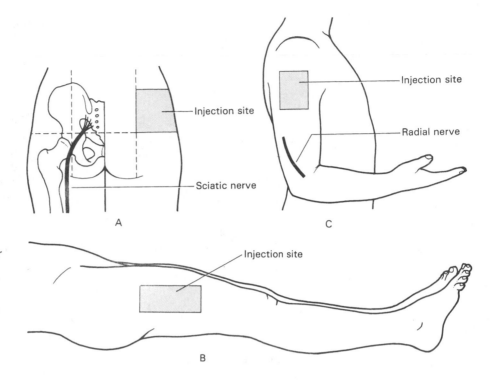

Figure 1.1
Administration of medicines: sites used for intramuscular injection
A Upper outer quadrant of the buttock
B Anterior lateral aspect of the thigh
C Deltoid region of the arm

dominant hand stretch the skin over the site; with the dominant hand insert the needle two-thirds in, at an angle of 90°, *to ensure that the needle is inserted into the muscle.*

Subcutaneous injection

Sites for subcutaneous injection are shown in Figure 1.2. Using the non-dominant hand gently grip the skin over the site. With the dominant hand introduce two-thirds of the needle at a 45° angle. Release the skin once the needle is in position *to ensure that the drug is given into the subcutaneous tissue.*

For more information on insulin therapy *see* Administration of insulin, page 8.

All injections

- withdraw the piston of the syringe. If blood is drawn up into the syringe withdraw the needle and syringe from the patient's tissue. Replace the needle and start the procedure again *to prevent the drug being injected into a blood vessel*
- if no blood is withdrawn into the syringe inject the solution slowly *to reduce patient discomfort*
- withdraw the needle smoothly and quickly. Apply pressure to the site of the injection using a cotton wool ball or swab. If bleeding occurs apply a small adhesive plaster *to prevent blood leakage*
- continue as for All forms of medicine administration.

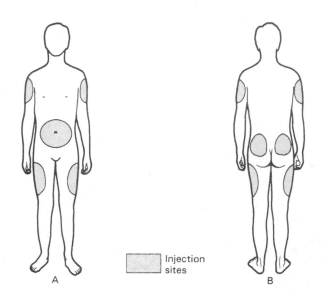

Figure 1.2
*Administration of
medicines: sites used for
subcutaneous injection
A Anterior aspect
B Posterior aspect*

Some medicines require a specialised technique (for example subcutaneous injection of goserelin implant). Specialised administration instructions provided by the manufacturer should always be followed.

The nurse should always be aware of the possibility of anaphylaxis following administration of medicines.

Health authority policy should be followed regarding the length of time for which the patient should be monitored following administration of medicine. This is particularly important for patients receiving medicines in the community. For further information *see* Anaphylaxis, page 12.

Administration of insulin

Insulin may be given via special insulin syringes or by an insulin pen device. For patients who are self-administering insulin the pen system is often more practical as the vial in the pen holds enough insulin for several doses. Insulin is given via the subcutaneous route. Some pen systems have a needle which is of a shorter length than the standard one normally used for subcutaneous injections. Some manufacturers advise that their pen be introduced at 90° angle. However there has been debate as to whether this technique causes insulin to be injected into the muscle rather than the subcutaneous tissue (in patients who have less than 10 mm of subcutaneous tissue) and thus increases absorption rate (Sykes 1991, Spence 1992). Patients injecting insulin should be taught the technique advised by the diabetic specialist within the health authority.

Intradermal route

This route is used only for selective vaccinations such as BCG. The nurse must meet the criteria for immunisation prior to administering this or any other vaccine via this route. The injection of a medicine into the dermis is a skilled injection technique. The sites where the injections can be given may vary according to the type of vaccination being administered: local health authority policy should therefore be followed. More detailed information on this technique is provided by the Department of Health (1992).

Topical application

There is a growing trend for certain medicines to be administered via the transdermal route (Kelly 1994). This usually takes the form of a 'skin patch'. Some drugs which can be given by this method include hormone replacement therapy and certain analgesics. Patches should normally be applied to clean dry skin. The length of time the patch should be worn is dependent on the drug, therefore the manufacturer's instructions should be followed. The site of the patch should be rotated to reduce risk of a skin reaction. Further information on drugs delivered via this route is available from individual manufacturers.

3   Immunisation

Nurses working in both community and institutional settings are increasingly undertaking immunisation.

This may include child immunisation regimes, vaccinations for travel abroad, administration of flu vaccines and the giving of anti-tetanus injections within accident and emergency units or treatment rooms.

Jones (1994) examines some of the legal and professional aspects of immunisation by nursing staff and discusses the use of protocols for this practice.

Nurses participating in any immunisation programme must meet the following criteria (Department of Health 1992):

- undertake additional training on immunisation
- undertake training on the management of anaphylaxis
- be competent in the practice of immunisation and able to recognise contraindications for vaccination
- be accountable for their practice.

4   Syringe driver pump

Indications and rationale for use of a syringe driver

A patient who requires a continuous dose of medicine may be given it via a syringe driver pump. A pump may be used:

- *when the patient is unable to tolerate oral medication* (for example because of a pathological lesion, unresolved nausea or vomiting or reduced level of consciousness)
- *when adequate pain control is unable to be achieved by oral medication*
- *when a medicine is required to be administered via the subcutaneous route over a period of time.*

Outline of the procedure

The syringe driver administers a continuous amount of a prescribed medicine via the subcutaneous route over a set period of time (for example 24 hours). The syringe driver may be used when a continuous infusion of a medicine is required, for example to manage postoperative pain or to control symptoms in the terminal stage of an illness. More than one medicine may be administered at any one time via this route. It is especially of benefit for patients being nursed in the community as it enables more accurate titration of drug doses and therefore more effective symptom control.

In many settings this practice requires to be undertaken by two people although policy may vary in a community setting. Within an institutional setting the medicine may already be made up in the syringe by the pharmacist or doctor. In a community setting the medicine is likely to be made up by the district nurse in the patient's own home. Health authorities may have a different policy which should be followed.

Different models of syringe driver with differing operating instructions are available. It is essential that any nurse working with syringe driver pumps is fully familiar with the specific manufacturer's instructions. It is therefore only possible to provide general guidelines, which should be followed in conjunction with health authority policy and manufacturer's instructions.

Equipment

Syringe driver and battery (if required)

Manufacturer's instructions for syringe driver

Patient's medicine prescription and recording documents

Trolley, tray or suitable work surface for equipment

Medication to be administered (including diluent)

22 gauge butterfly cannula and giving set

Syringes (type and size as instructed by manufacturer of syringe driver)

Sterile needles

Disposable gloves

Cotton wool

Semipermeable adhesive film dressing

Sharpsbox

Receptacle for soiled material

Adhesive label.

Guidelines and rationale for this practice

The following steps should be undertaken in conjunction with local policy and the instructions of the manufacturer of the syringe driver.

- as for All forms of medicine administration (p. 2) to the guideline 'check that the medicine has not already been administered'. If a controlled drug is to be administered then the guidelines given under Controlled drugs (p. 3) should be followed

- check that the syringe driver is functioning by following the checking procedure advised by the manufacturer and health authority. Normally this would involve inserting the battery or attaching the pump to the mains supply and ensuring that the indicator light was lit. Where applicable a check on the inbuilt alarm system should also be carried out *to perform any recommended safety checks*
- in an institutional setting: collect the ready prepared syringe containing the prescribed medicine and check the details on the syringe (name of patient, hospital number, date, medicine name(s) and diluent, dosage, total volume of fluid in syringe, starting time of administration, expiry date). This information should be checked with the details given on the patient's prescription sheet *to ensure that the medicine details on the syringe match those on the prescription sheet*
- in a community setting: prepare the medicine for administration as per the patient's prescription sheet (although the medicine dosage will be the same irrespective of the pump, the amount of diluent may differ). A label should be attached to the barrel of the syringe giving information on the contents of the syringe (date, name and dosage of the medicine, volume of drug and diluent, starting time of administration and signature of nurse) *in order that the contents are clearly identified*
- attach the giving set to the syringe and prime the tubing *so that all air is expelled from the tubing*
- elicit the duration of administration *as this will affect the rate of administration*
- set the prescribed rate according to the manufacturer's instructions *to ensure correct infusion rate*
- select the site for infusion (the same as Subcutaneous injection, p. 7) and, using the same method as when giving a subcutaneous injection, insert the needle of the infusion set at a 45° angle
- secure the needle with the semipermanent adhesive dressing *to prevent it from becoming dislodged and to enable the entry site to be clearly visible*
- secure the syringe into the driver, ensuring the plunger mechanism is correctly positioned and that any securing straps are in place to enable administration of the medicine and *to ensure that the syringe does not become dislodged from the pump*
- start the syringe driver and observe for the time specified by the health authority *to ensure that the driver is functioning*
- place the driver in a safe position (a carrying case is normally available for patients who are mobile) and ensure that it is kept away from water *to prevent the infusion set being dislodged from the syringe driver and to avoid damage to the machine*
- the syringe driver should be checked regularly and recordings such as fluid volume length documented (length of fluid in syringe barrel, measured normally in mm) (the checks to be carried out and their frequency may vary according to health authority policy) *to ensure that it is continuing to function correctly*
- check the infusion site regularly and report any signs of localised pain, inflammation or swelling. In the community the patient/carer may be taught

how to check the site. Any problems necessitate resiting of the infusion set. Doyle & Benton (1994) advise that the site should be changed routinely every 3–4 days *to identify and rectify at an early stage any localised skin reaction.*

- observe the patient's symptoms *to monitor the effectiveness of the drug therapy*

Regular maintenance and calibration of the pump by the health authority or manufacturer is essential.

5 Anaphylaxis

Outline of the procedure

This potentially fatal reaction, although rare, can occur at any time. It is essential that any nurse involved in the administration of medicines is familiar with the symptoms of an anaphylactic reaction. It is particularly important that nurses working in a community setting have the competence to both recognise and treat anaphylaxis (additional training will be given to staff in order that they can undertake this procedure). A reaction to a medicine may occur at any time following administration: it is not possible to give a time limit (Department of Health 1992). Brueton et al (1991) advise that a reaction frequently occurs within minutes of the patient receiving the injection (although it can also occur follow oral ingestion of medicines or certain foods), but may also be delayed up to several hours following administration.

The information provided in this section is based on the guidelines given by the Department of Health (1992) but individual health authorities may provide additional guidance for staff.

Signs and symptoms

- extreme anxiety and feeling of 'impending doom'
- skin itching/flushing/urticaria
- tachycardia followed by bradycardia
- hypotension
- airway obstruction presenting as wheezing from bronchospasm, dyspnoea and stridor.

If untreated the patient may eventually suffer respiratory and cardiac arrest.

Management of anaphylaxis

- place the patient in the left lateral position and insert an airway *to maintain an airway*
- in an institutional setting: remain with the patient but get help urgently from other medical and nursing staff (within most units it will be necessary to call the cardiac arrest team). When help arrives inform senior staff of the medication which the patient received prior to collapse *to initiate treatment and sustain life*
- in a community setting: remain with the patient and start treatment as soon as possible. Where possible send someone for medical help

Administer adrenaline 1/1000 (solution) by deep intramuscular injection ('unless

Table 1.1   **Adrenaline dosage: Adrenaline 1/1000 (1 mg/ml)**

Age	Dose of adrenaline
0–1 year	0.05 ml
1 year	0.1 ml
2 years	0.2 ml
3–4 years	0.3 ml
5 years	0.4 ml
6–10 years	0.5 ml
adults	0.5 ml–1 ml

Department of Health 1992 *Immunisation against Infectious Disease* (reprinted with permission of HMSO)

there is a strong central pulse and the patient's condition is good' Department of Health 1992:16). A maximum of 3 doses may be administered, with the second dose being given 10 minutes after the first dose (see Table 1.1 for dosage amounts), *to reverse the effects of the anaphylactic reaction* (see Brueton et al 1991 for further information on physiological changes associated with anaphylaxis).

Other medications may be given (Department of Health 1992) depending on health authority policy.

- commence resuscitation procedure if the patient has suffered a respiratory and/or cardiac arrest (*see* Cardiopulmonary resuscitation, p. 75) *to initiate treatment as quickly as possible and sustain the patient's life*
- any patient suffering an anaphylactic reaction should be admitted to hospital as soon as possible *in order that his condition may be monitored.* Fisher (1995) advises that a secondary reaction may occur up to 72 hours following the initial anaphylactic incident.

6   Patient controlled analgesic devices

Devices which enable the patient to self-administer his own analgesic are becoming increasingly popular. The device works via a pump system which enables the patient to administer small doses of the prescribed analgesic. An inbuilt safety mechanism prevents overdose of the drug. The main administration routes used are intravenous, subcutaneous or epidural. The benefits of this system are that the patient is more empowered and less anxious about effective pain control (Mc Donald 1994). The devices may be used by patients in both institutional and community settings (Roberts & Seaby 1995).

Patient controlled analgesia (PCA) may be prescribed for patients:

- following surgical procedures eg: Hysterectomy, Hip Replacement *It allows the patient to administer frequent small boluses of analgesia for pain relief without becoming over sedated. Good pain control enables the patient to mobilise earlier and enhances her post-operative recovery* (Clark et al 1989).

- for pain relief as part of palliative care in terminal illness. This may be at home, in an institutional or hospice setting *and allows the patient to be alert and aware of her surroundings with adequate pain control* (Roberts & Seaby 1994).

Equipment

- Venous or subcutaneous access
- Specialised PCA infusor (see manufacturer's instructions)

The infusor consists of a reservoir balloon or a reservoir syringe which is prepared with the prescribed analgesic medication by the nursing staff. The fluid from the reservoir flows through a filter and a control nozzle on the demand button via associated tubing (see Fig. 1.3). Many devices are available and the individual manufacturer's instructions should always be followed. Willis (1995) provides a summary of the devices currently on the market.

The patient administers her own dose of analgesia by pressing the demand button. This may be in the form of a wrist button or a small hand held demand

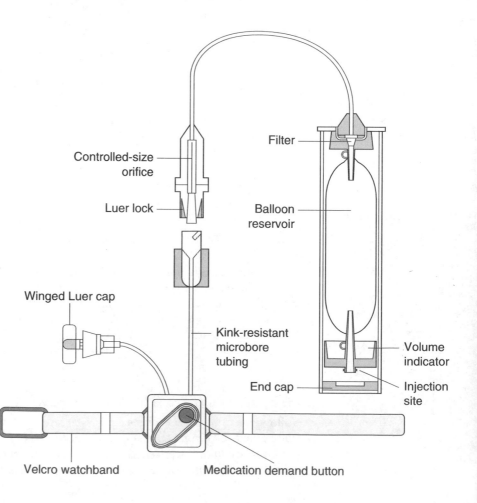

Figure 1.3 *Patient controlled analgesia infusor*

set. When the patient requires further analgesic the demand button is pressed and a small amount of medication is delivered (0.5 ml–1 ml). There is a safety mechanism built in to the equipment which only allows a certain amount of fluid to be infused during one hour, so that there is no possibility of a medication overdose. The strength of the individual bolus will be prescribed by the medical practitioner after assessing the patient's pain (Doverty 1994).

The amount transfused each hour should be recorded, monitored and documented for evaluation of the patient's pain control).

7   Patient compliance devices

There are many types of devices on the market to assist the patient to administer his medicines. They may comprise individual trays for each day of the week. The trays have different compartments for the different times of the day when the patient requires to take his medication. The trays are usually filled with all the patient's medicines up to one week in advance (this may be done by the patient, carer or pharmacist). If the nurse is required to fill these devices then UKCC guidelines (*Standards for the Administration of Medicines* 1992 and *Administration of Medicines: Standards for the use of Monitored Dosage Systems — Position Statement* 1994) and health authority policy should be followed. All patients should be fully assessed before a medicine device is given and checks made that the medicines are able to be stored in these devices. Interactions between medicines should also be checked; it is essential therefore that a pharmacist is involved at all stages. Increasingly, packs prepared by the pharmacist which provide a 7-day supply of medicines in blister packaging are being used.

Relevance to the activities of living

Maintaining a safe environment

The nurse in charge of the ward, department, unit or treatment room at any time of the day or night is responsible for maintaining the safe and correct storage of all medicines. The storage requirements are enforced by law through the Misuse of Drugs Act 1971. Medicines kept in the patient's own home are his responsibility, but the community nurse has an important role in the education of patients on all aspects of the regime. All protocols and records pertaining to medicine administration must be maintained, adhering to health authority legal requirements.

A learner nurse should be supervised by a qualified member of staff while administering medicines. A nurse can only administer a medicine on the written instruction of a medical practitioner (unless provided for in a specific agreed protocol). The UKCC (1992) *Standards for the Administration of Medicines* and health authority policy should be followed in respect of this practice. The medicine prescription should be written in indelible ink giving the date, patient's full name and age, the medication name (preferably generic title), dosage to be given and time of administration, and it must be signed by a medical practitioner. The whole prescription should be legible. In the future selected community nurses who have undertaken additional training may be able to prescribe items from a nurses' formulary. At the time of publishing nurse prescribing is being carried out at a small number of pilot sites.

The nurse is responsible for the correct administration and documentation of a prescribed medication. Recording of the administration may only be performed once the nurse is satisfied that the patient has received the prescribed medication. Should any error occur during administration this must be reported so that the appropriate action can be implemented.

The manufacturer's recommendations for the storage environment and expiry date should be adhered to otherwise the medicine composition may be altered. Vaccines in particular require to be stored under very stringent conditions (recommendations are provided by both the manufacturer and health authority).

The nurse should be familiar with the use, action, common side-effects and therapeutic dose of the medicine being administered. This will help in the education of patients and assists in identifying any adverse reaction which they may develop.

Administration of oral medicine does not require an aseptic technique but all equipment should be clean or disposable and all precautions be taken to prevent cross-infection. The nurse should wash her hands (and where indicated wear gloves) before commencing and on completion of oral medicine administration.

When a patient has difficulty in swallowing an oral preparation the nurse may request the medicine to be supplied in another form. The pharmacist should be consulted before any tablet is crushed or halved (as this may affect the composition or absorption of the medicine). Pills, capsules and cachets should be supplied in the dosage stated on the prescription sheet.

Liquids for oral administration should be shaken well to disperse the medicine thoroughly in the liquid base before pouring the prescribed amount. Spillage on the outside of the bottle should be wiped off to prevent disfiguration of the label.

An injection is an invasive procedure, so all principles of asepsis should be maintained. The equipment should be disposed of safely and immediately following the injection to reduce the potential hazards. Needles should never be resheathed. Certain medications (such as some medicines used in the treatment of cancer) can be hazardous to staff during preparation and administration, therefore disposable gloves and/or other protection may be required.

An intramuscular injection should only be administered into the areas shown in Figure 1.1 as this reduces the risk of damage to underlying tissue such as nerves and/or blood vessels.

If a patient is receiving subcutaneous injections over a period of time the site of injection should be rotated to reduce subcutaneous tissue irritation and maintain the medicine absorption rate.

Oral medications are dispensed in child-resistant containers unless a specific request is made for a screw-top container. It is therefore necessary for the nurse to assess the patient's ability to remove medicines from the container (this is especially important for elderly or disabled people).

Communicating

The nurse should help to reinforce any information given to the patient by the medical practitioner about the prescribed medicine and its effect within the patient's body.

Information about any known allergy to medicine, food or topical application (such as tape) should be requested during the initial patient assessment.

Observation of the effectiveness of a medicine is important, such as following administration of an anti-emetic or analgesic. Any sign of the development of a side-effect, non-effectiveness or dependence should be reported to the medical practitioner.

Most medicines are known to have some form of side-effect which can vary from minor upset to a life-threatening event; the nurse should have a knowledge of the side-effects of the medicine being administered. When a side-effect is not life-threatening it may be necessary for the patient to adjust to a change in his activity of living. The nurse therefore has a role as an educator and facilitator during the adjustment.

Eliminating

The patient should be informed if the medicine is likely to discolour the urine. Some medicines such as opiates may cause constipation; education should therefore be given on diet and, where necessary, a laxative prescribed.

Patient education: key points

Whatever the care setting the nurse should use every opportunity to educate the patient on all aspects of his medication regime. A study carried out by Whyte (1994) found that a personal medication record card significantly increased the amount of information elderly patients were able to recall about their medication regimes. A more structured programme may involve a self-administration system implemented whilst the patient is still in institutional care (Fuller 1995).

Education is needed to ensure that medicines are kept safely within the patient's own home.

Patients and carers can be taught how to administer medicines such as insulin as well as to report any side-effects from medication. This is particularly important for patients receiving chemotherapy, where a structured education programme of therapy is essential.

References

Brueton MJ, Lortan JE, Morgan DJ, Sutters CA 1991 Management of anaphylaxis. Hospital Update, May: 386–390

Clark E, Hodson N, Kenny G 1989 Improved postoperative recovery with patient controlled analgesia. Nursing Times 85(9): 54–55

Department of Health 1992 Immunisation against infectious diseases. HMSO, London

Doverty N 1994 Making pain assessment your priority. Practitioner led management of pain in trauma injuries. Professional Nurse 9(4): 230–237

Doyle D, Benton T F 1994 Palliative medicine: pain and symptom control. St Columba's Hospice, Edinburgh

Fisher M 1995 Treatment of acute anaphylaxis. British Medical Journal 311 September 16: 731–733

Fuller D 1995 Simplifying the system. Professional Nurse 10(5): 315–317

Jones M 1994 Vaccination: the facts. Primary Health Care 4(1): 16–17

Kelly J 1994 Understanding transdermal medication. Professional Nurse 10(2): 121–125

Lawrence J C, Lilly H A, Kidson A 1994 The use of alcoholic wipes for disinfection of injection sites. Journal of Wound Care 3(1): 11–14

McDonald S 1994 Controlled environment. Nursing Times 90(47): 42–44

Roberts K, Seaby L 1995 Empowering patients. Journal of Community Nursing 9(6): 4–6

Spence A 1992 Getting to the point. Journal of Community Nursing 6(2): 16

Stilwell B 1991 Injections. Community Outlook 1(1): 21–22

Sykes J 1991 Insulin injections. Diabetic Nursing 2(1): 3–4

UKCC 1992 Standards for the administration of medicines. UKCC, London

Whyte L A 1994 Medication cards for elderly people: a study. Nursing Standard 8(48): 25–28

Willis J 1995 Patient-controlled analgesia devices. Professional Nurse 10(9): 579–583

Further reading

Burton S 1988 Handling of cytotoxic drugs. Professional Nurse 3(12): 496–498

Engstrom L 1994 Technique of insulin injection: is it important? Practical Diabetes 11(1): 39

Freeman E 1990 Making sense of cytotoxic chemotherapy. Nursing Times 86(36): 45–47

Howard M, Tiziani A 1994 A nursing guide to drugs, 4th edn. Churchill Livingstone, Edinburgh

Latham J 1987 Syringe drivers in pain control. Professional Nurse 2(7): 207–209

Newton M, Newton D, Fudin J 1992 Reviewing the 'big three injection routes'. Nursing 2(9): 34–42

Sutcliffe B 1990 Pen style devices used in diabetes care. Diabetes Care 1(3): 3–5

Williams A 1990 Breaking the chain reaction (common errors in administration). Nursing Times 86(44): 39–41

2 Apical–Radial Pulses

Learning outcomes

By the end of this section you should know how to:
- prepare the patient for this nursing practice
- locate, assess, measure and record the apical–radial pulses.

Background knowledge required

Revision of the anatomy and physiology of the cardiovascular system.

Revision of pulse (*see* p. 81).

Indications and rationale for assessing the apical–radial pulses

The rate at the apex of the heart and the radial pulse rate are counted simultaneously and compared to ascertain if there is a deficit in the rate. It may be assessed *to estimate the degree of dysfunction on admission and the effect of treatment on:*
- patients who have cardiac impairment
- patients who are receiving medication to improve heart action
- patients who have vascular disease.

The assessment elicits a pulse apex deficit and helps in the decision about the necessity for treatment.

Equipment

Watch with a seconds hand

Stethoscope.

Guidelines and rationale for this nursing practice

Two nurses are required to carry out this practice *so that simultaneous recordings can be obtained of the radial pulse and the apex of the heart*
- explain the nursing practice to the patient *to gain consent and cooperation. Patients should be encouraged to be active partners in their care*
- ensure the patient's privacy *to maintain dignity and sense of 'self'*
- collect the equipment *for efficiency of practice*
- assist the patient to a comfortable position *so that there is easy access to the chest wall*
- observe the patient throughout this activity *to detect any signs of discomfort*
- place the diaphragm of the stethoscope over the apex of the heart (Fig. 2.1). This is usually located at the 5th intercostal space and 12 cm left of the midline (nurse 1)
- locate the radial pulse (nurse 2)

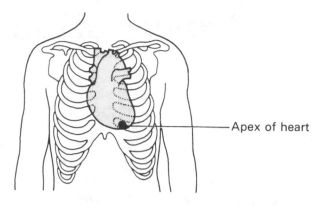

Figure 2.1 *Position of the apex of the heart*

Apex of heart

- ensure that the watch is visible to both nurses, who begin counting the rates simultaneously for 1 minute
- document the results appropriately, compare past recordings, and report abnormal findings immediately.

Relevance to the activities of living

Breathing

The patient who has a radial pulse deficit because of heart disease may have an elevated respiratory rate, because the inefficient heart action eventually leads to pulmonary oedema which causes respiratory distress.

The rate at the apex and at the radial artery should be compared. If there is a deficit in the radial pulse it should be reported as it may indicate left ventricular failure.

Controlling body temperature

An impaired blood supply to the limbs as a result of heart disease will probably result in complaints of cold hands and feet. The wearing of gloves and socks should be encouraged. Because sensation is also impaired, caution should be exercised in the use of hot applications.

Mobilising

This may be limited because of cardiac impairment and respiratory distress.

Working and playing

The patient with a radial pulse deficit may be unable to continue in previous employment and hobbies.

Sleeping

The patient's normal sleeping pattern may be altered because of some of the physical features of cardiac impairment. Assisting the patient into a fairly upright position with plenty of pillows may help to relieve any discomfort.

Patient education: key points

Explanations given before, during and after the practice will help the patient understand more about his or her health problems.

Further reading

Alexander M, Fawcett J, Runciman P 1994 Nursing care. Hospital and home. The adult. Churchill Livingstone, Edinburgh

Brunner L, Suddarth D 1989 The Lippincott Manual of medical-surgical nursing, vol 2. Harper & Row, London

Roper N, Logan W, Tierney A 1996 The elements of nursing, 4th edn. Churchill Livingstone, Edinburgh

3 Bathing and Showering

Learning outcomes

By the end of this section you should know how to:
- prepare the patient for this nursing practice
- Collect and prepare the equipment
- help the patient with an immersion bath or shower, at home or in an institutional setting.

Background knowledge required

Revision of the anatomy and physiology of the skin with special reference to its function as a barrier to infection.

Review of health authority policy relating to lifting and handling, both in an institutional and community setting.

Review of local policy regarding preoperative skin preparation.

Review of health authority policy regarding cleaning bathroom equipment and control of infection.

Indications and rationale for immersion bath or shower

An immersion bath or shower enables the patient to have a total body wash, and may be indicated:
- to maintain personal hygiene *and promote a feeling of well-being*
- to clean the skin prior to surgery *in order to help prevent infection in the wound area during the operation* (Rogers 1994)
- to clean the skin following surgery *to prevent infection and promote healing*.

Equipment

Soap

Face cloth

Bath towel

Clean clothing

Chosen toiletries, e.g. deodorant, perfume, aftershave

Suitable bath or shower

Chair or shower stool

Disposable floor mat

Bathing/showering equipment aids as appropriate.

Guidelines and rationale for this nursing practice

Bathing

- discuss the arrangements for his bath with the patient *to gain consent and cooperation and encourage participation in care.* In the community the patient should have a bathing assessment carried out; *this will assess the need for equipment available from occupational therapy, and whether help with bathing and showering should be given by nursing or social services' staff* (refer to health board policy)
- help the patient collect and prepare the equipment *so that everything is ready for use*
- help the patient to the bathroom; this may include the use of mechanical lifting aids or a wheelchair *if the patient has any difficulty with mobilising* (Barker et al 1994)
- ensure the patient's privacy as far as possible, *to respect individuality and maintain self esteem*
- prepare the water in the bath maintaining a safe temperature and gain the patient's approval *as bathing is a very personal activity*
- help the patient to undress *if he needs help, but encourage him to be as independent as possible*
- observe the patient throughout this activity *to observe any adverse effects*
- help the patient into the bath. For some patients, two nurses may be needed *to help the patient,* or mechanical aids may be used according to the manufacturer's instructions as appropriate (RCN 1993)
- help the patient to wash himself, commencing with washing and drying his face and neck (*see* Bed bath, p. 30) *so that clean water is used first on these areas*
- help to wash the patient's hair *if required* (*see* Hair care p. 153)
- help the patient out of the bath. He may sit on a chair which is protected with a towel *to prevent any unsteadiness and danger of falling*
- help the patient to dry himself *as required and encourage independence*
- help the patient to dress himself as required. He should choose what he wants to wear *to promote his self esteem and independence*
- allow the patient time to clean his teeth or dentures at the basin, *to promote oral hygiene,* giving help as required
- help to brush or comb the patient's hair *to help his self esteem*
- help the patient to a chair or bed as he chooses, or as his condition allows *for a period of rest after the exercise of bathing*
- ensure that the patient is left feeling as comfortable as possible *to promote relaxation*
- clean the bath *to promote a safe environment*
- dispose of equipment safely *to prevent any transmission of infection*
- document the nursing practice appropriately, monitor after-effects and report abnormal findings immediately *to ensure safe practice and enable prompt appropriate medical or nursing intervention to be initiated.*

Showering

- discuss the arrangements for the shower with the patient *to gain consent and cooperation*
- help collect and prepare the equipment *so that everything is ready for use*
- help the patient to the shower room. This may include the use of mechanical lifting aids or a wheelchair *if the patient has any difficulty with mobilising*
- help the patient to undress as required *maintaining privacy to respect her individuality* (Glen & Townley 1995)
- help the patient to sit on the shower chair or stool *so that there is no danger of falling*
- adjust the flow of water from the shower *to maintain a safe water temperature and gain the patient's approval*
- help the patient to wash herself while showering as required *so that she may have an enjoyable body wash*
- help the patient to wash her hair if required *to promote her self esteem* (Carter 1995)
- help the patient to dry herself
- proceed as for Guidelines for bathing.

Relevance to the activities of living

Observations and further rationale for this nursing practice will be included within each activity of living as appropriate.

Maintaining a safe environment

The nurse should ensure that the patient has appropriate assistance to help him bath or shower safely.

A chair should be available so that he can sit to dry or dress himself to prevent any danger of falling.

The water temperature should be checked to ensure that there is no danger of scalding. The ability to judge temperature may be impaired in elderly patients or those with diabetic neuropathy, so the water temperature should always be checked by a nurse or a responsible adult. The use of a bath thermometer will help with this.

The bath or shower area should be cleaned after each use. If the nurse is not confident that this has been done the bath should be cleaned before preparing it for the patient, to prevent any cross-infection.

Communicating

As far as possible the choice and timing of a bath or shower should be arranged according to the patient's preference. The patient's condition and the ward or community situation may affect this, however, and appropriate arrangements should be discussed with the patient to gain his cooperation.

The development of a caring relationship between the nurse and the patient is often enhanced during the patient's bath or shower. The opportunity for communication is increased so the nurse can encourage the patient to talk about himself, his family or his worries, and this information may contribute to the nursing assessment. The time can also be used for patient education in personal hygiene, using good communication skills (Conway 1994).

Eliminating

The patient should be given the opportunity to use the toilet or commode before bathing or showering.

Personal cleansing and dressing

While bathing the patient, the nurse should observe the condition of the skin for any abnormalities. Any redness, rashes, bruises, sores or lumps should be noted and reported (*see* Bed bath, p. 30).

The skin should be dried carefully after bathing or showering, especially in the creases of the body, e.g. under the breasts and in the groin. This helps to maintain the skin in good condition as a barrier to infection. A light dusting with talcum powder may help to keep the skin dry, but too much may collect in the body creases and cause soreness.

If possible the patient should be encouraged to wear his own clothes after a bath or shower to help retain his individuality.

Controlling body temperature

The bath or shower room should be at a comfortable room temperature of 18–21°C. This will prevent loss of body heat after a bath, when the patient may be exposed during drying and dressing.

Mobilising

Mechanical lifting aids should be used appropriately, according to the manufacturer's instructions, to help the patient in and out of a bath or shower (Professional Development Unit 1995). In the community this will be in accordance with the individualised community bathing assessment.

Expressing sexuality

If the patient is left alone to bath and shower, it is often difficult to ensure the safety of his environment and so complete privacy can not be assured; the patient will usually accept the presence of the nurse if the implications for his safety are explained. The nurse's attitude and communication skills should help acceptance of this invasion of privacy and prevent embarrassment. Apart from necessary attendant helpers, privacy should be ensured during this activity.

Male patients should be encouraged or helped to shave before or immediately after bathing or showering. They may like to apply some pleasant aftershave lotion to enhance their self image.

Women may be encouraged to apply make-up and perfume after bathing to help their individuality and self-esteem.

Patient education: key points

The nurse should emphasise the importance of personal hygiene in the prevention of infection.

The importance of a safe water temperature for bathing and showering should be explained, and the height of controls or taps may need to be adapted for safe use.

The use of aids, both simple and mechanical, should be explained to the patient. This helps maintain a safe environment by preventing accidental falls and also ensures safe lifting and handling techniques for nurses and carers.

Advice and teaching about the availability of aids and the adaptation of the patient's home should be part of the responsibility of the community nursing team and the occupational therapist.

The patient should understand the importance of reporting any redness, swelling or breakdown of the skin to the nurse or medical practitioner so that further deterioration in the condition of the skin can be prevented.

References

Barker A, Cassar S, Gabbett J et al 1994 Handling people: equipment, advice and information. Disabled Living Foundation, London

Carter A 1995 The use of touch in nursing practice. Nursing Standard 9 (16): 31–35

Conway J 1994 Reflection: the art and science of nursing and the theory – practice gap. British Journal of Nursing 3(3): 114–118

Glen S, Townley S 1995 Privacy: A key nursing concept. British Journal of Nursing 4(2): 69–72

Professional Development Unit 1995 12.2 Lifting and handling, the role of the nurse. Nursing Times (suppl) 91(2): 1–4

RCN 1993 Code of practice for the handling of patients. RCN advisory panel for back pain in nurses. Royal College of Nursing, London

Rogers S 1994 The patient facing surgery. In: Alexander M, Fawcett J, Runciman P (eds) Nursing practice, hospital and home, the adult. Churchill Livingstone, Edinburgh, pp 781–786

Further reading

Gilchrist B 1990 Washing and dressing after surgery. Nursing Times 86(50): 71

Kalideen D 1990 Preparing skin for surgery. Nursing 4(15): 28–29

RCN and BASW 1995 Bathing—an essential service: statement on current issues in nursing and social work. Royal College of Nursing and British Association of Social Workers

Roper N, Logan W, Tierney A 1996 The elements of nursing, 4th edn. Churchill Livingstone, Edinburgh, pp 231–264

Walsh M, Ford P 1989 Nursing rituals; research and rational actions. Heinemann Nursing, Oxford, pp 16–18, 114

Webster R et al 1988 Patients' and nurses' opinions about bathing. Nursing Times (occasional paper) 84(37): 54–57

4 Bed Bath

Learning outcomes

By the end of this section you should know how to:
- prepare the patient for this nursing practice
- collect the equipment
- carry out a bed bath.

Background knowledge required

Revision of the anatomy and physiology of the skin tissue.

Revision of Skin care (*see* p. 289) and Mouth care (*see* p. 209).

Indications and rationale for a bed bath

Bed bathing assists a bedfast patient *to maintain personal hygiene during a period of bedrest*. A patient may require a bed bath:
- postoperatively following major surgery when mobility is restricted
- following an acute illness, e.g. myocardial infarction
- while in an unconscious state
- following trauma, e.g. a patient in traction
- when extremely weak and debilitated due to the prolonged effects of a disease, trauma or treatment being administered.

Equipment

Basin of hot water (35–40°C)

Lotion thermometer

Soap, preferably the patient's own

Patient's toiletries such as deodorant, talcum powder

Bath towels, preferably the patient's own

Two face cloths or sponges

Disposable paper towel or similar

Patient's brush and comb

Nail scissors and nail file if required

Clean nightdress or pyjamas

Clean bed linen

Trolley or adequate surface

Equipment for catheter care (*see* p. 94) if required

Equipment for skin care (*see* p. 290)

Equipment for mouth care (*see* p. 210)

Receptacle for soiled patient clothing

Receptacle for soiled bed linen

Receptacle for soiled disposables.

Guidelines and rationale for this nursing practice

- explain the nursing practice to the patient *to gain consent and cooperation*
- collect and prepare the equipment *to ensure all equipment is available and ready for use*
- ensure the patient's privacy *to reduce anxiety*
- observe the patient throughout this activity *to note any signs of distress*
- check the bed brakes are in use *to prevent the patient or nurse sustaining an injury due to sudden uncontrolled movement of the bed*
- help the patient into a comfortable position *permitting easy comfortable access to the patient for the nurse*
- arrange the furniture around the patient's bed space *to allow easy access to equipment on the trolley/surface*
- remove excess bed linen and bed appliances if in use *allowing easy access to the patient*, but leaving the patient covered with a bed sheet *to maintain modesty*
- help the patient remove his pyjamas or gown *to reduce exertion as this can be a strenuous activity for a person who is in a weakened state*
- check the temperature of the basin of water using the lotion thermometer and ask the patient to test the water temperature *ensuring the water is neither too hot nor too cold*
- check with the patient if he uses soap on his face *ensuring individualised care*
- wash, rinse and dry the patient's face, ears and neck; when possible assist the patient to do this for himself *to encourage independence*
- expose only the part of the patient's body being washed *to maintain the patient's modesty and self esteem*
- change the water as it cools, or becomes dirty or immediately after washing the patient's pubic area *preventing cooling of the patient and reducing the risk of cross-infection respectively*
- wash, rinse and dry thoroughly the patient's body in an appropriate order such as the upper limbs, chest and abdomen, back and lower limbs *preventing excessive exertion by the patient*
- change the water immediately after perineal hygiene or leave this action to last, *reducing the risk of cross-infection from the normal skin flora of the perineal region to the rest of the skin*
- when washing the patient's limbs, wash first the limb furthest away from you. *This will allow the assistant to dry that limb as the other limb is washed, thus reducing the time the patient's body is exposed to the cooling effect of the environment.* When possible assist the patient to immerse his feet and hands in the basin of water (Fig. 4.1)
- as each part of the patient's body is washed, observe the skin for any blemish, redness or discoloration *which can alert the nurse to the potential problem of pressure sore development* (see Skin care p. 290)

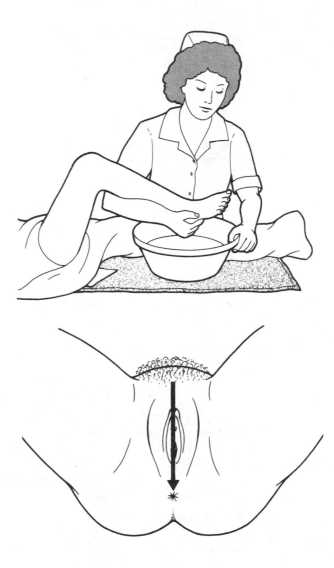

Figure 4.1   *Foot immersion: the patient's foot and leg should be supported. Upper limbs can be supported in a similar way*

Figure 4.2   *Perineal hygiene: wash in one direction only from front to back of perineum*

- apply body deodorants and/or talcum powder as desired by the patient *ensuring individualised care*
- assist the patient to wash, rinse and dry his pubic area using the extra face cloth/sponge or the disposable paper towel, washing from the front of the perineal area to the back *to prevent cross-infection from the anal region* (Fig. 4.2)
- carry out catheter care if required *which may prevent infection* (see p. 94)
- help the patient to dress in his clean pyjamas or gown *to reduce exertion by the patient*
- *to prevent injury, reduce the risk of cross-infection and promote self esteem* assist the patient to cut and clean his finger- and toenails if required, unless otherwise instructed

- *to promote patient comfort* remove any soiled or damp bed linen and remake the patient's bed
- assist the patient with his mouth care (see p. 210) *to promote a positive body image*
- assist the patient to brush or comb his hair into its usual style *promoting independence and self esteem*
- ensure that the patient is left feeling as comfortable as possible *maintaining the quality of this nursing practice*
- rearrange the furniture as wished by the patient *so that articles he requires are within easy reach and the patient is given control of the environment*
- dispose of the equipment safely *to reduce any health hazard*
- document the nursing practice appropriately, monitor after-effects and report any abnormal findings immediately *providing a written record and assisting in the implementation of any action should an abnormality or adverse reaction to the practice be noted.*

Relevance to the activities of living

Maintaining a safe environment

It is necessary to wash at regular intervals to keep the natural flora of microorganisms within manageable limits. When a patient is confined to bed, a bed bath is one of the nursing practices used to reduce the potential problem of cross-infection or infection of the patient himself during the period of vulnerability due to illness (Roper et al 1996).

The nurse must check that the temperature of the water is at a safe level prior to starting the bed bath and maintain this temperature throughout the bath to assist with patient comfort. The water should be changed as it becomes dirty, cooler or immediately following perineal hygiene. When assisting the patient with perineal hygiene, wash from front to back to reduce the problem of cross-infection from the anal region.

All equipment used should be clean or disposable and all precautions must be taken to prevent cross-infection. The nurse should wash her hands before commencing and on completion of a bed bath.

At home or in hospital it is preferable that the patient has a personal washbasin during his period of confinement to bed. The nurse should wash the basin and trolley with a detergent and water solution, drying thoroughly prior to and following a bed bath. The basin should be clean and dry when not in use (Greaves 1985) and stored in an easily accessible area for sole use by that patient.

The patient's face cloth or sponge should be rinsed in clean water and returned to the patient's locker or bathroom along with the other toilet items used and any soiled personal patient clothing which relatives wish to take home for laundering during hospitalisation. Any appliances removed during the bed bath, such as a bedcage, bed table or cot sides, should be returned to their previous position.

In some health authority areas bathing at home is no longer a responsibility of the community health service (Johnston 1994), but has become the task of social care workers (Nazarko 1995). However, where the bed bath is part of an overall package of care, such as for a terminally ill patient, the community nurse would be involved in the management of delivery of care.

Communicating

The nurse and patient should engage in verbal communication during a bed bath but this may have to be kept to a minimum when a patient is acutely ill. When a patient is acutely ill or unconscious, non-verbal cues can be used as a method of communication between the nurse and patient; touch becomes of increased importance.

The nurse should check that the patient who is suffering pain has had recent pain relief prior to starting a bed bath, as the movement during the bath may exacerbate the pain.

Breathing

Patient movement during a bed bath should be kept to a minimum, especially when a patient suffers from dyspnoea; for example, changing the bottom sheet should be planned to minimise movement and effort if the patient is acutely ill. When oxygen therapy is being administered, the mask/cannulae can be removed for facial cleansing, hair care and mouth care at separate intervals during the bed bath.

Eliminating

The patient should be offered facilities to empty his bladder prior to commencement of a bed bath.

Personal cleansing and dressing

A patient who does not wash on a regular basis may require some assistance and education by the nurse as to the benefit of this practice during his period of incapacity.

In hospital it is usual to have disposable toiletries available in ward areas for patients who may have been admitted as an emergency, until their own personal equipment is brought from home.

Soap should be used with caution as it has a drying effect on the skin. A patient who has dry skin may have an emollient prescribed by a medical practitioner which is added to the water for washing. The patient's skin must be rinsed well and thoroughly dried during the bed bath to reduce the potential problem of skin irritation.

When possible the patient should be dressed in his own bed clothing for his comfort and to help maintain his individuality.

A patient who has the power, movement or sensation of a limb altered temporarily or permanently, such as by the position of an intravenous infusion or following a cerebral vascular accident, will require some assistance and education on how to dress and undress during a bed bath. The weak or affected limb is dressed first and undressed last.

The nurse should carry out Skin care (*see* p. 290) during a bed bath.

The patient should be assisted to keep his finger- and toenails clean and manicured. A chiropody service may not be available for all patients, but should be used when special care has to be taken of a patient's nails, for instance a diabetic patient or a patient suffering from peripheral vascular disease, to prevent injury to the nail or nailbed. The nurse may assist the patient to apply nail polish if desired.

When a patient is confined to bed the friction between his head and pillow can cause the hair to become tangled and matted. A patient's hair should be brushed and combed into the usual style during a bed bath and at regular intervals throughout the day to prevent the hair becoming tangled and causing the patient discomfort. The patient can have his hair washed while in bed (*see* p. 153) to maintain its cleanliness. Should a patient be confined to bed over a prolonged period a hairdresser or barber may be required to cut his hair and style it to improve morale.

Mouth care (*see* p. 210) may be required during a bed bath.

Controlling body temperature

Before commencing the bed bath the nurse should check that the environment around the patient's bed space is at a comfortable temperature and no draughts are evident. During the bed bath the nurse should ensure that the patient is kept warm, as excessive loss of body heat could lead to the patient becoming hypothermic (Childs 1994).

Expressing sexuality

In western society, feeling fresh and clean is known to create a positive body image and maintain self esteem. Therefore, as well as feeling more comfortable, a patient confined to bed will also benefit psychologically from a bed bath.

The provision of privacy during this nursing practice is very important in the maintenance of the patient's self esteem and individuality (Glen & Townley 1995).

When possible, assist the patient to maintain individuality and independence by allowing him to wash and dry any part of his body such as his face, hands and pubic area. As the patient has no choice in the method used for cleansing, allow him to make choices that are available, such as which clothing he wishes to wear. The use of a body deodorant, perfume and make-up are personal preferences, and the nurse should be guided by the patient in their application.

**Patient education:
key points**

The carer may be taught how to perform this nursing practice.

The prevention of infection by the maintenance of skin hygiene by bed bathing should be explained to the patient and his carers.

Advice on the direction of washing to reduce the risk of cross-infection from the anal region to the rest of the perineal area should be given to the patient and other carers.

References

Childs C 1994 Temperature control. In: Alexander M, Fawcett J, Runciman P (eds) Nursing practice: hospital and home – the adult. Churchill Livingstone, Edinburgh

Glen S, Townley S 1995 Privacy: a key nursing concept. British Journal of Nursing 4(2) 69–72

Greaves A 1985 We'll just freshen you up dear . . . . Nursing Times Journal of Infection Control Nursing 81(10): 3–8 (Investigation into the misuse of patient wash bowls)

Johnston C 1994 Health care and social care boundaries. Nursing Times 90(26): 40–42

Nazarko L 1995 Community care deskilling. Nursing Management 2(4): 9–10

Roper N, Logan W, Tierney A 1996 The elements of nursing, 4th edn. Churchill Livingstone, Edinburgh, pp 231–264

Suggested reading

Ayliffe G, Lowbury E, Geddes A, Williams J 1992 Control of hospital infection — a practical handbook. Chapman & Hall Medical, London

Croton C 1990 Duvets on trial. Nursing Times 86(26): 63–67

Davidson L 1989 Patient clothing: time for a change. Nursing Times 85(48): 26–29

Gooch J 1987 Skin hygiene. Professional Nurse 2(5): 153–154

Webster R, Thompson D, Bowman G, Sutton T 1988 Patients' and nurses' opinions about bathing. Nursing Times 84(37): 54–57

Wright L 1990 Bathing by towel (describes new technique). Nursing Times 86(4): 36–39

5 Blood Glucose Monitoring

Learning outcomes	By the end of this section you should know how to: • collect and prepare the equipment • prepare the patient for this nursing practice • carry out blood glucose measurement.
Background knowledge required	Anatomy and physiology of the endocrine system with special reference to the regulation of blood glucose Clinical knowledge of insulin-dependent diabetes and non-insulin-dependent diabetes Knowledge of normal range of blood glucose Manufacturer's information on selected reagent strip Knowledge of different devices used to obtain blood sample and to measure blood glucose levels Health authority policy for this procedure Principles of infection control in respect of blood-borne infection.
Indications and rationale for blood glucose estimation	Blood glucose estimation is the measurement of the level of blood glucose using a chemical reagent strip. This investigation may be carried out to: • assist in the diagnosis of diabetes mellitus due to pancreatic disease or other hormonal disorders *through measurement of the level of glucose in the blood* • monitor blood glucose levels in patients with established diabetes *in order to facilitate acceptable blood glucose levels* • monitor patients receiving parenteral nutrition (*see* Section 33) *to ensure blood glucose levels are kept within an acceptable range.*
Equipment	Sterile lancet or pricking device Cotton wool balls Blood testing strip Disposable gloves Tray for equipment Watch with a seconds hand Sharpsbox Receptacle for soiled material Patient documentation and personal diabetic diary (if appropriate) Glucose meter device.

Guidelines and rationale for this nursing practice

- discuss the procedure with the patient *to inform the patient about the procedure and to discuss any concerns or queries*
- obtain consent from the patient to undertake the procedure *to ensure that the patient is aware of her rights as a patient*
- select a suitable clean surface and lay out equipment. If undertaking the procedure in the patient's own home then protect the surface with a waterproof cover *to provide a suitable protected work surface and ensure that the equipment is ready for patient use*
- cleanse hands using a bactericidal solution *to reduce risk of cross-infection* (Gould 1995)
- help the patient into a comfortable position (either sitting or lying in a supine position) *to ensure patient comfort and prevent injury if the patient feels faint during the procedure*
- ask or assist the patient to wash her hands with soap and warm water, ensuring that all traces of soap have been rinsed off and that the hands are dried thoroughly *to ensure that the skin surface is clean and that there is no residual soap which may affect the accuracy of the reading* (Siegal 1993). *Heat will help to dilate the small blood vessels in the finger tips*
- select an appropriate puncture site (normally the soft flesh at the top of the fingers). If blood glucose monitoring is a regular procedure then the sites should be rotated *to avoid overuse of any one site and thus reduce discomfort for the patient*
- put on gloves *to protect the patient and nurse from potential blood-borne infection*
- using the lancet or pricking device (the latter is now the preferred option unless the patient objects to its use) prick the patient's finger *to pierce the skin with minimal discomfort*
- gently massage the finger to obtain an adequate drop of blood. *Obtain a suitable amount of blood to cover the reagent strip*
- allow the drop of blood to come in contact with the reagent strip without smearing and spreading the blood *to ensure even coverage of the strip*
- note the time *to ensure an accurate reading*
- apply a clean cotton wool ball with firm pressure to the skin site for approximately 30–60 seconds or until bleeding has stopped (the patient may be able to undertake this activity) *to prevent any further bleeding after the sample has been obtained and prevent haematoma formation*
- after the correct time has elapsed as recommended by the manufacturer, carefully and firmly wipe the blood off the reagent strip using a clean cotton wool ball (certain glucose meter devices do not require the blood to be wiped off the strip — if using this type of device refer to the manufacturer's instructions) *to ensure an accurate result is obtained*
- allow the second period of time to elapse as recommended by the manufacturer *to ensure an accurate result is obtained*
- compare the colour of the reagent strip with the manufacturer's scale, usually found on the reagent strip container, *or*
  use a glucose meter device following the manufacturer's instructions *to*

obtain blood glucose level (Drug and Therapeutics Bulletin 1993, Laux 1994)

- note and document the results in both nursing/medical notes and the patient's personal diabetic diary (where applicable). Informing the patient of the result should only be carried out in consultation with the medical practitioner who authorised the investigation. Opportunity should be given for the patient/carer to discuss anxieties or issues about any newly diagnosed disease *to ensure that results are communicated to other health care professionals and the patient. It may not be appropriate for the nurse to give the result to the patient at this point if further investigations are required before an accurate diagnosis can be made*
- report any abnormal results to a medical practitioner as soon as possible. If the procedure is being carried out in the patient's own home then the nurse may be required to remain with the patient until the glucose level has stabilised *to ensure that prompt appropriate treatment may be initiated. Some health authorities may have a medically agreed treatment protocol to be followed when abnormal glucose readings are detected by nursing staff*
- dispose of any contaminated equipment according to health authority policy *to prevent transmission of infection*
- remove gloves and dispose of as above. Wash hands or cleanse with bactericidal solution *to prevent cross-infection*
- ensure that patient is not feeling unwell following the procedure (this is especially important if the procedure is carried out in the patient's own home) *to ensure that the patient does not feel unwell as a result of the procedure*
- discuss the points raised under 'Patient education: key points'. If the patient is unable to participate in follow-up self care then this should be undertaken by the nurse or an appropriate adult carer *to ensure that the patient/carer/nurse is aware of, and understands, follow-up self care.*

The frequency of blood glucose monitoring will be advised by the medical practitioner.

Relevance to the activities of daily living

Maintaining a safe environment

All containers of reagent strips should be stored in a locked cupboard or drawer when not in use to comply with health and safety at work regulations. The nurse in the community should encourage patients to keep all equipment in a safe place away from children. The manufacturer's recommendations for the conditions of storage and blood glucose monitoring technique must be observed, otherwise inaccurate results may be obtained from the reagent strips.

The nurse should assess the blood glucose level at the specific time requested by the medical practitioner.

Contamination of the reagent pad or the patient's blood could lead to inaccurate results. The patient's finger should not be cleansed with an alcohol-saturated wipe as the alcohol would act as a contaminant and cause the skin to harden with constant use. Any reagent strip accidentally contaminated by the nurse or the patient must be discarded.

The nurse must be aware of the theory underpinning glucose monitoring procedure, and have knowledge of the normal range of blood glucose levels in order that any abnormal readings may be immediately recognised and treatment initiated according to health authority policy. Blood glucose levels are measured in mmol/l. The normal range of blood glucose level is between 3.7 mmol/l and no greater then 10 mmol/l after a meal. The acceptable range for each individual patient (particularly with long-standing diabetes) may vary slightly but should be identified by the medical practitioner and recorded in all patient documentation. Hypoglycaemia is the term used to describe an abnormally low blood glucose. Hyperglycaemia describes an excessively high blood glucose. Both require urgent treatment.

Communicating

The experienced nurse should be able to detect potential problems of a patient with fluctuating blood glucose level and communicate that information to other colleagues involved in the care of that patient.

The nurse should be aware of what information the patient needs about the procedure of blood glucose estimation. The nurse should encourage the patient to discuss her understanding of why blood glucose estimation is being carried out and be responsive to the patient's need for information about the reason for blood glucose estimation (this should be carried out in consultation with the medical practitioner who authorised the investigation).

The nurse should initiate a patient education programme at a time which best suits the needs of the patient and her ability to learn. Patient education may need to continue on transfer from hospital, therefore good communication is essential for its continuity.

Health promotion may be carried out in relation to an underlying disease, for example in a diabetic patient attending for blood glucose monitoring.

Breathing

Development of tachycardia or palpitation by the patient can be suggestive of hypoglycaemic coma.

Eating and Drinking

The most common reason for estimating blood glucose is for diabetes mellitus. A patient will usually be given advice on a diet to suit her needs. The patient will require on-going support and education to help her cope with any changes in eating pattern.

Eliminating

Blood glucose estimation provides a more accurate assessment of blood glucose level than assessing the level of glucose in urine. Each patient's renal threshold (the level at which the blood glucose spills over into the urine) can vary, therefore measurement of glucose in the urine can be an inaccurate guide to the effectiveness of hormonal control of the glucose level in the body.

Patient education: key points	• Blood sample results. If the results are not given immediately following the procedure then the patient should be informed of when they will be available, and of the process for obtaining them • For newly diagnosed diabetic patients the teaching of blood glucose estimation should be part of an individual education package on disease and symptom management. Teaching the patient about blood glucose estimation should incorporate the following main stages: — education on the procedure (including rationale and treatment of abnormal readings) using verbal and written information — demonstration of blood glucose monitoring technique — supervision of the patient carrying out blood glucose estimation — regular monitoring of the technique as part of the ongoing management programme of care for the patient with diabetes • Patient education is likely to be shared between institutional and community staff • Patient education material is available from many of the manufacturers who produce reagent strips and devices (Alexander et al 1994) • Glucose meters can be purchased from the community pharmacist.

References

Alexander M F, Fawcett J N, Runciman P J 1994 Nursing practice — hospital and home: the adult. Churchill Livingstone, Edinburgh, pp 154–185
Drug and Therapeutics Bulletin 1993 Meters for measuring blood glucose at home. 31(8): 30–32
Gould D 1995 Now please wash your hands. Practice Nurse 10(3): 188–190
Laux L 1994 Visual interpretation of blood glucose test strips. Diabetes Education 20(1): 41–44
Siegal J 1993 Teaching infection control in blood glucose monitoring. Diabetes Education 19(6): 489–492, 495

Further reading

Heenan A J J 1995 Devices for measuring blood glucose levels. Professional Nurse 11(1): 53–54
Mills E, Jones K, Roberts J 1991 Blood glucose monitoring: establishing a standard training programme and implementing a quality assurance scheme Diabetic Nursing 2(1): 9–10
Newton R 1987 Testing testing.... Nursing Times Community Outlook 83(2): 16–18
Reading S 1986 Blood glucose monitoring — teaching effective techniques. Professional Nurse 2(2): 55–57
Steel L G 1994 Identifying technique errors. Self-monitoring of blood glucose in the home-setting. Journal of Gerontology 20(2): 9–12
Tsang W, Griffen H 1988 Making sense of blood glucose estimation. Nursing Times 84(25): 40–41
Weeden L, Curry M 1994 Diabetes monitoring for all? Practical Diabetes 11(1): 24–26

6 Blood Pressure

Learning outcomes	By the end of this section you should know how to:
	- prepare the patient for this nursing practice
	- collect and prepare the equipment
	- assess, measure and record blood pressure.

Background knowledge required	Revision of the anatomy and physiology of the cardiovascular system.

Indications and rationale for blood pressure	Blood pressure is the force exerted by the blood as it flows through the blood vessels. It is the arterial blood pressure which is normally recorded and this may be indicated:
	- *to aid the diagnosis of disease*
	- *to aid in the assessment of the cardiovascular system during and following disease*
	- preoperatively *to assess the patient's usual range of blood pressure*
	- *to aid in assessment of the cardiovascular system following surgery/trauma.*

Equipment	Sphygmomanometer (Fig. 6.1A)
	Stethoscope.
	Electronic sphygmomanometers (Fig. 6.1B)
	Increasingly, electronic sphygmomanometers are being used to monitor patients' blood pressure in general ward areas. Should the nurse encounter any of these machines she should have some instruction on the use of each specific make of sphygmomanometer, as there are variations.

Guidelines and rationale for this nursing practice	- explain the nursing practice to the patient *to gain consent and cooperation*
	- wash the hands *to reduce the risk of cross-infection*
	- ensure the patient's privacy *to reduce anxiety and/or embarrassment*
	- collect the equipment *to assist in the planning and implementation of the practice*
	- observe the patient throughout this activity *to note any signs of distress*
	- help the patient into a suitable position, either sitting or lying, and remove

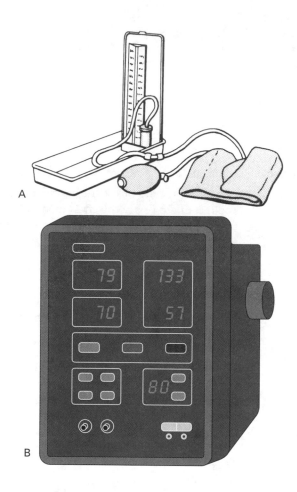

Figure 6.1 *A Mercury sphygmomanometer: used for blood pressure measurement B Electronic sphygmomanometer*

restrictive clothing from the arm. Avoid tightly rolled-up sleeves *as these prevent constriction of the vessels of the limb immediately before the practice and may lead to an inaccurate recording*

- position the sphygmomanometer at approximately heart height, ensuring that the mercury level is at zero and the mercury column can be easily read. *This will reduce the incidence of over/underestimation of blood pressure* (Petrie et al 1990a)
- apply the cuff 3–5 cm above the point where the brachial artery can be palpated. The cuff should be applied smoothly and firmly, covering 80% of the arm circumference (Croft & Cruickshank 1990), with the middle of the rubber bladder directly over the brachial artery *to permit access to the brachial artery by the stethoscope and even pressure around the circumference of the limb. A bladder which is too large or small will result in under/overestimation respectively of the blood pressure* (O'Brien 1995)
- ask the patient to rest his arm on a suitable firm surface *to ensure patient comfort and prevent movement of the limb which may lead to inaccurate results*

- connect the cuff tubing to the manometer tubing and close the valve of the inflation ball *creating a sealed unit within the equipment*
- palpate the radial pulse and inflate the cuff until the pulse is obliterated. Inflate a further 20 mmHg. Release the valve slowly, taking note of the reading on the mercury column when the radial pulse returns. The mercury is read at the top of the meniscus. Allow all air to escape from the cuff. *This will provide an initial assessment of the systolic pressure*
- palpate the brachial pulse, place the stethoscope over the site and inflate the cuff to 20 mmHg above the previous reading. Release the valve of the inflation ball at the rate of 2–3 mmHg per second. When the first pulse is heard, the mercury level should be noted — this is the systolic pressure (Petrie et al 1990b). *This provides an accurate assessment of the systolic pressure without excessive discomfort to the patient*
- continue to deflate the cuff, and the pulse will change to muffled sounds until finally it disappears; the mercury level should be noted — this is the diastolic pressure (Petrie et al 1990b). *This provides an accurate assessment of the diastolic pressure*
- continue controlled deflation until the point 20 mmHg below the diastolic pressure is reached *as this will eradicate the chance of a 'silent interval' leading to a false recording*
- completely deflate the cuff, disconnect the tubing and remove the cuff from the patient's arm *to prevent further compression of the limb*
- ensure that the patient is left feeling as comfortable as possible *to ensure the quality of this nursing practice*
- if a communal stethoscope has been used, clean the ear pieces with an alcohol-saturated swab *to reduce cross-infection between staff*
- dispose of the equipment safely *to comply with health and safety criteria and prolong the use of the equipment*
- document the nursing practice appropriately comparing past recordings; note differences, detect trends, monitor after-effects and report abnormal findings immediately. *This provides a written record and assists in the implementation of any action should an abnormality or adverse reaction to the practice be noted.*

Relevance to the activities of living

Maintaining a safe environment

It is recommended that a sphygmomanometer should be calibrated at regular intervals by trained personnel to maintain the accuracy of the equipment.

The size of the cuff is important in achieving accurate recordings (Croft & Cruickshank 1990). Different cuffs are available for use on a baby, child, or obese person or for recordings on the patient's thigh.

By listening for sounds 20 mmHg above and below the points of appearance and disappearance, the possibility of a 'silent interval' falsifying the reading is overcome.

Repeated measurements, i.e. more than twice in 5 minutes, should be avoided as venous congestion can cause a rise in pressure.

All equipment should be clean and all precautions be taken to prevent cross-infection. The nurse should wash her hands before commencing and on completion of the nursing practice. When a communal ward stethoscope has been used the ear pieces should be cleaned with an alcohol-saturated swab before commencing and on completion of blood pressure assessment. A nurse may wish to purchase her own stethoscope which would prevent any ear cross-infection.

Communicating

Blood pressure measurements can be recorded on a graded chart or abbreviated by placing the systolic pressure reading over the diastolic pressure reading, i.e.

$$\frac{130}{80}$$

Hypertension is the term used when the systolic or diastolic blood pressure is elevated beyond the normal range.

Hypotension is the term used when the blood pressure is lower than the normal range.

Stressful situations such as admission to hospital or a visit to a health care professional are known to have an effect on a person's blood pressure. The nurse should allow the patient to relax before the recording is taken.

Patient education: key points

Results of blood pressure measurement Inform the patient of the results and any action required should an abnormality be detected.

Risk factors affecting blood pressure Information regarding the common lifestyle factors which are known to affect blood pressure should be discussed with the patient. This may allow the patient to make an informed choice about whether or not to continue such practices.

References

Croft P, Cruickshank J 1990 Blood pressure measurement in adults: large cuffs for all? Journal of Epidemiology and Community Health 44: 170–173
O'Brien E 1995 Blood pressure measurement. In: O'Brien ET, Beevers DG, Marshall HJ (eds) ABC of hypertension, 3rd edn. BMJ Publishing, London
Petrie JC, O'Brien ET, Littler WA, de Swiet M, Dillon MJ, Padfield PL 1990a Recommendations on blood pressure measurement, 2nd edn. BMJ Publishing, London
Petrie J, Jamieson M, O'Brien E, Littler W, Padfield P, de Swiet M for the Working Party on Blood Pressure Measurement 1990b Blood pressure measurement (videotape). BMJ Publishing, London

---

Further reading

Brunner L, Suddarth D 1992 The textbook of adult nursing. Chapman Hall, London, pp 316–317
Marieb E 1989 Human anatomy and physiology. Benjamin Cummings, New York, pp 628–630

O'Brien D, Davison M 1994 Blood pressure measurement: rational and ritual actions. British Journal of Nursing 3(8): 393–396

Roper N, Logan W, Tierney A 1996 The elements of nursing, 4th edn. Churchill Livingstone, Edinburgh, pp 156–158

Walsh M, Ford P 1989 Nursing rituals — research and rational actions. Heinemann Nursing, Oxford, pp 55–57

7 Blood Transfusion

Learning outcomes

By the end of this section you should know how to:

- prepare the patient for this nursing practice
- collect and prepare equipment
- assist the medical practitioner with the safe insertion of an intravenous cannula
- maintain a blood transfusion for a period of time.

Background knowledge required

Revision of the anatomy and physiology of the blood, with special emphasis on blood groups.

Revision of Intravenous therapy (*see* p. 165).

Revision of Aseptic technique (*see* p. 383).

Review of health authority policy in relation to blood transfusion.

Indications and rationale for a blood transfusion

A blood transfusion is the introduction of prepared compatible donor blood into the circulation of a recipient patient. A blood transfusion may be indicated for the following reasons:

- *to restore circulatory blood volume following haemorrhage*
- *to maintain adequate circulatory blood volume during and following surgical procedures*
- *to maintain adequate levels of haemoglobin which have been reduced by blood disorders,* e.g. anaemia, leukaemia (Higgins 1995).

Blood for transfusion is prescribed and ordered by a medical practitioner.

Blood is cross-matched in the blood transfusion laboratory for compatibility, *to correspond with the blood group of the individual recipient,* and labelled accordingly.

Each unit of blood ordered is stored in the blood bank at 1–6°C for use within 48 hours. *This ensures that the blood remains safe for transfusion use whenever it is needed within that time span. After 48 hours the condition of the blood begins to deteriorate* (Dodworth 1995).

Equipment

As for intravenous infusion (*see* pp. 166–167).

Additional equipment

- Grouped and cross-matched unit of prescribed blood

- Sterile blood administration set
- Sterile blood filter as appropriate
- Non-sterile gloves which should be worn when handling all blood products.

In emergency situations

- Pressure bag (Fenwal bag)
- Blood warming equipment.

Guidelines and rationale for this nursing practice

This procedure will be initiated by a medical practitioner using aseptic technique. Blood should be transfused by an intravenous route separate from all other infusions. This may necessitate a separate peripheral intravenous line for the duration of the blood transfusion only (*see* Intravenous therapy, p. 165). *This prevents contamination of the blood by other infusion fluids during the transfusion; some fluids may be incompatible with blood, e.g. dextrose/glucose causes 'clumping' of red blood cells.*

- help to explain the nursing practice to the patient *to gain consent and cooperation and encourage participation in care*
- ensure the patient's privacy *to respect individuality and maintain self esteem*
- collect and prepare the equipment *making efficient use of time and resources*
- help the patient into a comfortable position as required *so that he will find it easier to accept the transfusion*
- observe the patient throughout this activity *to monitor any adverse affects* (Bradbury & Cruickshank 1995)
- obtain the prescribed unit of blood from the blood bank immediately prior to use. *Blood is only safe for use for 4–6 hours after removal from the blood bank; it deteriorates quickly after that*
- check that the blood is compatible for that particular patient, *incompatible blood causes adverse reactions.* This is because the blood cells of incompatible blood 'clump' together (Higgins 1994)
- prime the administration set with normal saline (Fig. 7.1). *Only normal saline (sodium chloride 0.9%) is compatible with blood; no other intravenous fluid should be used*
- assist the medical practitioner as required with the insertion of an intravenous cannula (*see* Intravenous therapy, p. 165). Gloves should be worn *to prevent contamination with body fluids*
- commence the transfusion of blood at the rate prescribed by the medical practitioner *as part of the patient's individual treatment*
- help the patient into a comfortable position following the commencement of the transfusion *to help the patient accept the transfusion for a period of time*
- regulate the flow rate *to maintain the flow of blood at the prescribed rate*
- record accurately the volume of blood transfused. *Note:* the volume of one unit of whole blood is 500 ml; the volume of one unit of concentrated red cells is 300 ml. *Any adverse effects may be related to the amount transfused*
- ensure that the patient is left feeling as comfortable as possible *to help reduce anxiety*

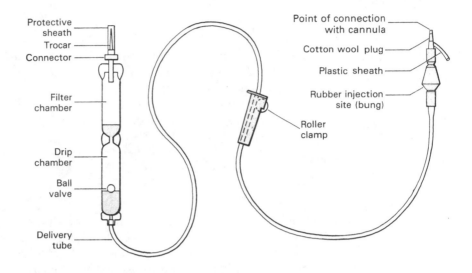

Figure 7.1
Administration set for blood transfusion. An extra filter may be introduced between the blood pack and the blood administration set

- dispose of the equipment safely *to prevent transmission of infection*
- document this nursing practice appropriately, monitor after-effects, and report abnormal findings immediately *to ensure safe practice and enable prompt appropriate medical and nursing intervention to be initiated as soon as possible.*

Guidelines and rationale for withdrawal of blood from the bank

- refer to health authority policies for access to the blood bank and local procedure *as there may be slight variations in documentation*
- withdraw blood from the blood bank one unit at a time immediately before transfusion for an individual patient *so that each unit of blood is stored at the correct temperature until immediately before use*
- check information on the label of the blood container against appropriate documentation for that particular patient *as incompatible blood causes adverse reactions*
- complete documentation of withdrawal for the blood transfusion service and the patient's medical records *ensuring accurate record keeping* (UKCC 1993).

Guidelines and rationale for checking blood for transfusion

Blood for transfusion is checked by two people, one of whom must be a medical practitioner or a registered nurse. *This is safe professional practice for ensuring that the correct patient receives a compatible unit of blood.*

- identify the prescription for blood transfusion and check the following information:
  — the date and time of commencement
  — the name of the patient
  — the unit or hospital number of the patient
  — the type of blood prescribed, e.g. whole blood or concentrated red cells
  — the number of units prescribed

> — the rate of transfusion ordered
> — the signature of the medical practitioner

- check the following information against the patient's own documentation and each labelled unit of blood:
  - the name of the patient
  - the unit or hospital number of the patient
  - the age and date of birth of the patient
  - the address of the patient
  - the blood group of the patient
  - the rhesus factor of the patient
  - the expiry date of the blood pack
  - the unit number of the blood pack
- establish the patient's identity by appropriate means, e.g. identification bracelet
- sign the label on the checked blood unit; this is signed by the two people involved *acknowledging professional responsibility*
- transfer the duplicate unit pack number to the patient's records according to health authority policy; *if adverse effects occur, the blood unit transfused can be investigated to identify any problems* (DOH 1994).

Relevance to the activities of living

Observations and further rationale for this nursing practice will be included within each activity of living as appropriate.

Maintaining a safe environment

Gloves should be worn at all times when handling blood products and associated equipment to prevent cross-infection from blood-borne viral infections such as hepatitis B or HIV/AIDS and to protect staff from invasive contact (*see* Isolation nursing, p. 185).

All precautions for the prevention of infection and the prevention of air emboli should be maintained (*see* Intravenous infusion, p. 165).

Accurate checking of individual units of blood will help to ensure that only compatible blood is transfused.

Despite careful cross-matching some patients develop a transfusion reaction, accurate observations will help to detect this as early as possible. All observations should be continued for at least 4 hours after the last unit of blood has been transfused, and thereafter as appropriate (Glover 1995).

If a transfusion reaction is suspected, the transfusion is discontinued and the medical practitioner informed immediately. The haematologist should also be informed, and used blood containers returned to the blood transfusion laboratory for testing.

Communicating

Any complaint of pain should be reported, e.g. headache, loin pain. These may indicate emboli caused by a transfusion reaction.

Breathing

Pulse, respiration rate and blood pressure should be monitored, normally hourly, during the transfusion. Respiratory function should not be affected unless a transfusion reaction occurs or the blood is transfused at a rate which causes fluid overload (*see* Intravenous infusion, p. 165).

Patients who have congestive cardiac failure should be transfused at an appropriately slower rate to prevent fluid overload with associated pulmonary oedema and dyspnoea; diuretics are sometimes prescribed to cover the duration of the transfusion to prevent this complication. The use of concentrated red cells instead of whole blood helps to prevent fluid overload.

Eating and drinking

An accurate chart of fluid intake should be maintained.

The patient may need help with placing and preparing food if one hand is immobilised (*see* Intravenous infusion, p. 165).

Personal cleansing and dressing

Skin colour should be noted and abnormalities reported, e.g. pallor, flushing, rash, which may indicate transfusion reaction.

The patient may need some help with personal cleansing and dressing if one arm is immobilised.

The need for light clothing to allow access to the transfusion site should be explained.

Eliminating

Urine output should be accurately measured to maintain fluid balance charts.

Diuresis may occur if diuretic medication is ordered; this should be explained.

If any incompatibility occurs the kidneys may be the first organs to be affected, because emboli form in the renal capillaries due to clumping of incompatible blood. The patient may complain of back pain and there may be frank haematuria, which should be reported immediately.

The patient may need help, when using a commode, to support the administration tubing while the transfusion is in progress.

Controlling body temperature

Body temperature should be monitored hourly or as ordered; one of the early signs of an adverse reaction may be a sudden rise in body temperature. Often this is associated with rigor, and either chilling or flushing is experienced by the patient.

Appropriate clothing and covering will help the patient to feel more comfortable.

Donor blood only remains stable at 1–6°C and should not be warmed prior to transfusion. In emergencies when a rapid transfusion is needed, special blood warming equipment is used, as ordered by the medical practitioner. This is usually confined to transfusions occuring in accident and emergency units, the operating theatre, and intensive care areas.

In non-acute situations transfusions are normally prescribed at a flow rate of one unit every 4 hours. This slower rate of transfusion allows the body to adjust to the initially low temperature of the donor blood.

Maintaining an accurate flow rate will help the patient to control body temperature.

Mobilising

The degree of mobility may depend on other factors. Initially it may be appropriate for the patient to rest comfortably; this allows more accurate recordings and observations to be maintained.

The patient may move around the bed, sit in a chair and use a commode with help, as his condition allows.

Sleeping

Any change in the patient's general state of consciousness, e.g. confusion, restlessness, or disorientation should be noted, as it may indicate a transfusion reaction.

The patient may find it difficult to lie in his normal sleeping position because of the transfusion lines. Help may be needed in adjusting to a suitable comfortable position.

Necessary observations may waken the patient. Temperature recordings may need to be maintained. Continuous recording with an electronic probe may be less disturbing than intermittent recording with a mercury thermometer. The blood pressure may be recorded less frequently during the sleeping period, as the patient's condition allows, if the less disturbing pulse recording is continued.

Patient education: key points

- Explain the reason for the transfusion as part of the patient's treatment, and state the time expected for completion of each unit. This makes it easier for the patient to tolerate the practice.
- Explain the importance of maintaining the cannula and lines safely in situ and the need for keeping the cannulated limb as still as possible. The dangers of disconnection should be emphasised so that the lines and dressing are not dislodged.
- The patient should understand the importance of reporting immediately any soreness or redness at the site of the transfusion, which may be a sign of local infection, even after completion of the transfusion.
- He should understand the importance of reporting any headache, sweating, dizziness or feeling of distress to the nursing staff who will be monitoring his progress, as this may indicate an adverse reaction to the blood being transfused.

- Patients who have had a blood transfusion will have had their blood group identified. They should be given information about this, preferably documented, for future reference.

References

Bradbury M, Cruickshank J P 1995 Blood and blood transfusion reactions: 2. British Journal of Nursing 4(15): 861–868
Department of Health 1994 Guidelines for blood transfusion services. HMSO, London
Dodworth H 1995 Making sense of . . . . blood and blood products. Nursing Times 91(1): 25–29
Glover G 1995 Blood transfusion. Nursing Standard 9(33): 31–35
Higgins C 1994 Blood transfusions: risks and benefits. British Journal of Nursing 3(19): 986–991
Higgins C 1995 Haematology blood testing for anaemia. British Journal of Nursing 4(5): 248–253
UKCC 1993 Standards for records and record keeping. United Kingdom Central Council for Nursing, Midwifery and Health Visiting, London

Further reading

Bradbury M, Cruickshank J P 1995 Blood and blood transfusion reactions: 1. British Journal of Nursing 4(14): 814–817
Contreras M (ed) 1992 ABC of transfusion. BMJ Publications, London
Duke F 1994 Blood disorders. In: Alexander M, Fawcett J, Runciman P (eds) Nursing practice—Hospital and home: the adult. Churchill Livingstone, Edinburgh, pp 415–419
Miller J A 1989 Transfusion of blood and blood products. Professional Nurse 4(11): 560, 562–565

8 Body Temperature

Learning outcomes	By the end of this section you should know how to: ▪ prepare the patient for this nursing practice ▪ collect and prepare the equipment ▪ measure and record the body temperature at the axilla, in the oral cavity or in the rectum, both in a community or institutional setting.
Background knowledge required	Revision of the anatomy and physiology of the skin in relation to the control of body temperature and of the temperature-regulating centre, and related body mechanisms associated with heat production and heat loss. Revision of the anatomy of the area where the temperature is to be measured.
Indications and rationale for recording body temperature	A temperature recording is a measurement of body temperature in degrees Celsius (°C) using a calibrated clinical thermometer, a disposable thermometer or an electronic probe. The axilla, the oral cavity or the rectum may be the chosen site for the recording. For each patient the site chosen for measuring the temperature should be used consistently, *so that any changes in temperature can be accurately monitored*. The normal range of body temperature is 36–37.5°C. The upper and lower limits of survival are not known exactly, but are thought to be at body temperatures of 44°C and 27°C respectively (Fig. 8.1). The recording of body temperature may be required: ▪ *to establish a baseline temperature*, e.g. when patients are admitted to hospital or clinic ▪ *to monitor fluctuations in temperature*, e.g. for patients during the postoperative period, *as temperature fluctuations can indicate developing infection or the presence of a deep venous thrombosis* ▪ *to monitor signs of incompatibility when patients are receiving a blood transfusion* ▪ *to monitor the temperature of patients being treated for an infection* ▪ *to monitor the temperature of patients recovering from hypothermia.* The frequency of the recording *will depend on the reason for monitoring body temperature, and on the patient's condition* (Gould 1994).
Equipment	Tray Appropriate thermometer, e.g.

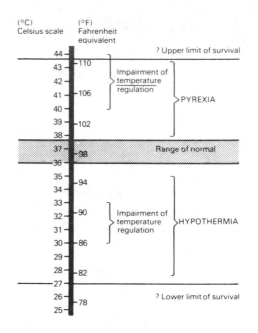

Figure 8.1   *Range of normal/abnormal body temperature (oral) (Reproduced with permission from Roper N, Logan W, Tierney A 1990 The elements of nursing, 3rd edn. Churchill Livingstone, Edinburgh)*

— clinical thermometer
— disposable thermometer
— electronic thermometer plus probe

Alcohol-impregnated swabs, e.g. Mediswabs

Watch with a seconds hand

Tissues

Receptacle for disposables.

Additional equipment as required

▪ Disposable sleeve for clinical thermometer, e.g. Steritemp sleeve
▪ Disposable probe cover for electronic probe
▪ Lubricant for rectal thermometer, e.g. petroleum jelly.

Clinical thermometers

These thermometers have a glass bulb filled with mercury; the mercury expands along a calibrated glass tube in response to contact with the warmer temperature of human body tissues. The tube has a constriction above the bulb to prevent the mercury from returning to its original position when removed from the site of the recording, thus allowing the temperature measurement to be accurately read. Before commencing a recording, the mercury in the tube should be shaken down to give a reading level with the lowest calibrated figure on the thermometer. The clinical thermometer should remain in position for at least 4 minutes to prevent a false low result. Research has shown that thermometers should be in situ for 4–9 minutes (Blumenthal 1992). There are various types of clinical thermometer (Fig. 8.2):

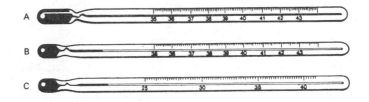

Figure 8.2   *Clinical glass thermometers A Oral/axillary B Rectal C Low reading*

Oral/axillary thermometer This is used for measuring the oral or axillary temperature. It has an oval-shaped clear glass-covered mercury bulb and is calibrated between 35°C and 43.5°C.

Rectal thermometer This is used for measuring the rectal temperature. It has a blue-coloured, more rounded mercury bulb and is calibrated between 35°C and 43.5°C.

Low reading thermometer This is specially calibrated to record temperature readings between 25°C and 40°C and is used to record the temperature of patients suffering from hypothermia (Toulson 1994).

Disposable thermometers (Fig. 8.3)

These have rapid-reacting heat-sensitive chemicals in the recording head, so that a recording can be made in 60 seconds. They are used for oral recording and are discarded after one use. Similar equipment is available for measuring skin temperature (Fig. 8.4).

Electronic thermometers

These have probes which must be protected by a disposable cover before being placed at the recording site. They are connected to equipment which gives an electronic readout of the temperature in 25–35 seconds. Various types of

Figure 8.3   *Disposable thermometer with rechargeable, battery-operated readout unit A Thermometer in situ B Recording the oral body temperature with the readout unit C Disposable thermometer*

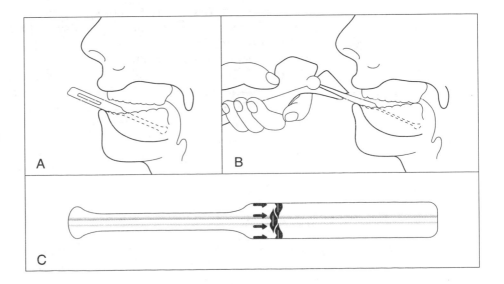

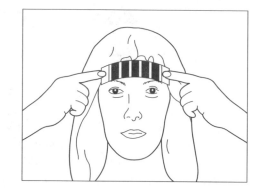

Figure 8.4 *How to take temperature using a simple disposable thermometer. Refer to manufacturer's instructions for reading the colour changes.*

electronic temperature/recording equipment are available. Some probes are designed for oral or axillary temperatures, others for rectal recordings (refer to the manufacturer's instructions).

Guidelines and rationale for this nursing practice

Guidelines are given for temperature recording in three sites using a clinical thermometer, but the principles can be adapted for any type of thermometer (Fulbrook 1993).

Axilla

- explain the nursing practice *to gain consent and cooperation and encourage participation in care.* Ensure that the patient has not recently had a hot bath or been engaged in strenuous exercise *as these will cause a temporary rise in body temperature*
- ensure the patient's privacy *to respect her individuality*
- help the patient into a comfortable position with the back and shoulders well supported, *so that she may remain in that position for a few minutes.* She may be either sitting or lying
- help the patient to remove or adjust her clothing *to expose one axilla*
- observe the patient throughout this activity *to monitor any adverse effects*
- dry the skin of the axilla by wiping with a tissue. *A film of moisture between the skin and the thermometer bulb can cause an inaccurate reading*
- check the thermometer reading and shake the thermometer *to return the mercury column to 35°C for accuracy of recording*
- clean the thermometer by wiping it with an alcohol solution (e.g. Mediswab) and allow the alcohol solution to evaporate *to prevent any cross-infection*
- place the bulb end of the thermometer in the axilla where the skin surfaces will surround it *to gain an accurate temperature reading*
- help the patient to hold her arm across her chest *to retain the thermometer in the correct position*
- leave the thermometer in position for the required time *to allow the maximum temperature to be measured — a minimum of 4 minutes* (Cutler 1994)

- remain with the patient if required *to reassure the patient and ensure the thermometer remains in the correct position*
- remove the thermometer *when the optimum time for accurate recording is reached*
- read the temperature measured by the thermometer *for an accurate recording to be monitored and documented*
- wipe the thermometer with alcohol solution *to maintain a safe environment*
- shake the thermometer to return the mercury to the bulb and leave a reading of 35°C on the thermometer *in preparation for any further recording*
- ensure the patient is left feeling as comfortable as possible *to reassure the patient and reduce anxiety*
- dispose of equipment safely *to prevent cross-infection*
- document the temperature reading in the patient's records, compare the reading with previous recordings and report abnormal findings immediately. *This will ensure safe practice and enable prompt appropriate medical and nursing intervention to be initiated.*

Oral cavity

- explain the nursing practice *to gain consent and cooperation.* Ensure that the patient has not recently had a hot or cold drink, or a hot bath, or been engaged in strenuous exercise *as this may temporarily raise the body temperature*
- help the patient into a comfortable position *so that he will more readily tolerate the thermometer in his mouth*
- prepare the thermometer as for an axillary temperature recording
- apply a disposable sleeve if required *to prevent transmission of infection*
- place the thermometer under the patient's tongue so that the bulb lies adjacent to the frenulum at the junction of the floor of the mouth and the base of the tongue, on either the right or left side. *A maximum temperature recording will be obtained from one of these two 'heat pockets' in the mouth* (Fig. 8.5) This is also the position for disposable oral thermometers
- explain to the patient the importance of closing only the lips round the thermometer, and not biting it, *so that oral temperature is maintained and not distorted by inspiration of air through the mouth*
- leave the thermometer in position for the required time *for accurate recording to occur* (Closs 1992)
- remove the thermometer and proceed as for an axillary temperature recording.

Rectum

- explain the nursing practice to the patient *to gain consent and cooperation*
- ensure the patient's privacy *to respect individuality and maintain self esteem*
- help the patient into a comfortable position lying on his side with knees bent *so that access is easier and the patient is least distressed*
- prepare the thermometer as for an axillary temperature recording
- apply a disposable sleeve *to prevent transmission of infection*

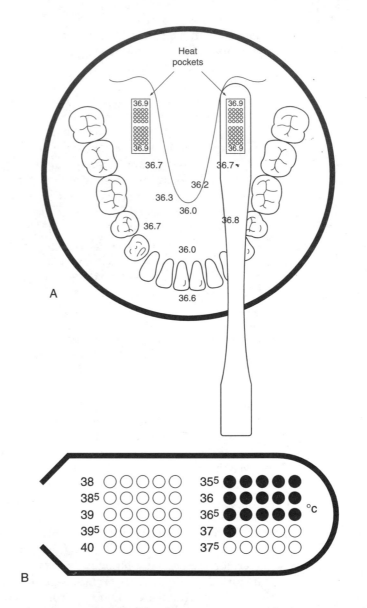

Figure 8.5   *A Heat pockets in the oral cavity B Recording area of a disposable thermometer*

- lubricate the protected end of the thermometer *to make insertion easier and to prevent any damage to the mucosa*
- gently insert the thermometer into the patient's anus for 2–4 cm and hold the thermometer in position for the required time *for accurate recording of the temperature to occur* (Jensen et al 1994)
- remove the thermometer, dispose of the protective sleeve and proceed as for an axillary temperature recording.

Relevance to the activities of living

Observations and further rationale for this nursing practice will be included within each activity of living as appropriate.

Maintaining a safe environment

Temperature recording is a non-invasive practice; however, the nurse should wash her hands before and after the recording to prevent cross-infection. The equipment should be kept clean; rectal thermometers should be stored separately from other thermometers. Clinical thermometers should be handled and stored with care; broken glass and mercury vapour can cause harm to both patients and staff.

Oral temperature recording should only be used for adult patients who are alert, well-orientated and able to cooperate in carrying out the procedure.

Rectal temperature recordings should be used for infants. Children and all adults who are unable to cooperate, e.g. due to breathlessness, confusion or unconsciousness, should have an axillary or rectal temperature recorded. Electronic probes are more suitable and less traumatic than clinical thermometers for recording rectal temperature, and are increasingly, being used as are disposable thermometers (Rogers 1992).

The probe or bulb of a rectal thermometer should be covered by a disposable cover or sleeve before lubrication and insertion. This not only prevents cross-infection, but also prevents damage to the surrounding mucosa. When no specialised cover is available, the probe can be inserted into the finger of a plastic glove before insertion, the rest of the glove remaining outside the body and easily removable.

In a general ward, fans should not be used to cool patients who have a pyrexia caused by infection. The increased movement of air may increase the risk of cross-infection in the area.

Communicating

While the oral temperature is being recorded the patient should not speak. Apart from the danger of breaking the thermometer, the passage of air through the mouth while talking affects the temperature reading, and this should be explained to the patient.

Eating and drinking

Patients with a raised body temperature are prescribed an increased fluid intake to compensate for the increased loss of fluid due to perspiration. Fluid intake should be encouraged and accurately recorded. Fluid balance charts should be maintained for all patients with a pyrexia, to monitor hydration.

Eliminating

Fluid output should be recorded, and fluid balance charts accurately maintained for all patients with other than normal body temperature.

Pyrexia may result in decreased output of urine, which may be concentrated and dark in colour. This may be a result of dehydration caused by increased fluid loss from perspiration.

Personal cleansing and dressing

Clothing may have to be adjusted for the recording of both axillary and rectal temperatures. The nurse should gain the patient's help and co-operation during this nursing practice.

The amount of clothing and bed covers may be adjusted depending on the patient's reaction to a change of body temperature. A patient with a pyrexia may feel very warm or very cold.

Occasionally the patient may be sponged with tepid water to try to reduce a raised body temperature. This may be prescribed for patients who have damage to the temperature-controlling centre in the hypothalamus, causing hyperpyrexia (Sidebottom 1992) (*see* Tepid sponging, p. 319).

A bed bath should be given as frequently as required to ensure the patient's comfort, as patients with a raised body temperature perspire profusely.

Patients with a pyrexia may become dehydrated due to excess insensible fluid loss. Frequent mouth care should be given to maintain a healthy mucosa, and to help alleviate the 'dry mouth' effect associated with pyrexia.

Controlling body temperature

Any change in body temperature may indicate the patient's response to an adverse environment. Under normal conditions the body's internal temperature remains remarkably constant at around 37°C. The range of normal recordings in the adult is 36–37.5°C (see Fig. 8.1). Children have a correspondingly higher range of body temperature than adults due to their increased metabolic rate.

For a healthy person the axillary temperature is at the lower range of normal, the rectal temperature is at the upper range of normal, and the oral temperature lies somewhere in between. For each patient the site chosen for the temperature recording should be used consistently to enable changes in body temperature to be accurately monitored.

Both core temperature and peripheral temperature may be recorded for seriously ill patients suffering from, for example, cardiogenic, bacteraemic or haemorrhagic shock. Under normal conditions, there should not be more than 3°C difference between the core temperature and the peripheral temperature.

The core temperature should be recorded at a site where the reading will be as near as possible to the temperature of the blood. An electronic probe may be inserted into the rectum or the oesophagus and attached to an electronic monitor to give a continuous core temperature reading.

The peripheral temperature may be recorded by a small flat probe taped to the patient's big toe to give a continuous readout of the peripheral temperature on the electronic monitor.

Pyrexia is the term given to a rise in body temperature above 37.5°C; this should be reported.

Hyperpyrexia is the term given to a body temperature above 40°C. Body temperature above 41°C or prolonged hyperpyrexia may cause damage to brain cell function and result in associated fits or rigors. Hyperpyrexia should be treated as an emergency and reported immediately.

Hypothermia is the term given to a fall in body temperature below 35°C. Warming a patient suffering from hypothermia should be done gradually (a rise of 0.5°C per hour is suggested) under medical guidance. Sudden heating of the periphery of the body can divert the blood from the vital centres and cause further shock.

Expressing sexuality

The recording of a rectal temperature can be an uncomfortable and undignified procedure. The reason for this choice of site should be explained to the patient. A nurse who has good communication skills can help to maintain the patient's dignity.

Sleeping

When an electronic thermometer is in situ, there is no need to disturb a patient who is sleeping. When other types of thermometer are used, clinical judgement is needed to decide whether or not to waken a patient, especially during the night, in order to record his temperature.

Patient education: key points

- Explain the importance of monitoring the body temperature for evaluating progress and treatment of the patient's condition
- The patient should understand the importance of the thermometer remaining in position for the correct period of time
- Explain the importance of reporting headache, excess sweating, shivering or general feelings of distress which may indicate changes in body temperature
- Patients with pyrexia should understand the importance of drinking adequate amounts of fluid to prevent dehydration
- Elderly patients should be given advice on how to prevent heat loss at home and told of the dangers of hypothermia. This should be reinforced with written advice and specific information about the resources available, and should involve family and carers as applicable.

References

Blumenthal I 1992 Should we ban mercury thermometers? Discussion paper. Journal of the Royal Society of Medicine 85: 553–555

Closs J 1992 Monitoring the body temperature of surgical patients. Surgical Nurse 5(1): 563, 565–568

Cutler J 1994 Recording a patient's temperature: are we getting it right? Professional Nurse 9(9): 608–616

Fulbrook P 1993 Core temperature measurement: a comparison of rectal, axillary and pulmonary artery blood temperature. Intensive and Critical Care Nursing 9(4): 275–286

Gould D 1994 Controlling patients' body temperature. Nursing Standard 8(35): 29–31

Jensen N, Jepperson P, Mortensen R et al 1994 The superiority of rectal thermometry to oral thermometry with regard to accuracy. Journal of Advanced Nursing 20(4): 660–665

Rogers M 1992 A viable alternative to the glass/mercury thermometer. Paediatric Nursing 4(9): 8–11

Sidebottom J 1992 When it is hot enough to kill (hyperthermia, heat related illness), Registered Nurse 55 (8): 48–57

Toulson S 1994 Treatment and prevention of hypothermia. British Journal of Nursing 3 (13): 662–666

Further reading

Childs C 1994 Temperature control. In: Alexander M, Fawcett J, Runciman P (eds) Nursing practice — hospital and home: the adult. Churchill Livingstone, Edinburgh, pp 679–695

Walsh M, Ford P 1989 Nursing rituals — research and rational actions. Heinemann Nursing, Oxford, pp 50–53

Yiu Tsu Vyvian M 1992 Making sense of . . . hypothermia. Nursing Times 88(49): 38–40

9 Bone Marrow Aspiration

Learning outcomes	By the end of this section you should know how to:
	• prepare the patient for this procedure
	• collect and prepare the equipment
	• assist the medical practitioner during bone marrow aspiration.

Background knowledge required	Revision of the anatomy and physiology of the blood with special reference to the source and development of the red blood corpuscles.
	Revision of Wound care technique (*see* p. 381).

Indications and rationale for bone marrow aspiration	Bone marrow aspiration is the aspiration of a specimen of red bone marrow:
	• *to aid diagnosis in some anaemias and leukaemias*
	• *to aid assessment of the effect of treatment during the course of a disease.*

Outline of the procedure	This procedure is carried out by a medical practitioner using aseptic technique. The patient may have some form of sedation prescribed prior to the procedure. After washing his hands the medical practitioner administers the local anaesthetic into the chosen site. He then prepares his hands for the application of the sterile gloves. The patient's skin is cleansed using the antiseptic, a small stab incision may be made and the marrow needle is inserted into the red bone marrow cavity. The needle is specially designed and is fitted with an adjustable protective guard to control the level of penetration by the needle, thus preventing injury to underlying vital organs (Fig. 9.1). The stilette of the needle is removed and the syringe attached to the hub of the marrow needle. Following aspiration of a specimen of red bone marrow, the syringe is disconnected, the stilette is replaced and the needle withdrawn. The microscope slides are prepared by the medical practitioner or a haematology technician if present. As the microscope slides are prepared, pressure should be applied to the puncture site until bleeding ceases. The puncture site should be covered with a sterile adhesive dressing.
	The position of the patient during the procedure is dependent on the chosen site for aspiration of the red marrow. The main sites are:
	The sternum The patient lies supine with one pillow at his head.
	The iliac crest This can be either an anterior or posterior approach. If the anterior approach is used the patient can lie prone or on his side. When the

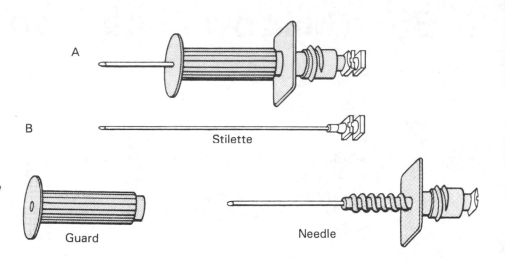

Figure 9.1 *Bone marrow aspiration needle (disposable) showing adjustable guard A Complete needle B Needle taken apart*

posterior approach is used the patient must lie on his side. The iliac crest has the advantage that there are no vital organs near the puncture site.

Equipment

Sterile gloves

Sterile dressings pack

Alcohol-based antiseptic for cleansing the skin

Local anaesthetic and equipment for its administration

Sterile disposable scalpel or similar equipment

Sterile marrow aspiration needles

Sterile 20 ml syringe for aspiration of the marrow

Plastic spray dressing

Sterile adhesive dressing

Disposable plastic aprons

Trolley for equipment

Receptacle for soiled disposables

Microscope slides, appropriately labelled, coverslips and slide fixative if haematology technician service not available Sterile specimen containers appropriately labelled with a completed laboratory form and plastic specimen bag for transportation.

Guidelines and rationale for this nursing practice

- help the medical practitioner to explain the procedure to the patient *to gain consent and cooperation*
- wash the hands *to reduce the risk of cross-infection* (Horton 1995)
- give the patient sedation if prescribed *to assist in the reduction of anxiety*
- prepare the equipment and trolley as required *to ensure that all equipment is available and ready for use*

- ensure the patient's privacy *to assist in the reduction of anxiety*
- help the patient into the correct position depending on the chosen site *as this will permit easy access to the site and promote a positive outcome of the procedure*
- observe the patient throughout this activity *to note any signs of distress*
- assist the medical practitioner as necessary during the procedure *to ensure safe and competent completion of the procedure*
- remain with the patient and help maintain his position as required during the procedure *giving physical and psychological support during an uncommon experience*
- ensure that the patient is left feeling as comfortable as possible, *maintaining the quality of this nursing practice*
- dispose of the equipment safely *to reduce any health hazard*
- dispatch the labelled specimens to the laboratory immediately with the completed laboratory forms *to allow microscopic examination of fresh body cells*
- document the nursing practice appropriately, monitor after-effects, and report abnormal findings immediately. *This provides a written record and assists in the implementation of any action should an abnormality or adverse reaction to the practice be noted.*

Relevance to the activities of living

Maintaining a safe environment

As this is an invasive procedure all precautions and observations to prevent infection should be maintained. The adhesive dressing can be removed 2–3 days following the procedure unless a complication has arisen.

For safe transportation of the specimen collected, *see* page 301.

If the patient received sedation prior to the procedure, the effects of this should have worn off before he is allowed to mobilise. The patient may attend as an outpatient, day patient or inpatient for this procedure if his daily lifestyle is not significantly affected by the undiagnosed condition (Duke 1994).

Communicating

It is important that an easily understood explanation is given to the patient beforehand. This is primarily given by the medical practitioner, but the nurse may be required to repeat the explanation. If the sternal site is used, the thought of a needle being introduced into one's chest can be extremely alarming; if the patient is very anxious, the doctor may prescribe light sedation prior to the procedure.

The patient should be told to expect a momentary sharp pain during the procedure due to the suction created as the syringe piston is withdrawn (Long et al 1995).

The patient may require mild analgesia once the effect of the local anaesthetic has worn off.

Breathing

The patient's blood pressure, pulse and respiration rates may be taken following bone marrow aspiration. The puncture site should be observed for continued bleeding or haematoma formation as some patients may have a bleeding disorder.

Any sudden change in the patient's general condition, especially in breathing if the sternal site is used, should be reported as this may signify injury to underlying vital organs (Booth 1983, Duke 1994).

Mobilising

The patient should be allowed to rest quietly for approximately an hour following the practice. Thereafter he can resume his previous form of mobilising. If sedation is given prior to the practice, allow the effects to wear off before the patient is mobilised.

Patient education: key points

The medical practitioner and the nurse should provide information regarding the necessity for this procedure. The patient and relatives will need time to ask questions and discuss any aspect of the planned procedure.

Before the procedure the nurse should give information and the rationale about the position the patient requires to adopt during and following the aspiration, and the aftercare which will be delivered.

Should the patient be for discharge after the procedure, give information regarding the care of the puncture site, what level of discomfort may be experienced, who to contact should any adverse reaction occur, when the results will be available and the date and time of the next outpatient appointment (Duke 1994).

References

Booth J 1983 Handbook of investigations. Harper & Row, London, pp 49–51
Duke F 1994 Blood disorders. In: Alexander M, Fawcett J, Runciman P (eds) Nursing practice — hospital and home: the adult. Churchill Livingstone, Edinburgh
Horton R 1995 Handwashing: the fundamental infection control principle. British Journal of Nursing 4(16): 926–933
Long B, Phipps W, Cassmeyer V (eds) 1995 Adult nursing — a nursing process approach. Mosby-Times Mirror International Publishers, London

Further reading

Brunner L, Suddarth D (eds) 1992 The textbook of adult nursing. Chapman & Hall, London, ch10
Molassiotis A 1995 Psychological care in bone marrow transplantation. Nursing Times 91(37) 36–37
Rowswell M 1992 Caring for the patient with a haematological disorder. In: Royle J, Walsh M (eds) Watson's medical–surgical nursing and related physiology. 4th edn Bailliere Tindall, London
Knowle S, Hoffbrand A 1980 Bone marrow aspiration and trephine biopsy. British Medical Journal 281(6234): 204–205
Roper N, Logan W, Tierney A 1996 The elements of nursing, 4th edn. Churchill Livingstone, Edinburgh, p 141–168

10 Bowel Washout

Learning outcomes	By the end of this section you should know how to: • prepare the patient for this nursing practice • collect and prepare the equipment • carry out a bowel washout.
Background knowledge required	Anatomy and physiology of the lower alimentary tract. Solutions that may be safely used for bowel washout.
Indications and rationale for a bowel washout	A bowel washout is the introduction of fluid through a tube into the rectum and siphoning of the contents to help empty the rectum and sigmoid colon. It is used in the following circumstances: • prior to special radiological examinations *to clear the bowel so that a good radiological picture can be obtained* • prior to sigmoidoscopy *so that a clear view of the lining of the intestine can be obtained* • prior to surgery on the rectum or descending colon *to help reduce the risk of infection from faecal matter and intestinal flora around the area of surgery* • *to empty the bowel in certain cases of faecal impaction*, e.g. when there is no peristalsis because of nerve damage.
Equipment	Trolley or tray Protective covering for the bed and floor Disposable gloves and apron Disposable bowel irrigation set (see Fig. 10.1) Sterile rectal tube — usually Jacques catheter no. 21 Lubricant — KY jelly Solution as ordered — usually plain water or sodium chloride 0.9% at room temperature Medical wipes/tissues Bucket to receive return flow Receptacle for soiled disposables Bedpan or commode.

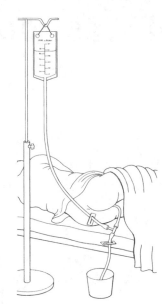

Figure 10.1
*Disposable bowel
irrigation set*

**Guidelines and
rationale for this
nursing practice**

- explain the nursing practice to the patient *to gain consent and cooperation*
- collect and prepare the equipment *for efficiency of practice*
- assist the patient into the left lateral position in bed, with his buttocks exposed *but ensuring that he is adequately covered and has as much privacy as possible to reduce embarrassment*
- observe the patient throughout this activity *for signs of discomfort or distress*
- place the protective covering on the bed, under the patient's buttocks, and the other protective covering on the floor at the side of the bed, under the bucket which receives the return flow. *This will help prevent any leakage from the anal sphincter soiling the bed*
- join the Jacques catheter to the connecting tubing
- don the disposable gloves
- lubricate the end of the catheter to ease insertion into the rectum. *The insertion of the tube can be very uncomfortable if the patient has haemorrhoids*
- run some of the solution through the tubing and catheter *to expel the air. The introduction of air into the rectum can add to discomfort and the release of flatus from the rectum will embarrass the patient*
- clamp the end of the catheter before all the solution has run out and then introduce the catheter into the rectum in an upwards and backwards direction for 10–12 cm *to follow the curve of the rectum*
- administer 120–150 ml fluid then close the inlet gateclip and open the outlet gateclip to allow fluid to run into the bucket (see Fig. 10.1)
- observe the character of the return flow, e.g. colour, blood streaks
- repeat the practice until the return flow is clear or until all the solution ordered has been used

- gently withdraw the catheter. Offer the patient a bedpan or commode or access to a toilet *as there may still be some slight leakage of fluid from the anal sphincter*
- dry the perineal area carefully *as faecal matter can cause skin breakdown*
- remove the protective covering
- ensure the patient is left feeling as comfortable as possible; a protective pad may be placed under the patient if he is worried about any leakage
- dispose of the equipment safely *for the protection of others*
- document this nursing practice, monitor after-effects and report abnormal findings immediately *to provide a written record and assist in the implementation of any action should an abnormality or adverse reaction to the practice be noted.*

Relevance to the activities of living

Maintaining a safe environment

Although this does not require aseptic technique, all the equipment should be clean or disposable. The nurse should wash her hands before commencing and on completion of the practice. Gloves and apron should be worn for protection.

This nursing practice is not usually advised when the patient has rectal bleeding, as the rectal tube may seriously damage an already friable mucosa.

Communicating

A careful explanation of the necessity for this nursing practice should be given to the patient, to help reduce embarrassment.

Eating and drinking

This procedure is often carried out prior to surgery on the bowel. After the procedure the patient may be limited to fluids or to a low residue diet.

Eliminating

Ensure access for the patient to a bedpan, commode or toilet after this nursing practice.

Mobilising

The effectiveness of the washout may be increased if the patient can move around in bed to distribute the solution.

Expressing sexuality

This is a very embarrassing practice for the patient, so an adequate explanation should be given and as much privacy as possible should be provided. Ideally it should be carried out in a treatment room away from other patients and convenient for a toilet.

Patient education: key points

A clear explanation of the necessity for this practice must be given to the patient.

A warning to expect some leakage of fluid after the procedure and the supply of some sort of protection for the patient must be given.

Further reading

Lawler J 1991 Behind the screens. Churchill Livingstone, Edinburgh
Ratcliffe P 1988 Whole gut irrigation: an acceptable risk? Nursing Times 84(18): 33–34
Roper N, Logan W, Tierney A 1996 The elements of nursing, 4th edn. Churchill Livingstone, Edinburgh
Royle J, Walsh M 1992 Watson's Medical surgical nursing, 4th edn. Bailliere Tindall, London
Walsh M, Ford P 1989 Nursing research, rituals and rational action. Heinemann, Oxford

11 Cardiopulmonary Resuscitation

Learning outcomes

By the end of this section you should know how to:
- diagnose cardiac arrest quickly
- call the emergency team promptly
- initiate resuscitation effectively
- locate the necessary equipment.

Background knowledge required

Revision of the anatomy and physiology of the cardiovascular and respiratory systems.

Review of the health authority policy pertaining to the procedure of cardiopulmonary resuscitation.

Indications and rationale for cardiopulmonary resuscitation

Cardiopulmonary resuscitation is a dramatic, emergency exercise *to restore effective circulation and ventilation following cardiac arrest.* Of the three levels of skill detailed under the Activity of Living of communicating (*see* p. 79), the second is the level of knowledge expected of a nurse.

Cardiac arrest is the abrupt cessation of cardiac function; it may be induced by any of the following:
- respiratory failure, as the cardiovascular and respiratory systems are interdependent
- cardiac arrhythmias caused by cardiac disease or electrolyte imbalance
- surgery
- asphyxia
- accidents such as drowning or electrocution.

Diagnosis of cardiac arrest is confirmed by:
- sudden loss of consciousness
- absence of the carotid pulse
- absence of respirations
- pallor, often associated with cyanosis
- dilation of the pupils
- convulsions, which may or may not be present.

Immediate cardiopulmonary resuscitation consists of three procedures. The mnemonic 'ABC' acts as an aide memoire:

A — **Airway:**   providing and maintaining a clear airway.

B — **Breathing:**   supplying oxygen to the blood by means of expired air respiration or artificial ventilation.

C — **Circulation:**   forcing the blood out of the heart into the arterial system by means of external chest compression.

Equipment

Suction equipment

Oral pharyngeal airway, e.g. Guedel airway

Disposable face mask, e.g. Laderal pocket mask (community use)

Ambubag and face mask or similar equipment

Oxygen equipment

Emergency cardiac medications

Defibrillator

Receptacle for soiled disposables.

Guidelines and rationale for this nursing practice

- once cardiac arrest has been diagnosed, note the time. *Knowledge of the elapse of time is very important as brain cells will begin to die due to lack of oxygen within 4–6 minutes*
- in hospital, order someone to alert the cardiac arrest team and bring emergency equipment, or, in the community, order someone to contact the emergency services *to make best use of the elapsing time and gain support from skilled personnel*
- place the patient in a supine position on a firm surface *to permit easy access to the patient's airway and chest*
- in an institutional setting remove the bedhead from the patient's bed *to further enhance access to the airway.*

Support for breathing and circulation must be carried out simultaneously to be effective.

A — airway

- use suction if available to clear the airway or clean the mouth of obstructing debris *to remove any obstruction.* Dentures should remain in situ if well fitting *as this creates a good seal during assisted ventilation*
- tilt the head backwards and pull the mandible forwards *to open the airway.* Maintain this position (Fig. 11.1). If an injury to the cervical spine is suspected, open the airway using the jaw thrust technique *as this will reduce movement of the cervical spine*
- insert an oral airway if available *to maintain the airway in an open position by preventing the tongue falling back onto the oropharynx* (Baskett 1993)

B — breathing

- ventilations at 2 seconds per breath should be administered using an airway

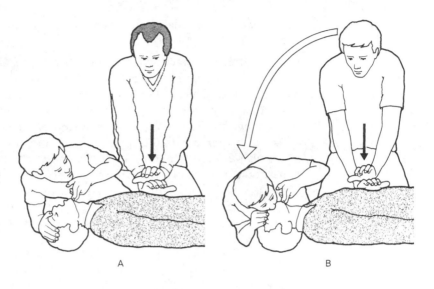

Figure 11.1
Cardiopulmonary resuscitation
A Two resuscitators
B One resuscitator

A   B

or disposable face mask *to provide supportive breathing* (European Resuscitation Council 1992)
- note the rising of the chest wall *to confirm ventilation*
- ventilate at a rate of at least 12 per minute *as this imitates the physiological rate of an average breathing pattern* (Baskett 1993)

C — circulation

- if the cardiac arrest is witnessed, give one sharp blow over the mid-sternal area. *This may cause the heart to restart* (Resuscitation Council UK 1989)
- check the carotid pulse *to note the effectiveness of the precordial thump*; if the pulse is absent, continue
- place the heel of one hand over the lower half of the sternum, place the other hand on top and, while keeping the arms straight and elbows locked, depress the sternum 4–5 cm towards the spine (Fig. 12.1). *This compresses the heart between the spinal column and posterior of the sternum, creating circulation*
- repeat this movement at a rate of one depression per second *as this imitates the physiological rate of the average heart function*
- continue chest compression and artificial ventilation at the rate of five chest compressions to one lung inflation when two people are resuscitating a patient. If only one person is carrying out the practice the ratio is 15:2, with a faster chest compression of 80 per minute because of the breaks for lung ventilation (European Resuscitation Council 1992). *These rates will provide a very modest level of oxygenation of the brain tissue* (Baskett 1993)
- check for the return of the pulse and breathing after one minute and thereafter every three minutes *to check for return of spontaneous circulatory function.*

With the arrival of skilled personnel the role of the nurses may alter. Breathing support is usually taken over by a medical practitioner or, in the community, a paramedic, but external chest compression is not always taken over. Staff may thereafter:

- assist a medical practitioner/paramedic with the passage of an endotracheal tube *through which ventilation is continued*
- assist a second medical practitioner or paramedic with the commencement of an intravenous infusion *to aid correction of the acid – base balance in the body and provide a route for administration of emergency medications*
- assist if required with the application of limb or chest electrodes *to provide continuous monitoring of cardiac function*
- assist the medical practitioner to draw up emergency cardiac medications as needed. These medications may assist with the correction of the acid – base balance of the body or have a direct effect on the heart. A brief record of all medications administered should be kept, *permitting written prescriptions to be made at a later time*
- a defibrillator may be used by a medical practitioner/paramedic during cardiopulmonary resuscitation *to help establish cardiac function or correct a cardiac arrhythmia.* The defibrillator transmits an electric current through the patient's chest wall. All personnel must stand clear of the bed while the patient is being defibrillated as they would act as a 'ground' for the electric current, cancelling its usefulness and endangering the lives of the staff present (Thompson & Hopkins 1987)
- ensure the patient is left feeling as comfortable as possible following successful resuscitation *maintaining the quality of this nursing practice*
- in the community, ensure safe transportation of the patient to hospital *maintaining the quality of this nursing practice*
- dispose of equipment safely *to reduce any health hazard*
- document the nursing practice appropriately, monitor after-effects and report abnormal findings immediately *providing a written record of the practice which should accompany the patient.*

| **Relevance to the activities of living** | ***Maintaining a safe environment*** |

The brain tissue is most sentitive to the lack of blood and oxygen; if an adequate cerebral circulation is not restored within three minutes, irreversible brain damage will occur. A nurse, when commencing work in a new ward, should quickly familiarise herself with the position of the equipment used in that ward during cardiopulmonary resuscitation.

Following cardiopulmonary resuscitation procedures, and at regular intervals, e.g. weekly, the equipment should be checked to ensure that it is in working condition and that stocks are replenished.

In the community the nurse should carry a disposable face mask for emergency use. In the United Kingdom the emergency services provided by ambulance and paramedical personnel commonly deal initially with cardiac arrest situations outwith health care institutions. Once a patient is stabilised, he or she will then be transported to an acute hospital environment.

The European Resuscitation Council (1992) has published recommended protocols for advanced life support which have been adopted by staff in the United Kingdom health care setting (see Fig. 11.2).

Communicating

It is now accepted that three levels of skill in cardiopulmonary resuscitation should be taught (Chamberlain 1989). The first is 'basic life support', which the population as a whole should learn. No equipment is necessary as the victim's airway is maintained, and breathing and circulation supported, by simple skills which can be easily taught.

The second level is 'basic life support with adjuncts', which all nurses should learn. The basic principles of life support are utilised with the additional use of an airway, Ambubag and mask. Nursing personnel working in high patient dependent units frequently assume an extended nursing role by receiving further education and practice in the use of a defibrillator (Last et al 1992).

The third level is 'advanced life support', which all cardiopulmonary resuscitation teams should be competent in delivering. This involves the implementation of internationally recognised recommendations for treatment regimens following a cardiac arrest (European Resuscitation Council 1992).

Other patients or bystanders witnessing any part of cardiopulmonary resuscitation will be alarmed and distressed. During the procedure, nurses who are not involved can give comfort and reassurance to these patients/bystanders and, wherever possible, continue with the normal work pattern.

Following this emergency the patient's next of kin should be contacted and informed.

When resuscitative measures are successful the patient will require a brief, easily understood explanation as to what has happened, and the reasons for the equipment in use.

Following such a dramatic emergency procedure, junior nursing staff may be distressed, and can be helped by supportive colleagues.

Resuscitation is essentially a practical skill which requires regular practice to maintain skill level (Ferguson 1990).

The nurse has a responsibility to ensure that she maintains her level of skill in resuscitative practices; this will involve regular practice at simulation sessions (Wynne 1990).

Breathing

Ribfracture may result from external chest compression. If the patient experiences pain on inspiration following external cardiac massage, this should be reported immediately.

Eating and drinking

During cardiac arrest and resuscitation procedures a patient may vomit and create problems for the maintenance of a clear airway. When appropriate, sheets

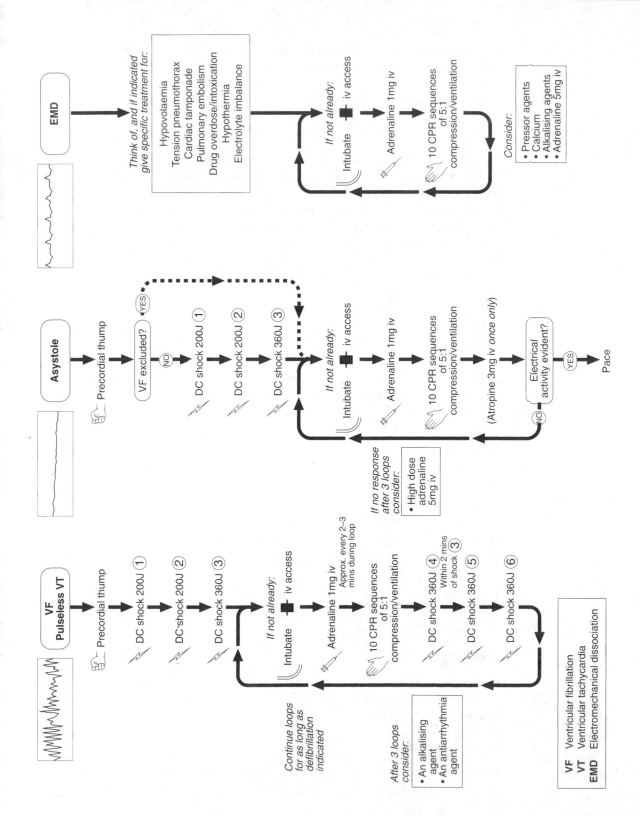

Figure 11.2 *(facing page) Revised advanced resuscitation protocols (Reproduced with kind permission from the European Resuscitation Council 1992)*

and clothing should be changed as soon as possible for the patient's comfort and dignity.

Eliminating

There may be incontinence of urine or faeces immediately following a cardiac arrest, which adds to the patient's distress, and sheets and clothing should be changed as soon as possible for his comfort and dignity.

Personal cleansing and dressing

As cardiopulmonary resuscitation is an emergency procedure, during which immediate exposure of the patient's chest and limbs is required, some damage to the patient's clothing may occur, and this should be explained to the patient at a later time.

Immediately following successful resuscitation the patient will require nursing intervention related to this activity of living to ensure that he is as comfortable as possible.

Sleeping

Following resuscitation and regaining consciousness a patient may have difficulty in resuming his normal sleep pattern due to the fear of suffering a further cardiac arrest, and the nurse should take appropriate measures to help to induce sleep.

Dying

As cardiac arrest is an emergency and may not be reversible, the patient's next of kin may suddenly have to be told of their relative's death and will display any of the many grief reactions; the nurse's empathy and support are then required.

Patient education: Key points

Following a successful resuscitation the patient and relatives must be given information about the event and permitted to discuss their feelings and anxieties about the emergency.

Other patients within the clinical area will require to be given an explanation for the events to assist in relieving some of their anxieties.

The nurse has a role in encouraging and teaching the general population to develop skills in basic life support as suggested by the Resuscitation Council UK (1989).

References

Baskett P 1993 Resuscitation handbook, 2nd edn. Wolfe, London
Chamberlain D 1989 Advanced life support. British Medical Journal 299(6696): 446–448
European Resuscitation Council 1992 Guidelines for basic and advanced life support. Resuscitation 24(2): 103–123

Ferguson A 1990 Cardiopulmonary resuscitation — a teaching guide. Nurse Education Today 10: 50–53

Last T, Self N, Kassab J, Rajan A 1992 Extended role of the nurse in ICU. British Journal of Nursing 1(13): 672–675

Resuscitation Council UK 1989 Basic and advanced life support guidelines of the Resuscitation Council UK. Resuscitation Council UK, London

Thompson D, Hopkins S 1987 Making sense of defibrillation. Nursing Times 83(49): 54–55

Wynne G 1990 Training and retention of skills. In: Evans T (ed) ABC of resuscitation, 2nd edn. British Medical Journal, London

Suggested reading

Ellis F 1990 Think pink (describes learning of cardiopulmonary resuscitation). Nursing Times 86(34): 52–53

Evans A 1989 To resuscitate or not. Surgical Nurse 2(1): 9–11

Flanders A 1994 A detailed explanation of defibrillation. Nursing Times 90(18): 37–39

Marsden A 1989 Basic life support. British Medical Journal 299(6696): 422–445

Newbold D 1987 The physiology of cardiac massage. Nursing Times 83(25): 59–62

Newbold D 1987 External chest compression. Nursing Times 83(26): 41–43

Roper N, Logan W, Tierney A 1996 The elements of nursing, 4th edn. Churchill Livingstone, Edinburgh, pp 141–168

Stewart K, Raj G 1989 A matter of life and death. Nursing Times 85(35): 27–29

Thom A 1988 Who decides? (opinions about the decision to resuscitate). Nursing Times 85(2): 35–37

Wynne G 1990 Revised guidelines for life support. Nursing Times 86(3): 70–75

Wynne G, Kirby S, Cordinglya A 1990 No breathing ... no pulse. Professional Nurse 5(10): 510–513

12 Care of the Deceased Person

Learning outcomes	By the end of this section you should know how to: • care for a deceased person
Background knowledge required	Review of the health authority policy pertaining to care of a deceased person. Review of the religious/spiritual rites of care of a deceased person. Revision of Bed bath (*see* p. 29) and Mouth care (*see* p. 210).
Indications and rationale for care of a deceased person	Before transfer to the mortuary or undertaker's premises a deceased patient requires care which may be delivered by a professional carer, undertaker or the appropriate person identified by the spiritual beliefs of the deceased. This care may also be referred to as 'Last Offices'.
Equipment	Disposable gloves Equipment as for Bed bath (*see* p. 29) Equipment as for Mouth care (*see* p. 210) Incontinence pad or disposable napkin Dressings pack Waterproof dressing for open wounds if necessary Hypoallergenic tape Shroud Disposable bowl 2 patient identification bands Patient identification cards and/or notification of death cards ⎬ appropriately completed with the patient's full name and other details as requested Mortuary sheet or clean white sheet Gauze bandage Trolley for equipment Receptacle for patient's clothing Patient clothing list book Patient valuables list book Receptacle for patient's valuables

Receptacle for soiled linen

Receptacle for soiled disposables

Guidelines and rationale for this nursing practice

- inform the medical practitioner when a patient is thought to have died *to confirm the diagnosis of death and comply with the legal requirements before the issue of a death certificate* (Parliament of Great Britain 1953)
- *to prevent further distress of those persons present,* ensure the patient's privacy and the privacy of relatives
- ensure that the patient's relatives are notified of the death, if they are not present. *This will allow expressed wishes of the deceased to be implemented and funeral arrangements initiated*
- assist and support bereaved relatives *as the professional carer is in a key position at this time* (Kindlen 1994)
- inform the nursing officer or deputy, and portering staff or, in the patient's home, assist the carer to contact the undertaker *to allow initial arrangements for transfer of the body to the mortuary*
- collect and prepare the equipment *to ensure all equipment is available*
- wash the hands *for general hygiene*
- remove all upper bed linen, leaving a sheet to cover the patient *to give easy access to the body*
- lay the patient flat, face up with his limbs in a natural position and his arms by his side. *Rigor mortis occurs 2–4 hours following death; after this time positioning of the body would be very difficult*
- remove any mechanical aids, e.g. heel pads or rubber rings *as they may cause marking of the tissues*
- gently close the eyelids *to protect the tissues should the deceased or relatives give permission for corneal donation and also to improve the facial appearance* (Green & Green 1992)
- clean the patient's mouth and replace any dentures *to enhance the aesthetic appearance of the deceased and maintain hygiene*
- support the mandible in a closed position using a light pillow. An hour may elapse prior to the continuation of the practice but this interval is not essential. *This will allow rigor mortis to develop prior to the completion of the practice*
- apply the gloves and, using the disposable bowl, manually express the urinary bladder *as any body fluid leakage would act as a health hazard to staff who come in contact with the deceased*
- remove all tubes and drains, unless otherwise instructed, *to reduce the health hazard*
- re-dress all wounds with a waterproof dressing *thereby reducing the potential problem of leakage of body fluids*. When drains or tubes are left in position these should also be covered with a padded waterproof dressing
- wash the patient as for Bed bath (*see* p. 29) *for general hygiene purposes*
- a male patient should be shaved *for aesthetic reasons*
- all jewellery, once removed, should be listed in the patient valuables book in the presence of two nurses *to maintain the security of the deceased's*

belongings. In the community, personal belongings should not be removed by the nurse unless a witness is present. Any action should be documented and signed
- apply identification bands and cards to the appropriate limbs and parts of the body *to ensure continued identification of the deceased*
- apply an incontinence pad or disposable napkin *which will reduce the health hazard for staff who are in contact with the body*
- place the shroud, or at home fresh bedclothes, in position *to enhance the appearance should relatives wish to view the deceased.*

Institution

- wrap the body in the sheet, ensuring complete coverage, and secure the sheet with adhesive tape or the gauze bandage *to prevent exposure of the deceased during transfer to the mortuary*
- fix an identification card or notification of death card to the sheet using adhesive tape *for ease of future identification*
- list the patient's clothing *thus creating a receipt for future use*. Place this clothing and the patient's valuables in a secure place *to ensure safe-keeping until removal by the relatives*
- dispose of equipment safely *to reduce any health hazard*
- inform portering staff that the body is ready for collection; *this will permit the body to be cooled as soon as possible after death, thus slowing the decomposition process*
- on arrival of portering staff with the mortuary trolley, ensure the privacy of the other patients *in an attempt to prevent further distress*
- document the nursing practice appropriately *to provide a written record of the care given.*

Community

- cover the patient with a sheet *for aesthetic purposes*. Unless requested otherwise by the carer, leave the face uncovered
- remove any portable nursing material/ equipment *to reduce the 'clinical' appearance of the room*
- following removal of the body, arrange for the collection of any residual equipment *thereby returning the home environment to 'normal'*
- document the nursing practice appropriately *to provide a written record of the care given.*

Relevance to the activities of living

Although the patient is deceased, a consideration of the activities of living is important in relation to the family and for the protection of staff.

Maintaining a safe environment

All equipment should be clean or disposable and all precautions be taken to prevent cross-infection. The nurse should wash her hands before commencing and on completion of the practice. Disposable gloves should be worn when the nurse is handling soiled pads or body fluids from the deceased. On the death of a patient with a contagious disease, such as hepatitis B or Acquired Immune Deficiency Syndrome, isolation techniques should be maintained. The body is placed in a large polythene bag and sealed, usually with adhesive tape, prior to being wrapped in a sheet. These practices reduce the health hazard to staff who come in contact with the body.

If a patient dies unexpectedly, or within 24 hours of surgery, or within 24 hours of involvement in some form of trauma, the nurse may be requested to leave in position all drains, tubes and dressings during the practice (Green & Green 1992). This may help to establish the cause of death. A patient who dies suddenly and unexpectedly will require a postmortem examination.

Communicating

Communication with bereaved relatives can be stressful (Niven 1989). The nurse should not hide her own feelings of loss and sadness from the deceased's relatives, as the feeling of sharing may be of great support to them. Informing relations adequately and kindly about immediate practicalities is also crucial. For example, it is important that the next of kin understand what is written on the death certificate and know that it has to be registered locally, as only then can funeral arrangements be made.

Following the death of a patient the other patients may question the nurse about the deceased. The nurse should inform the patients kindly and honestly that the patient has died and give support when needed (Kindlen 1994).

The nurse may also need to assist and support her colleagues prior to, during, and following the nursing practice.

Dying

The details of the practice can vary according to the patient's cultural background and religious practices. The nurse must be aware of specific requirements prior to, during or following death: for example, for the body of the Orthodox Jew there is a ritual purification, no postmortem is permitted, and no organs may be removed for transplant.

The bereaved relatives will require sensitive and compassionate care. Morris (1988) suggests that nurses shy away from death as it acts as a reminder of our mortality. Little can be done to ease the relatives' distress but the nurse should be aware of the many reactions that may be demonstrated and remain calm and supportive. Any request to see the deceased should be arranged as soon as possible, as this may assist the relatives during the grieving process; care should be taken to ensure that the patient looks as peaceful as possible, that the environs are cleared of equipment, and that a chair is available.

The deceased person's clothing and valuables should be returned to the next of kin in a sympathetic manner. If clothing and valuables can not be returned to the next of kin, they should be transferred to the appropriate administrative department.

In the community the nurse may make a more gradual withdrawal from the family of the deceased by visiting after the funeral. Referral to other professionals or voluntary agencies who specialise in caring for the bereaved may be required.

References

Green J, Green M 1992 Dealing with death. Chapman Hall, London
Kindlen M 1994 The terminally ill patient. In: Alexander M, Fawcett J, Runciman P (eds) Nursing
    practice — hospital and home: the adult. Churchill Livingstone, Edinburgh
Morris E 1988 A pain of separation. Nursing Times 84(42): 54–56
Niven N 1989 Health psychology. Churchill Livingstone, Edinburgh
Parliament of Great Britain 1953 Births and Deaths Registration Act. HMSO, London

Further reading

Cathcart F 1989 Death: coping with distress. Nursing Times 85(42) 33–35
Green J 1991 Death with dignity — meeting the spiritual needs of patients in a multi-cultural society.
    MacMillan, London
Hughes S, Henley A 1990 Dealing with death in hospital: procedures for managers and staff. King's
    Fund, London
Malcolm D 1985 Letting Alan go (care study of the bereavement process). Nursing Times 81(29):
    30–31
Manley K 1988 The needs and support of relatives. Nursing 3(32): 19–22
Neuberger J 1994 Caring for dying people of different faiths, 2nd edn. Mosby, London
Roper N, Logan W, Tierney A 1996 The elements of nursing, 4th edn. Churchill Livingstone,
    Edinburgh, pp 395–420
Royal College of Nursing 1981 Verification of death and performance of last offices. Royal College
    of Nursing, London
Smith C 1995 Bereavement care in A&E departments. British Journal of Nursing 4(9): 485–486
Walsh M 1990 Sudden death. Surgical Nurse 3(4): 10–13
Walsh M, Ford P 1989 Nursing rituals — research and rational actions. Heinemann Nursing,
    Oxford, ch 10
Wilson-Barnett J, Raiman J (eds) 1988 Nursing issues and research in terminal care. J Wiley,
    Chichester

13 Catheterisation: Urinary

There are 4 parts to this section:

1 Catheterisation
2 Catheter care
3 Bladder irrigation
4 Bladder lavage

The concluding subsection 'Relevance to the activities of living' refers to the four practices collectively.

Learning outcomes

By the end of this section you should know how to:

- prepare the patient for these four nursing practices
- collect and prepare the equipment
- carry out catheterisation, catheter care, bladder irrigation and bladder lavage.

Background knowledge required

Revision of the anatomy and physiology of the urinary system and external genitalia.

Revision of Wound care technique (*see* p. 381).

1 Catheterisation

Indications and rationale for urethral catheterisation

Urethral catheterisation is the passing of a catheter through the urethral orifice to the bladder:

- *to re-establish a flow of urine in urinary retention*
- *to provide a channel for drainage when micturition is impaired*
- *to maintain a dry environment in urinary incontinence when all other forms of nursing intervention have failed*
- *to empty the bladder preoperatively*
- *to allow monitoring of fluid balance in a seriously ill patient*
- *to facilitate bladder irrigation procedures.*

Equipment

Good light source, such as spotlight or torch

Sterile gloves

Sterile catheterisation pack or dressings pack

Sterile water-based solution for cleansing the genitalia

Sterile anaesthetic gel if required, or water-soluble lubricant

Sterile receiver

Sterile catheter of type and size required

Appropriate equipment for catheter balloon inflation, e.g. syringe, needles and sterile water

Sterile closed drainage system if required

Hypoallergenic tape

Sterile specimen container appropriately labelled with a completed laboratory form and plastic specimen bag for transportation

Trolley or adequate surface for equipment

Receptacle for soiled disposables

Catheters

The reason for urinary catheterisation can dictate the type and size of catheter (Fig. 13.1) to be used, e.g.:

- round-ended catheter can be used when a retained catheter is not required
- Foley double lumen self-retaining catheter can be used when a short-term retained catheter is required

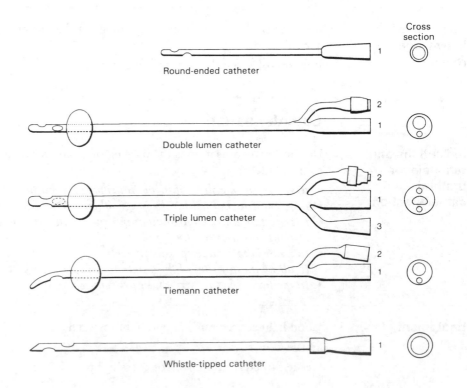

Figure 13.1
Catheterisation: examples of catheters (Key: 1 = channel for urine flow; 2 = channel for balloon inflation; 3 = channel for irrigating fluid flow)

- Foley triple lumen self-retaining catheter can be used when continuous bladder irrigation is required
- Tiemann catheter can be used when the urethral canal is narrowed, such as occurs when a male patient has an enlarged prostate gland: the shape of the catheter tip aids the passage of the catheter
- whistle-tipped catheter can be used postoperatively to allow the passage of blood clots, particularly when bladder irrigation is not being utilised
- silastic catheter can be used when a retained catheter is required for long-term use, as silastic is less irritant to the body tissue.

Sizes:

- 12 FG–14 FG is a suitable size of catheter for female and male patients (Lowthian 1995)
- larger-sized catheters may be used when the urine has an excess of sediment and/or blood
- catheters are manufactured in female and male catheter lengths.

Guidelines and rationale for this nursing practice

Female patient

- explain the nursing practice to the patient *to obtain consent and cooperation*
- collect and prepare the equipment *to ensure all equipment is available and ready for use*
- ensure the patient's privacy *to reduce anxiety*
- observe the patient throughout this activity *to note any signs of distress*
- prepare and help the patient into a supine position with knees bent, hips flexed, and feet resting on the bed approximately 0.7 m apart. *This position provides good access and visualisation of the genitalia*
- place an incontinence pad or similar waterproof sheet under the patient's buttocks *to prevent spillage of fluids onto the patient's bed linen*
- arrange the lighting *to assist with good visualisation of the genitalia* (Morrison et al 1994)
- wash the hands and put on the gloves *which will act as a barrier between the nurse's skin and the patient's tissues, thus reducing the incidence of contamination* (Horton 1995)
- open and arrange the equipment, maintaining sterility *to reduce contamination*
- cleanse the labia minora swabbing from above downwards *to reduce the danger of cross-infection from the anal region*
- using the non-dominant hand, separate the labia minora to reveal the urethral meatus. Hold this position until the completion of insertion of the catheter *to prevent re-contamination of the urethral meatus by the labia minora after cleansing*
- with the dominant hand cleanse the urethral meatus *to prevent introduction of microorganisms into the urethra and/or bladder* and position the sterile receiver *to collect the urine from the catheter*
- insert the lubricated catheter into the urethra in an upward and backward direction *which follows the anatomical route of the female urethra* (Marieb 1989)

- avoid contamination of the surface of the catheter until a flow of urine is established (Fig. 13.2), *to prevent the introduction of microorganisms* (Gould 1994)
- if it is not intended that the catheter should be left in situ, gently remove the catheter when the urine flow ceases
- if for retention, gently advance the catheter 4–5 cm and inflate the balloon according to the manufacturer's directions. *The inflated balloon will maintain the catheter's position*
- attach a drainage system and properly manage all potential entry points of infection *to prevent the development of ascending infection* (Swaffield 1994), (Fig. 13.3)
- anchor the catheter when appropriate by supporting the catheter and drainage tubing *to reduce trauma to the bladder neck and urethra which may lead to pressure sore development* (Lowthian 1994)

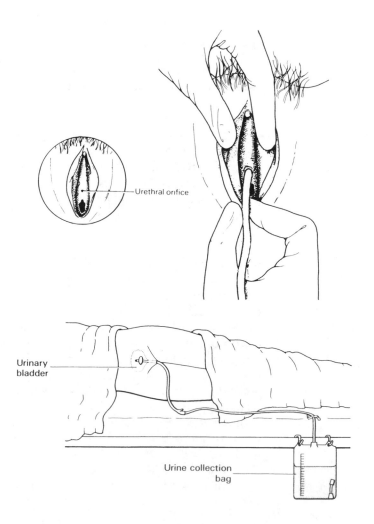

Figure 13.2
Catheterisation: inserting a catheter into the female urethra (Reproduced with permission from Roper N, Logan W, Tierney A 1985 The elements of nursing, 2nd edn. Churchill Livingstone, Edinburgh)

Figure 13.3   *Closed bladder drainage system showing the drainage bag below the level of the bladder*

- ensure that the patient is left feeling as comfortable as possible *maintaining the quality of this nursing practice*
- dispose of the equipment safely *to reduce any health hazard*
- document the nursing practice appropriately, monitor after-effects and report abnormal findings immediately *providing a written record and assisting in the implementation of any action should an abnormality or adverse reaction to the practice be noted.*

Male patient

This practice is usually carried out by a medical practitioner, a male nurse or a female nurse who has extended role responsibilities following additional education.

- explain the nursing practice to the patient *to obtain consent and cooperation*
- collect and prepare the equipment *to ensure all equipment is available and ready for use*
- ensure the patient's privacy *to reduce anxiety*
- observe the patient throughout this activity *to note any signs of distress*
- prepare and help the patient into a supine position. *This position provides good access and visualisation of the genitalia*
- place an incontinence pad or similar waterproof sheet under the patient's buttocks *to prevent spillage of fluids onto the patient's bed linen*
- arrange the lighting *to assist with good visualisation of the genitalia* (Morrison et al 1994)
- wash the hands and put on the gloves *which will act as a barrier between the nurse's skin and the patient's tissues, thus reducing the incidence of contamination* (Horton 1995)
- open and arrange the equipment maintaining sterility *to reduce contamination*
- withdraw the patient's foreskin with the non-dominant hand. Maintain this position until the completion of insertion of the catheter *to prevent re-contamination of the urethral meatus by the foreskin after cleansing*
- with the dominant hand cleanse the glans penis and urethral meatus *to prevent introduction of microorganisms into the urethra and/or bladder*
- insert the lignocaine gel and leave for 2 minutes *to allow the local anaesthetic to act*
- position the sterile receiver and with the non-dominant hand gently grasp the shaft of the penis, raising it straight up *as this will aid the passage of the catheter along the length of the urethra*
- *as the male urethra is longer* (Marieb 1989), insert the lubricated catheter into the urethral meatus for approximately 20–25 cm, until a flow of urine is established (Fig. 13.4)
- continue as for the Guidelines in the female patient until the anchoring of the catheter
- replace the patient's foreskin over the glans penis, *otherwise a paraphimosis may develop*
- anchor the catheter by either taping laterally to the thigh or abdomen or use a

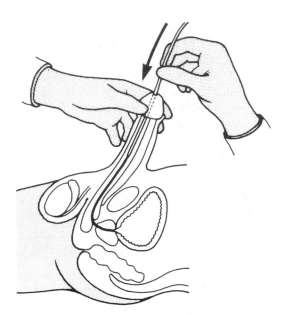

Figure 13.4
*Catheterisation: inserting
a catheter into the male
urethra*

supportive waistbelt *to reduce trauma to the urethra and bladder neck which
may cause the development of a pressure sore* (Lowthian 1994)
- ensure that the patient is left feeling as comfortable as possible *maintaining
the quality of this nursing practice*
- dispose of the equipment safely *to reduce any health hazard*
- document the nursing practice appropriately, monitor after-effects, and report
abnormal findings immediately *providing a written record and assisting in the
implementation of any action should an abnormality or adverse reaction to
the practice be noted.*

2   Catheter care

**Indications and
rationale for
catheter care**

Catheter care is the cleansing of the exposed part of a catheter which may:
- *help reduce the risk of ascending infection via the catheter to other parts of the
urinary system*
- *remove any crusts or discharge from the catheter as they can harbour
pathogenic microorganisms.*

Equipment

Sterile disposable gloves
Sterile swabs or cotton wool balls
Sterile gallipot
Sterile normal saline or fresh water and soap
Tray for equipment
Receptacle for soiled disposables

Guidelines and rationale for this nursing practice

- explain the nursing practice to the patient *to obtain consent and cooperation*
- collect and prepare the equipment *to ensure all equipment is available and ready for use*
- ensure the patient's privacy *to reduce anxiety*
- observe the patient throughout this activity *to note any signs of distress*
- help the patient into a suitable position *permitting easy comfortable access to the patient for the nurse*
- wash the hands *to reduce cross-infection* (Horton 1995), and arrange the equipment *allowing easy access during the practice*
- gently cleanse the external urethral meatus, using the swab only once and in only one direction, swabbing from above downwards in the female patient and away from the catheter–meatal junction *to reduce the risk of cross-infection* (Crow et al 1986)
- in a male patient retract the foreskin before cleansing *allowing clear access to the meatus*
- replace the foreskin following completion of this nursing practice *preventing the development of a paraphimosis*
- gently swab the shaft of the catheter away from the catheter–meatal junction, *to remove any discharge away from the urethral orifice* (Crow et al 1986)
- ensure that the patient is left feeling as comfortable as possible *maintaining the quality of this nursing practice*
- dispose of the equipment safely *to reduce any health hazard*
- document the nursing practice appropriately, monitor after-effects and report abnormal findings immediately *providing a written record and assisting in the implementation of any action should an abnormality or adverse reaction to the practice be noted.*

3 Bladder irrigation

Indications and rationale for bladder irrigation

Bladder irrigation is the continuous washing out of the bladder using sterile fluid.

Continuous bladder irrigation can be carried out through a three-way urethral catheter or through suprapubic and urethral catheters:

- *to prevent blood clot formation following surgery to the urinary tract*
- *to aid removal of blood clots and/or sediment in the bladder*
- *to clear an obstructed catheter.*

Equipment

Sterile dressings pack

Sterile normal saline

Sterile irrigating solution at 37.8°C, e.g. normal saline, chlorhexidine 0.02% in water

Sterile irrigation set

Sterile drainage bag with outlet tap

Trolley/adequate surface for equipment

Receptacle for soiled disposables

Guidelines and rationale for this nursing practice

- explain the nursing practice to the patient *to gain consent and cooperation*
- collect and prepare the equipment *to ensure all equipment is available and ready for use*
- ensure the patient's privacy *to reduce anxiety*
- observe the patient throughout this activity *to note any signs of distress*
- help the patient into a comfortable position *permitting easy comfortable access to the patient for the nurse*
- wash the hands *to reduce cross-infection* (Horton 1995), and arrange the equipment *allowing easy access during the practice*
- cleanse the irrigation inlet arm of the catheter with the antiseptic solution *to reduce cross-infection*
- insert the irrigation set connector into the cleansed inlet arm of the catheter *to permit the introduction of the irrigating fluid*
- attach the urine drainage bag if a drainage bag is not already in use. *This will act as a collection container for the returned irrigating fluid*
- empty the drainage bag *to allow accurate monitoring of the volume of returned irrigating fluid and urine output*
- open the valve of the irrigation set and regulate to the prescribed rate *complying with the medical practitioner's prescription*
- renew the irrigating fluid as stated on the patient's prescription and empty the drainage bag as required *to maintain the bladder irrigation*
- ensure that the patient is left feeling as comfortable as possible *maintaining the quality of this nursing practice*
- dispose of the equipment safely *to reduce any health hazard*
- document the nursing practice, monitor after-effects and report abnormal findings immediately *providing a written record and assisting in the implementation of any action should an abnormality or adverse reaction to the practice be noted.*

4   Bladder lavage

Indications and rationale for bladder lavage

Bladder lavage is the intermittent washing out of the bladder using sterile fluid:

- *to aid removal of sediment and/or blood clots*
- *to clear an obstructed catheter*
- *to allow administration of medicine into the bladder.*

Equipment

Sterile disposable gloves

Sterile dressings pack

Sterile normal saline solution

Sterile lavage fluid at 37.8°C, e.g. normal saline

Sterile 50 ml bladder syringe

2 sterile receivers

Sterile drainage bag

Large clean receiver for returned lavage fluid

Trolley/adequate surface for equipment

Receptacle for soiled disposables

Guidelines and rationale for this nursing practice

- explain the nursing practice to the patient *to gain consent and cooperation*
- collect and prepare the equipment required *to ensure all equipment is available and ready for use*
- ensure the patient's privacy *to reduce any anxiety*
- observe the patient throughout this activity *to note any signs of distress*
- help the patient into a comfortable position *permitting easy comfortable access to the patient for the nurse*
- wash the hands *to reduce cross-infection* (Horton 1995), and arrange the equipment *allowing easy access during the practice*
- disconnect the drainage bag and discard *to prevent ascending infection should this bag be reconnected*
- cleanse the end of the catheter with the antiseptic solution using the dressing forceps or a gloved hand. *This will reduce the number of microorganisms present on the catheter end and lessen cross-infection*
- place one sterile receiver under the catheter *to act as a collecting container for the returned lavage fluid*
- *to permit commencement of the lavage,* charge the bladder syringe with the lavage solution which has been poured into the second receiver
- release the clamp on the catheter and slowly introduce all the solution into the bladder. *Sudden, fast introduction of the lavage fluid may cause the patient extreme discomfort*
- allow this fluid to flow into the sterile receiver *to permit the lavage fluid and any debris to be returned prior to the introduction of the next volume of fluid.* Repeat until the prescribed volume of fluid has been used
- attach the sterile drainage bag *to act as a collection container for any residual lavage fluid and to return the patient's catheter to the former drainage system*
- ensure that the patient is left feeling as comfortable as possible *maintaining the quality of this nursing practice*
- dispose of the equipment safely *to reduce any health hazard*
- compare the volume, colour and consistency of fluid injected with the fluid returned *to assist in the assessment of the effectiveness of the bladder lavage;* discrepancies should be documented *as this would suggest some lavage fluid has been retained*
- document the nursing practice appropriately, monitor after-effects and report abnormal findings immediately *providing a written record and assisting in the implementation of any action should an abnormality or adverse reaction to the practice be noted.*

Relevance to the activities of living

Figure 13.5 *Points at which pathogens can enter a closed urinary drainage system:*
1 the urethral orifice
2 connection of catheter and drainage tube
3 where sample of urine is taken
4 connection of drainage tube and collecting bag
5 drainage bag outlet
(Reproduced with permission from Roper N, Logan W, Tierney A 1985 The elements of nursing, 2nd edn. Churchill Livingstone, Edinburgh)

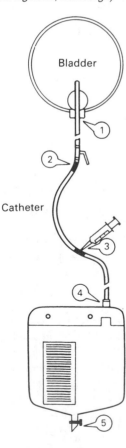

Maintaining a safe environment

Introducing a catheter into the bladder has the potential to allow pathogenic microorganisms to enter a sterile environment in a healthy individual and therefore the nurse must be vigilant in maintaining aseptic technique throughout the practice (Roper et al 1996). Anchoring the catheter reduces the potential problem of trauma to the internal and external urethral sphincters and bladder tissue (Brunner & Suddarth 1992, Lowthian 1994), and a self-retaining catheter with a small balloon may help reduce trauma to the bladder epithelium (Lowthian 1989).

The maintenance of a 'closed' drainage system and the use of appropriate infection control measures when emptying a drainage bag will help reduce the potential problem of ascending infection to the urinary system (Gould 1994) (Fig. 13.5). Lanara (1987) has suggested that the concept of the 'closed' drainage system as a method of preventing ascending infection is flawed as the system when being emptied is open to the air. The effectiveness of instillation of antiseptic solution through the outlet tap of the drainage bag to discourage the growth of pathogens and the benefit of catheter care in reducing the risk of ascending infection remain unclear, therefore the nurse should be guided by local policy (Roe et al 1986, Roper et al 1996).

During bladder lavage, the connection between the catheter and drainage bag is broken and this creates the problem that pathogens may be introduced to the urinary tract. Because of this danger, some health agencies do not advocate bladder lavage (Swaffield 1994).

To prevent blockage by blood clots and/or sediment, a catheter may require regular 'milking' of the tubing. Maintaining a clear flow of urine helps to prevent stagnation of urine, which can act as a precursor to the development of infection, and therefore prevents infection of the bladder and urinary tract.

Any patient with an indwelling catheter must know who to contact if a problem arises with the catheter or/and drainage system (Wright 1989).

A patient who uses intermittent self catheterisation as a method of bladder control will undertake the catheterisation using a clean technique (Winder 1995).

Communicating

The patient must be given an easily understood explanation about the reason for the commencement of any of the nursing practices listed. If these practices are to be used as part of a patient's postoperative care, the explanation should be given preoperatively, and this will help to reduce patient anxiety.

The patient's anxiety must be further reduced by explaining the reason for the appearance and colour of the drainage fluid during a bladder irrigation or lavage.

During bladder irrigation the patient may experience pain due to irritation of the raw areas of the bladder by the irrigating solution. Analgesia should be given as prescribed by the medical practitioner.

The patient with a long-term catheter, and his carers, will require an appropriate teaching programme; unfortunately this is not always seen as a priority in nursing practice (Roper et al 1996). A programme of teaching has been recommended by Wright (1989).

The nurse who is to teach a patient self catheterisation must have a good understanding of normal bladder function and dysfunction (Winder 1995).

Eliminating

Drainage of urine via a catheter is a deviation from the normal method of micturition but does not interfere with normal defaecation.

Before cleansing of the urethra the nurse should look for any urethral discharge. Any resistance felt during the passage of the catheter, and any bleeding from the urethra following insertion of the catheter, should be noted.

The nurse should note and record the quantity of urine drained from the patient's bladder. If the catheter has been inserted to re-establish urine flow in urinary retention, only 500 ml of urine should be drained in the first hour. The catheter should then be clamped and 200–300 ml of urine be drained every hour until the patient's bladder is empty. This will help to prevent loss of bladder muscle tone following acute retention of urine.

The colour of the urine should be noted. Pale pink to red through to brown is suggestive of blood in the urine — haematuria. Blood or sediment in the urine is suggestive of a malfunction of the renal or urinary systems due to disease or trauma, and should therefore be noted. It should be remembered that certain medicines such as rifampicin (an anti-tuberculosis medication) can colour the urine reddish-brown; this is not a cause for alarm.

Following the commencement of bladder irrigation the rate of infusion of the irrigating solution will usually be dependent on the appearance of the fluid returned into the urine drainage bag. After surgery such as a prostatectomy the patient may require an irrigating volume of 5–10 l in the first 12 hours, but this volume of fluid can usually be reduced to 3–5 l during the following 12–18 hour period. The amount and appearance of the fluid removed from the drainage bag should be recorded and, following surgery, fluid which appears to be rose in colour indicates an adequate irrigation rate (Morrison et al 1994). The patient's urinary output is calculated by subtracting the amount of drained fluid from the volume of infused irrigating solution. Any resistance or inability to introduce the irrigating or lavage fluid should be reported and documented appropriately.

Eating and drinking

Assistance should be given to the patient to increase his oral fluid intake. This will promote an increase in the volume of fluid passing through the urinary system and bladder which will help to prevent a urinary tract infection developing due to urinary stagnation. An accurate fluid balance chart must be maintained at all times. Should the patient have both an intravenous infusion and a bladder irrigation system in position, care must be taken not to confuse the urinary irrigation set and solution with the intravenous giving set and fluid.

A patient who practises intermittent self catheterisation may benefit from a reduction in oral intake during the evening, reducing the necessity of catheterisation during the night.

Personal cleansing and dressing

When a catheter is retained over a long period, it is important to ensure that perineal hygiene is maintained; this may involve some education of the patient and carers. He should be advised to wear loose underwear which is less likely to compress the catheter tubing. Showering rather than immersion bathing is preferable to reduce the incidence of ascending infection from the dirty water of a bath. The use of a leg drainage bag in conjunction with trousers or longer skirt lengths can benefit the patient's appearance.

Mobilising

If a catheter is retained, it and the drainage tubing may impede mobilising. Interference may be reduced by using leg drainage bags, which can be easily anchored to the patient's leg.

Catheter movement, which could lead to trauma of the urethra and/or bladder neck when mobilising, can be reduced by supporting the catheter (Lowthian 1994).

Expressing sexuality

Introduction of a catheter could be perceived by the patient as an 'assault' on body image. Adequate provision of privacy during catheterisation and catheter care is conducive to reducing the patient's anxiety and embarrassment.

The appearance of a retained catheter and urine drainage bag can cause a patient a great deal of embarrassment and anxiety. For the bedbound patient the discreet placement of the urine drainage bag out of the obvious sight of visitors will be greatly appreciated by the embarrassed patient (Roper et al 1990). Leg drainage bags are less visible and more comfortable for the chairbound or ambulant patient.

The use of a urinary catheter is a deviation from the normal mechanism of micturation and can thus have effects on the patient's self esteem and body image. The nurse and carer must be sensitive to the needs of the patient and assist and support the patient during the period of adaptation to this change. Advice should be given to the patient and the partner about sexual activity when a long-term catheter is in use.

Sleeping

A retained catheter may interfere with a patient's usual sleep pattern. As the patient moves during sleep the catheter and/or tubing may become trapped, causing the patient to awaken due to the discomfort caused by tension on the catheter; this possibility should be discussed with the patient in order to reduce alarm should it occur.

A patient at home will require information and education about when to renew and how to keep clean a night drainage bag (Roper et al 1996).

Patient education: key points

Provide verbal and written information on the reason for the use and care of the catheter while it is in situ for both the patient, carer and relatives.

When possible, give the patient an indication of the length of time the catheter will be in use.

Ensure that the patient knows what to do should a problem develop with the catheter.

A patient who has a catheter on a long-term basis will require extra information and education regarding the continued care and effect of the catheter on his activities of living.

The technique of self catheterisation may be taught to some patients as a method of coping with their particular urinary problem.

References

Brunner L, Suddarth L D 1992 The textbook of adult nursing. Chapman and Hall, London

Crow R, Chapman R, Roe B, Wilson J 1986 A study of patients with an indwelling urethral catheter and related nursing practice. Nursing Practice Research Unit, University of Surrey, Guildford

Gould D 1994 Keeping on tract. Nursing Times 90(40): 58–64

Horton R 1995 Handwashing: the fundamental infection control principle. British Journal of Nursing 4(16): 926–933

Lanara V 1987 Catching infection from catheters. Nursing Standard 1(1): 6

Lowthian P 1989 Catheters — preventing trauma. Nursing Times 85(21): 73–75

Lowthian P 1994 The 'WISSC' — a device to prevent pressure sores in the urethra and bladder neck. Journal of Tissue Viability 4(4): 133

Lowthian P 1995 An investigation of the uncurling forces of indwelling catheters. British Journal of Nursing 4(6): 328–334

Marieb E 1989 Human anatomy and physiology. Benjamin Cummings, Redwood City

Morrison M, Shandran T, Smithers F 1994 The urinary system. In: Alexander M, Fawcett J, Runciman P (eds) Nursing practice — hospital and home: the adult Churchill Livingstone, Edinburgh

Roe B, Chapman R, Crow R 1986 A study of the procedures for catheter care recommended by district health authorities and schools of nursing. Nursing Practice Research Unit, University of Surrey, Guildford

Roper N, Logan W, Tierney A 1996 The elements of nursing, 4th edn. Churchill Livingstone, Edinburgh, pp 199–230

Swaffield J 1994 Continence. In: Alexander M, Fawcett J, Runciman P (eds) Nursing practice — hospital and home: the adult. Churchill Livingstone, Edinburgh

Winder A 1995 Intermittent self catheterisation. Journal of Community Nursing 9(2): 24–28

Wright E 1989 Teaching patients to cope with catheters at home. Professional Nurse 4(4): 191–194

Further reading

Britton P, Wright E 1990 Catheters: making an informed choice. Professional Nurse 5(4): 194–198

Campbell J 1993 Bladder washouts. Community Outlook 3(6): 26–27

Gilbert V, Gobbi M 1989 Making sense of bladder irrigation. Nursing Times 85(16): 40–42

Glenister H 1990 Investigating infection acquired in hospitals. Nursing Times 86(49): 46–48

Pick D 1990 Standards of excellence (a standard for catheter care). Nursing 4(2): 17–18

Roe B 1990 Do we need to clamp catheters? Nursing Times 86(43): 66–67

Roe B 1990 Catheter prescribing and the use of antimicrobials. Nursing Times 86(14): 46–48

Thelwell S 1995 Systems for legbags. Nursing Times 91(16): 62–64

Walsh M, Ford P 1989 Nursing rituals — research and rational actions. Heinemann Nursing, London, pp 19–21

Winder A 1994 Supra-pubic catheterisation. Community Outlook 4(12): 25–27

14 Central Venous Pressure

There are 2 parts to this section:

1 **Insertion of a central venous catheter**
2 **Measuring and recording central venous pressure**

The concluding subsection 'Relevance to the activities of living' refers to both practices.

Learning outcomes

By the end of this section you should know how to:

- prepare the patient for this nursing practice
- collect and prepare the equipment
- assist the medical practitioner with safe insertion of the central venous catheter
- measure and record central venous pressure
- maintain the catheter in situ for a period of time.

Background knowledge required

Revision of the anatomy and physiology of the cardiovascular system, especially the heart, main vessels, and the veins of the neck and upper thorax.

Revision of Intravenous therapy, especially part 4 — Hickman catheter (*see* p. 175).

Revision of Aseptic technique (*see* p. 383).

Review of health authority policy in relation to central venous pressure.

Indications and rationale for monitoring central venous pressure

Central venous pressure (CVP) recording is the measurement of the pressure in the right atrium of the heart and is quantified in cmH_2O. The pressure recorded reflects the circulatory fluid volume; *assessment of this may be required for seriously ill patients where close monitoring of fluid balance is needed*. It may be indicated:

- for preoperative monitoring of patients who have haemorrhage or trauma *to monitor fluid balance closely*
- for postoperative monitoring following major surgery, especially when intravenous therapy or parenteral nutrition are being administered *to monitor fluid balance* (Daffurn et al 1994)
- for patients who have severe dehydration, e.g. following vomiting, diarrhoea or haemorrhage, *to monitor fluid replacement therapy*
- for patients who have cardiogenic, bacteraemic or hypovolaemic shock, *as this*

will adversely affect the circulatory system as the cardiac output falls (Hayes 1994)

- for patients who have cardiac disease, *to monitor fluid overload*
- for patients who have renal disease, *to monitor fluid overload*
- for patients who have acute renal failure during haemodialysis or ultra filtration procedures *to monitor fluid balance.*

1   Insertion of a central venous catheter

Outline of the procedure

This procedure is carried out by a medical practitioner using aseptic technique. The procedure involves the passage of a catheter through the veins to the superior vena cava, so that the tip of the catheter lies at the entrance of the right atrium of the heart (Fig. 14.1). The catheter is then connected to the manometer and giving set, and an intravenous infusion is commenced (*see* Parenteral nutrition, p. 247).

The position of the patient

The position of the patient is important during this procedure, and is dependent on the choice of the entry site for catheterisation. There are three main entry sites (the first two are used more frequently) (Stillwell 1992):

The subclavian vein   The patient lies supine with his arms by his side. The head of the bed is lowered by 10° *to prevent the danger of an embolus occurring.*

The internal jugular vein   The patient lies supine, with no pillow. The neck is extended. The head is rotated away from the site of entry, and well supported in position. The head of the bed is lowered by 10°. *This position is important to prevent the danger of an air embolus occurring.*

The median cephalic vein   The patient lies supine. The chosen arm is extended with the palm upwards and the elbow supported *to ensure easy access to the entry site.*

Ideally, this procedure should be performed in theatre. If it is performed in the ward, it should take place in the treatment room *to prevent any cross-infection.*

Equipment

As for intravenous infusion (*see* p. 166).

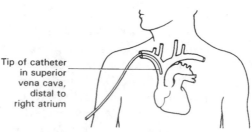

Tip of catheter
in superior
vena cava,
distal to
right atrium

Figure 14.1   *Central venous pressure: position of catheter in relation to the heart*

Additional equipment

- Theatre cap and mask
- Sterile gown
- Sterile gloves
- Minor operation sterile pack or sterile drape and towels
- Waterproof protection for the bed
- Alcohol-based antiseptic for cleansing the skin
- Venous pressure manometer set
- Non-viscous sterile intravenous fluid, e.g. normal saline, dextrose 5% (this will be prescribed by the medical practitioner)
- Appropriate sterile catheter depending on the site of entry used, e.g. single, double or triple lumen catheter (Fig. 14.2)
- Sterile needles and black silk sutures
- ECG monitoring equipment if required
- Local anaesthetic and equipment for its administration.

Guidelines and rationale for this nursing practice

Refer to the section on Intravenous therapy (*see* p. 169) for detailed guidelines.

- help to explain the procedure to the patient *to gain consent and cooperation and encourage participation in care*
- ensure the patient's privacy *respecting his individuality*
- prepare the equipment and prime the administration set with the prescribed infusion fluid *in preparation for commencement of infusion*
- help the patient into the correct position depending on the site of entry used *to ensure that access is safely achieved*
- observe the patient throughout this activity *to monitor any adverse effects*
- adjust the angle of the bed so that the patient's head is lowered if required *to prevent any air embolus occurring — any air entering the vein would track towards the heart if the head was not lowered*
- protect the bed with waterproof material *as some fluid or blood may spill*
- assist the medical practitioner as required *ensuring safe practice*
- remain with the patient *and help to maintain his position and to reduce his anxiety as far as possible*
- commence the infusion of prescribed fluid once the catheter is in position and connected to the manometer and administration set. If a double or triple lumen catheter is used, the line designated for CVP recording is connected to the appropriate administration set and manometer, and labelled accordingly *ensuring all personnel have accurate information*

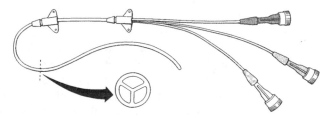

Figure 14.2 *Triple lumen catheter*

- ensure the patient is left feeling as comfortable as possible *so that he will tolerate the catheter in situ as long as necessary* (RCN 1992)
- dispose of the equipment safely *to prevent transmission of infection*
- document the procedure appropriately, monitor after-effects and report abnormal findings immediately *to ensure safe practice and enable prompt appropriate medical and nursing care to be initiated as soon as possible*
- monitor and adjust the flow rate *to maintain the infusion at the rate prescribed* (*see* Intravenous therapy, p. 165).

A portable chest X-ray is taken as soon as possible after catheter insertion *to check that the catheter is in the correct position.*

A temporary sterile dressing may be applied until this has been performed. The catheter is usually held in place with skin sutures *once it is judged to be correctly positioned,* and a sterile transparent dressing is applied over the site *to maintain asepsis* (Keenlyside 1993).

Occasionally arrhythmias may occur, *due to irritation of the heart by the passage of the catheter,* and observations may be supplemented by ECG monitoring. The rhythm usually returns to normal *once the catheter is in the correct position.*

2 Measuring and recording central venous pressure

The central venous pressure is measured in cm H_2O. The range of normal is between 3 and 10 cm H_2O.

The central venous pressure (CVP) may be measured hourly, 2-hourly or 4-hourly, depending on the patient's condition.

Equipment

A central venous catheter, intravenous fluid and associated lines in situ (Fig. 14.3)

A venous pressure manometer (Fig. 14.3)

A spirit level.

Guidelines and rationale for this nursing practice

- explain the nursing practice to the patient *to gain consent and cooperation and encourage participation in care*
- ensure the patient's privacy *to respect individuality and maintain self esteem*
- help the patient into the correct position (Fig. 14.3). It is preferable for the patient to lie flat *for absolute accuracy, as this position will prevent upward pressure of the abdominal organs affecting the reading.* However, *if lying flat causes the patient any distress* an acceptable reading can be obtained with the patient sitting comfortably at an angle of about 45°. His body should be straight, with his shoulders flat against the back of the bed; *the thorax must not be turned or twisted or a false reading may result* (Woodrow 1992)
- position the manometer. It should be supported on a pole *so that it is easily read,* while still allowing the patient freedom of movement in bed between

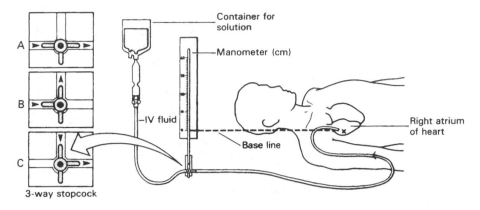

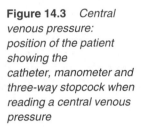

Figure 14.3 *Central venous pressure: position of the patient showing the catheter, manometer and three-way stopcock when reading a central venous pressure*

readings. There should be no strain on the lines or the catheter *to prevent any disconnection occurring*

- observe the patient throughout this activity *to monitor any adverse effects*
- assess the baseline. *The baseline is the pressure level above which measurement of central venous pressure is taken.* This is level with the patient's right atrium where the tip of the catheter is lying. The medical practitioner will note the level at an imaginary 90° angle between the sternal notch and the midline from the axilla. This can be marked on the patient's skin with his consent *to ensure consistency of baseline measurement*
- read the baseline. A spirit level is used to record the level on the manometer gauge which corresponds with the baseline level, which may be marked on the side of the patient's chest *this ensures that measurement is as accurate as possible*
- turn off all other infusions. Ideally only the CVP fluid should be infused through the CVP line, but on occasions other fluids are infused through the same line. *CVP is measured in cm of water, so only fluids of similar specific gravity should be used, i.e. normal saline.* The use of multiple lumen lines overcomes this problem. The tap of the three-way stopcock should be at position A between recordings and before commencing reading (Fig. 14.3)
- flush the line *to ensure patency and to clear all other infusions* (Leighton 1994)
- turn the tap on the three-way stopcock away from the patient, towards the infusion fluid to position B (Fig. 14.3); *this allows the manometer tube to refill with fluid*
- turn the tap towards the patient to position C (Fig. 14.3); *this allows a free flow of fluid between the manometer tube and the catheter to be established.* The fluid in the manometer tube will fall to a level *which corresponds to the pressure in the right atrium or superior vena cava.* The fluid fluctuates *in relation to the patient's respirations* once it falls to the level for recording
- read the level of the lower fluctuation on the manometer gauge once the fluid in the tube maintains a steady level with a fluctuation of 0.2–1.0 cm. *This relates to the pressure in the right atrium*
- subtract the baseline reading from this figure; *the resultant figure is the measurement of central venous pressure*

- turn the tap on the stopcock back to position A (Fig. 14.3) *to occlude the manometer and recommence the infusion fluid at the prescribed rate*
- ensure that the patient is left feeling as comfortable as possible *to help reduce anxiety and promote the healing process*
- document the nursing practice appropriately, monitor after-effects and report abnormal findings immediately. *This ensures safe practice and enables prompt appropriate medical and nursing intervention to be initiated.* A single reading is not as valuable as monitoring a series of recordings. *These will show whether the central venous pressure is rising, falling or remaining steady and give some indication of patient response to treatment* (UKCC 1993).

Pressure transducers

Pressure transducers are increasingly being used to monitor the central venous pressure. The principles of the practice, the care of the patient, and the care of the lines are exactly the same. The pressure transducer and the appropriate lines are substituted for the manometer set. The measurement is recorded on a bedside monitor screen. When a reading is taken, the height of the transducer, which is supported on a pole, is adjusted level with the assessed baseline, as previously described. The monitor may be programmed to assess the reading in mm of mercury (Hg). The normal recording parameters may have to be adjusted (see manufacturer's instructions).

Relevance to the activities of living

Observations and further rationale for this nursing practice will be included within each activity of living as appropriate.

As for intravenous infusion and in addition:

Maintaining a safe environment

A central venous catheter gives direct access to the heart so the dangers from infection are increased. Meticulous care to prevent infection must be maintained at all times. Aseptic technique should be used whenever dressings, infusions or lines are changed. Good hand washing technique should be used before touching the equipment for measuring the central venous pressure.

The nurse should ensure that the lines do not become disconnected, otherwise air may enter and create an air embolus. The lines should be observed for air bubbles and appropriate action taken. The danger from an air embolus is increased because of the direct access to the heart.

The nurse should ensure that the line remains patent and that the infusion is maintained at the required rate to help prevent clotting or occlusion of the line (*see* Intravenous therapy, p. 165).

Breathing

The central venous pressure is at the lower level of normal in young healthy adults. It increases slightly with age.

It is raised in patients who have respiratory disease, due to the increased intrapulmonary pressure.

It is significantly raised in patients with bronchospasm, e.g. asthma, as this increases the intrathoracic pressure and may mask any change in circulatory fluid volume.

It is raised in patients with congestive cardiac failure due to the increase in circulatory fluid volume.

A rare complication would be the development of a pneumothorax. This is more likely to occur at the time of insertion of the catheter. Any sudden change in the patient's general condition or respiratory function should be reported immediately.

Eating and drinking

The central venous pressure reflects the volume of circulating fluid and any fluid imbalance; it is lowered in patients who are dehydrated and raised in patients with fluid overload. Accurate recordings of fluid intake should be maintained during the period of monitoring central venous pressure.

Eliminating

Accurate recordings of fluid output should be maintained during the period of monitoring, for assessment of the patient's fluid balance.

The central venous pressure is raised in patients who have renal disease; it will show a temporary fall during a period of treatment with diuretic medication.

Personal cleansing and dressing

The patient may need appropriate help with personal cleansing while attached to the manometer. The need to wear light clothing to allow unrestricted access to the site of catheterisation should be explained to the patient.

Controlling body temperature

The dangers of infection are increased during this procedure, as the central line has direct access to the heart. The patient's temperature should be recorded 2-hourly or 4-hourly during the period of CVP monitoring, to observe any signs of developing infection. This should continue to be monitored 4-hourly for 48 hours after the central line has been removed.

Mobilising

The central venous pressure will not be affected by the patient moving around the bed between readings. He may be helped into a chair with the manometer and lines adequately supported, as his condition allows.

Patient education: key points

- The reason for central venous pressure monitoring and its importance for treatment and care should be explained to the patient. This practice will normally only take place in an institutional setting
- The importance of maintaining the catheter in situ should be emphasised, and the dangers of disconnection explained, so that the patient does not pull the lines or dislodge the dressing
- All patients should understand the importance of reporting to the nursing staff any redness, swelling or pain at the infusion site, even after the line has been removed, as this may indicate a developing infection.

References

Daffurn K, Hillman K, Baumn A et al 1994 Fluid balance charts: do they measure up. British Journal of Nursing 3(16): 816–820

Hayes E 1994 Shock (monitoring haemodynamic state). In: Alexander M, Fawcett J, Runciman P (eds) Nursing practice — hospital and home: the adult. Churchill Livingstone, Edinburgh

Keenlyside D 1993 Avoiding an unnecessary outcome. A comparative trial between I.V. 3000 and conventional film dressing to access rates of catheter related sepsis. Professional Nurse 8(5): 288–291

Leighton H 1994 Maintaining patency of transduced arterial and venous lines using 0.9% sodium chloride. Intensive and Critical Care Nursing 10(1): 23–25

RCN 1992 Skin tunnelled catheters. Guidelines for care. Royal College of Nursing, London

Stillwell B 1992 Skills update. Central venous lines (using Hickman lines). Community Outlook 2(5): 22–23

Woodrow P 1992 Monitoring CVP. Nursing Standard 6(33): 25–29

UKCC 1993 Standards for records and record keeping. United Kingdom Central Council for Nursing, Midwifery and Health Visiting, London

Further reading

Corbett K, Meehan L, Sackey V 1993 A strategy to enhance skills. Developing intravenous therapy skills for community nursing. Professional Nurse 9(1): 60–63

Darbyshire P 1988 Making sense of . . . central venous catheters. Nursing Times 84(6): 36–38

Gourlay D 1996 Central venous cannulation. British Journal of Nursing 5(1): 8–15

Raad I 1992 Impact of central venous catheter removal on the recurrence of catheter related sepsis. Infection Control and Hospital Epidemiology 13(4): 215–221

Speer E W 1990 Central venous catheterisation. Issues associated with the use of single and multilumen catheters. Journal of Intravenous Nursing 13(1): 30–39

15 Chest Drainage: Underwater Seal

There are three parts to this section:

1 Insertion of an underwater seal chest drain
2 Changing a chest drainage bottle
3 Removal of an underwater seal chest drain

The concluding subsection 'Relevance to the activities of living' refers to the three practices collectively.

Learning outcomes

By the end of this section you should know how to:

- prepare the patient for these three nursing practices
- collect and prepare the equipment necessary to insert a chest drain and connect it to underwater seal drainage, change a chest drainage bottle, and remove an underwater seal chest drain
- assist the medical practitioner in parts 1 and 3
- care for the patient who has a chest drain connected to underwater seal drainage.

Background knowledge required

Revision of the anatomy and physiology of the respiratory system.

Revision of Aseptic technique (*see* p. 383).

1 Insertion of an underwater seal chest drain

Indications and rationale for insertion of an underwater seal chest drain

Underwater seal chest drainage is a closed system of drainage which allows air or fluid to pass in one direction only, i.e. from the pleural space to the collecting bottle. It may be established in the following circumstances:

- *to bring about re-expansion of the lung* when there is air or fluid, e.g. blood or pus, in the pleural space as a result of injury, surgery or a respiratory disease or dysfunction.

Outline of the procedure

Using an aseptic technique, the medical practitioner washes and dries his hands, cleanses the patient's skin over the selected site of entry for the drain, injects a local anaesthetic and waits for it to take effect. He then makes a small incision with the scalpel, inserts the drain and introducer, removes the introducer and connects the drain to the equipment already prepared by the nurse. A purse-string suture is inserted round the entry site of the drain to seal off the site when the drain is eventually removed. A dressing is usually placed over the site to help prevent infection of the small wound (Fig. 15.1).

If there is air in the pleural space, the drain is usually inserted at the level of the 3rd or 4th intercostal space. The insertion site is lower if fluid has gathered in the pleural space, to promote maximum drainage.

Equipment

Trolley

Sterile dressings pack

Alcohol-based antiseptic for skin cleansing

Local anaesthetic and equipment for administration

Sterile scalpel and blade

Sterile black silk suture

Sterile chest drain and introducer

Sterile drainage equipment—either glass bottles or a disposable set, e.g. Pleurovac or Argyle Double Seal System

2 pairs tubing clamps

Receptacle for soiled disposables.

Guidelines and rationale for this nursing practice

- help to explain the procedure to the patient *to gain consent and cooperation. Patients should be encouraged to be active partners in care*
- ensure the patient's privacy *to help maintain dignity and sense of 'self'*
- administer a sedative if prescribed by medical staff. *This may help to reduce anxiety levels in the patient*
- collect the equipment *for efficiency of practice*
- help the patient into the position suggested by the medical staff *to allow best access to the site for insertion of the drain*
- observe the patient throughout this activity *to detect signs of discomfort or distress*
- ensure that the drainage equipment is assembled correctly and ready for connection to the drain when required, *for efficient practice*
- open the sterile equipment and help the medical practitioner as requested
- seal all connections *to ensure that they are airtight as this is necessary for the maximum efficiency of function*
- ensure that the collection equipment is always below the level of the patient's chest *so that there is no reflux into the pleural space* (Fig. 15.2)
- release the clamps when connected to the drain and the nurse is satisfied that there are no air leaks at the connections *to permit the apparatus to start functioning*
- check that the apparatus is functioning; the fluid should be oscillating in the long underwater tube in time with the patient's respirations. If positive suction is required, connect to a second drainage bottle by tubing from its long rod to the short rod of the first. The short rod of the second drainage bottle is then

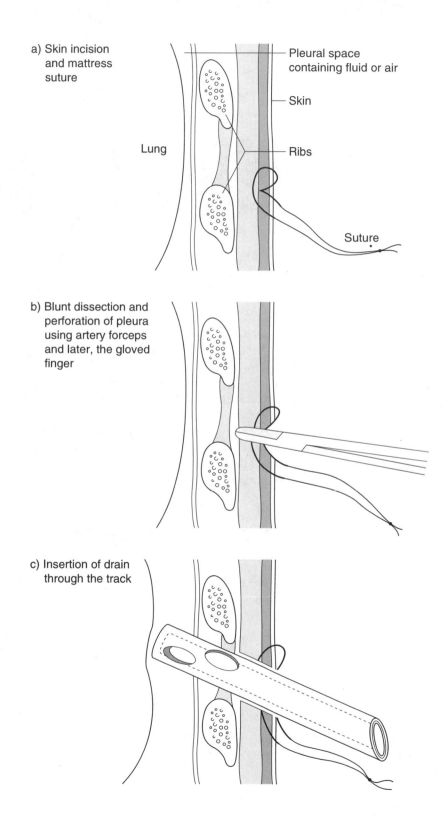

a) Skin incision
   and mattress
   suture

Pleural space
containing fluid or air

Skin

Lung

Ribs

Suture

b) Blunt dissection and
   perforation of pleura
   using artery forceps
   and later, the gloved
   finger

c) Insertion of drain
   through the track

Figure 15.1 *Insertion
of a chest drain*

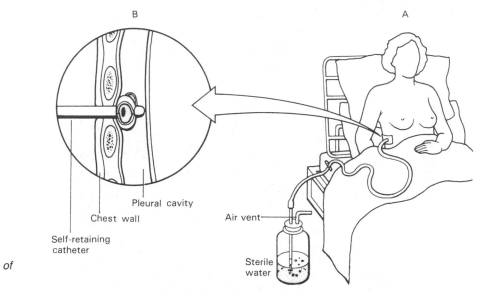

Figure 15.2
Underwater seal chest drainage
A Drainage system in position
B Detail of the position of the catheter

connected by tubing to a suction machine, the pressure of which has been decided by the medical practitioner (Fig. 15.3)
- apply a sterile dressing to the wound site *to help prevent infection*
- ensure the patient is left feeling as comfortable as possible *to maintain the quality of this practice*
- dispose of the equipment safely *for the protection of others*
- document the procedure appropriately, monitor after-effects and report abnormal findings immediately *to ensure safe practice and enable prompt appropriate medical and nursing intervention to be initiated.*

2　Changing a chest drainage bottle

Indications and rationale for changing a drainage bottle

As drainage from the pleural space accumulates and approaches the three-quarters full level, the drainage bottle has to be changed:
- *to enable the equipment to continue functioning efficiently.*

Equipment

Sterile drainage bottle, cap, glass or plastic rods and tubing or disposable set
500 ml sterile water or normal saline
Receptacle for soiled disposables.

Guidelines and rationale for this nursing practice

- collect and prepare the equipment *for efficiency of practice*
- explain this practice to the patient *to encourage active participation in care*
- observe the patient throughout this activity *to detect signs of discomfort or distress*

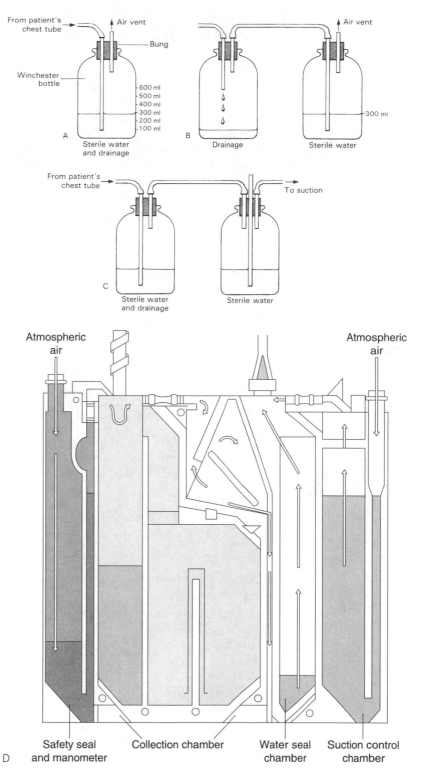

Figure 15.3
Underwater seal chest drainage system
A Using one bottle
B Using two bottles
C Using two bottles plus suction
D Disposable set

- clamp off the intercostal drain securely with the two pairs of clamps *to prevent any backflow of air or fluid*
- disconnect the tubing
- connect fresh tubing and apparatus
- ensure that all connections are airtight and that the drainage bottle is below chest level *so that it will function correctly*
- release the clamps and check the oscillation of fluid in the underwater tube *to confirm that the apparatus is functioning correctly*
- ensure the patient is left feeling as comfortable as possible *to maintain the quality of this practice*
- dispose of the equipment safely *for the protection of others*
- document this nursing practice and report abnormal findings immediately *so that actions can be taken to relieve any problems.*

3 Removal of an underwater seal chest drain

Indications and rationale for removal of an underwater seal chest drain

Underwater seal drainage is a temporary measure and is removed:

- *when radiological examination demonstrates that the patient's lung has fully re-inflated.*

Equipment

Trolley

Sterile dressings pack

Sterile stitch cutter

Water-based antiseptic for wound cleansing

Waterproof tape and scissors

Sterile artery forceps

Receptacle for soiled disposables.

Guidelines and rationale for this nursing practice

Two nurses, one of whom must be qualified, or the nurse and a medical practitioner are required to carry out this practice.

- explain the nursing practice to the patient *to gain consent and cooperation. Patients should be encouraged to be active partners in their care*
- ensure the patient's privacy *to maintain dignity and sense of 'self'*
- administer a sedative if it is prescribed by the medical practitioner. *This will help to reduce anxiety*
- collect the equipment *for efficiency of practice*
- prepare and assist the patient into a suitable position which is as comfortable as possible. *It is necessary to have clear access to the drain site*
- observe the patient throughout this activity *to detect any signs of discomfort and distress*

- remove the dressing from the drain site
- clean the drain site with the antiseptic *to cleanse the skin*
- clamp the ends of the purse-string suture with the artery forceps to facilitate tightening the suture *so that the wound is sealed off as quickly as possible*
- raise the drain slightly (performed by the assistant) while the qualified practitioner cuts and removes the retaining suture
- request the patient to breathe in; while he is breathing out the qualified practitioner holds folded swabs over the puncture site with one hand and with the dominant hand pulls the drain out quickly and smoothly. The assistant tightens the purse-string suture as the drain is removed
- remove the artery forceps from the end of the purse-string suture and knot the suture
- apply a sterile dressing and waterproof tape *to stop as much air as possible accessing the drain site*
- order a chest X-ray *to ensure that the lung is functioning normally*
- ensure the patient is left feeling as comfortable as possible *to maintain the quality of this practice*
- dispose of the equipment safely *for the protection of others*
- document the nursing practice, monitor after-effects and report abnormal findings immediately *to provide a written record and assist in the implementation of any action should an abnormality or adverse reaction to the practice be noted.*

Relevance to the activities of living	***Maintaining a safe environment***

A meticulous technique must be used for the prevention of infection. Thorough handwashing should be carried out, preferably using an antiseptic detergent.

Ensure that the tubing is not being compressed or kinked by the patient lying on it, as this will cause the equipment to function inefficiently.

It is imperative that the drainage bottle is kept below the level of the patient's chest, unless double clamped, or there may be a backflow of fluid into the pleural cavity.

When the drain is being removed, care must be taken to prevent a pneumothorax occurring (i.e. the entry of air into the pleural space).

Communicating

Because of breathlessness, the patient may have difficulty in talking. A pencil and paper may help communication with staff and visitors, and a bell should always be to hand to summon assistance if necessary. Analgesia may be prescribed to help relieve any pain or discomfort.

Breathing

If the equipment is functioning correctly, after the insertion of the drain the patient's respiratory rate should gradually return to his normal range.

The patient's respirations should be closely monitored after removal of the drain so that the potential complication of pneumothorax can be quickly detected.

Personal cleansing and dressing

Some assistance with washing and dressing may have to be given to patients who are attached to underwater seal drainage equipment as their mobility is reduced. Light, loose clothing should be worn so that breathing is not unduly impaired.

Mobilising

Movement will be restricted by the equipment but the patient should be encouraged to be as independent as possible.

Sleeping

The patient's normal sleeping pattern may be altered because of difficulty with breathing and because of the presence of the equipment, so the nurse should take measures which help to induce sleep.

Patient education: key points

Continuing information should be given to the patient to relieve anxiety. Education about mobility when a chest drain is in situ should also be given.

Further reading

Alexander M, Fawcett J, Runciman P 1994 Nursing care—hospital and home: the adult, Churchill Livingstone, Edinburgh
Campbell J 1993 Making sense of underwater sealed drainage. Nursing Times 89(9): 34–36
Walsh M 1989 Making sense of chest drainage. Nursing Times 85(24): 40–41
Yeaw E M J 1992 Good lung down. American Journal of Nursing 92(3): 27–29

16 Eardrops: Instillation of

Learning outcomes	By the end of this section you should know how to: • prepare the patient for this nursing practice • collect and prepare the equipment • instil drops safely and effectively into the patient's ear.
Background knowledge required	Revision of the anatomy of the ear. Revision of Administration of medicines, especially checking the medication with the prescription (*see* p. 1).
Indications and rationale for instilling eardrops	Instillation of eardrops involves dropping a prescribed solution into the external auditory canal from a dropper. This may be required: • *to soften wax before syringing.* If the wax has become impacted, syringing the external canal with solution will be ineffective and it is necessary to soften the wax first • *to reduce inflammation and relieve discomfort* • *to combat infection.*
Equipment	Prescribed eardrops Cotton wool balls Receptacle for soiled disposables.
Guidelines and rationale for this nursing practice	• explain the practice to the patient *to ensure understanding and gain consent and cooperation* • collect and prepare the equipment *for efficiency of practice* • ensure the patient's privacy *to preserve dignity and sense of 'self'* • assist the patient to sit in an upright position with the head tilted slightly away from the affected ear *so that the inserted drops will run the length of the canal* • observe the patient throughout this activity *to detect any signs of discomfort* • check the drug prescription with the eardrops label *to ensure the correct drops are administered* • check the expiry date of the bottle of drops *as expired medication may be ineffective* • verify which ear should receive the drops *to avoid errors*

- pull the pinna of the ear gently in an upward and backward direction in adults, and a downward and backward direction in children, *to straighten the external canal*
- insert the prescribed number of eardrops into the canal
- release the pinna of the ear
- position a piece of cotton wool at the entrance to the canal if this is local policy
- dispose of the equipment safely *for the protection of others*
- document this nursing practice appropriately, monitor after-effects and report abnormal findings immediately *to provide a written record and assist in the implementation of any action should an abnormality or adverse reaction to the practice be noted.*

Relevance to the activities of living

Maintaining a safe environment

To avoid the risk of cross-infection each patient should have an individual container of prescribed eardrops. The nurse should wash her hands before commencing and on completion of the practice.

Communicating

Any patient who is receiving medication by ear may experience difficulty with hearing, and this should be explained.

Should a patient complain of skin irritation, pain or a burning sensation following instillation of an ear medication this should be reported as it may be an indication of a drug allergy.

Mobilising

It aids the effectiveness of the eardrops if the ear in which the drops are inserted is kept level or tilted upwards for a period of time after insertion. This aids absorption.

Patient education: key points

If the patient is expected to self-administer the drops it will be necessary to teach this technique and ensure proficiency.

Further reading

McKenzie G, Chawla H, Gordon D 1986 The special senses, 2nd edn. Churchill Livingstone, Edinburgh, pp 9–47
Surkitt-Par D 1989 The removal of foreign bodies. Nursing 3(35): 11–14

17 Ear Syringing

Learning outcomes

By the end of this section you should know how to:
- prepare the patient for this procedure
- collect and prepare the equipment
- syringe a patient's ear.

Background knowledge required

Revision of the anatomy and physiology of the external and middle ear.

Review of health authority policy for this procedure.

Indications and rationale for syringing an ear

Syringing an ear is washing out the external auditory canal with a prescribed solution using a special syringe.

This may be required:
- *to clear the external canal of an obstruction which may be blocking it*
- *to wash out softened wax which may be impeding the transmission of sound waves to the tympanic membrane.*

Outline of the procedure

Using the auriscope, the external canal and eardrum are examined. If the eardrum is intact and no other abnormalities are detected, the practice of syringing the ear can be carried out. Sometimes it is not possible to visualise the tympanic membrane at this stage because of the impacted wax. In this case, if there is no history of ruptured eardrums, after preparing the equipment and solution as outlined below, insert some of the solution gently to dislodge some of the wax and then check the membrane. The syringe or tubing is primed with the solution, or ready prepared equipment assembled, care being taken to expel all the air. The protective covering is placed over the patient's shoulder and the receiver held in place under the ear. The pinna of the ear is gently pulled in an upward and backward direction to straighten out the canal, then the fluid is introduced through the syringe or tubing, which should point to the roof of the canal so that the solution flows along the roof and down and back out, washing any debris with it (Fig. 17.1). After the qualified practitioner has again examined the canal to assess the result of the syringing, the canal is carefully dried using the dressed applicators.

Equipment

Tray

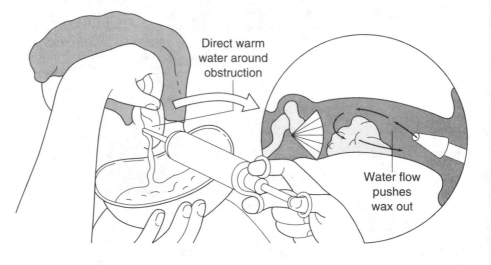

Figure 17.1 *Ear syringing showing fluid being directed to the roof of the aural canal (the nurse should pull the pinna of the ear gently upwards) (Reproduced with permission from Chilman A, Thomas M (eds) 1987 Understanding nursing care, 3rd edn. Churchill Livingstone, Edinburgh)*

Direct warm water around obstruction

Water flow pushes wax out

Waterproof protection for the patient

Container with prescribed amount of solution

Lotion thermometer

Aural (ear) syringe

or

Disposable ready prepared equipment

or

Electronically operated apparatus with which the operator can control the pressure of the fluid

Receiver for return flow

Auriscope

Dressed applicators

Receptacle for soiled disposables

Tap water is commonly used nowadays for ear syringing, although sodium chloride 0.9% or a solution of sodium bicarbonate (4 g to 600 ml water) may be ordered. About 500 ml of the solution is usually prepared

The temperature of the solution should be 38°C. Temperatures other than this are uncomfortable, may injure tissues and may cause the patient to feel dizzy and nauseated. This procedure is normally only carried out if the tympanic membrane is intact, in which case it is a socially clean procedure.

Guidelines and rationale for this nursing practice

- help explain the procedure to the patient *to ensure the practice is understood and to gain consent and cooperation*
- assemble and prepare the equipment *to increase the efficiency of the practice*
- ensure the patient's privacy *to help maintain dignity and sense of 'self'*

- assist the patient to sit in an upright position with the head tilted slightly to the affected side *to aid the return flow of the solution*
- observe the patient throughout this activity *to detect any signs of discomfort or distress*
- arrange the waterproof protection around the patient's neck and shoulders *to prevent the patient's clothes becoming damp or damaged*
- place the receiver for the return flow under the patient's ear and ask for the patient's assistance in holding it in place
- after examining the external canal, insert the equipment and direct the flow of solution in an upward direction
- continue until the return flow is clear of debris
- dry the patient's ear
- ensure the patient is left feeling as comfortable as possible and check for improved hearing
- dispose of the equipment safely *for the protection of others*
- document the procedure appropriately, monitor after-effects and report abnormal findings immediately *to provide a written record and assist in the implementation of any action should an abnormality or adverse reaction to the practice be noted.*

Relevance to the activities of living

Maintaining a safe environment

Although aseptic technique is not required, the equipment should be clean or disposable and the nurse should wash her hands before commencing and on completion of the procedure.

It is important to examine the patient's ear before carrying out this procedure as there is a danger of causing serious damage or introducing infection into the middle ear if the tympanic membrane has been ruptured.

The temperature of the solution should be 38°C: cold or hot solutions may stimulate the labyrinth and cause vertigo or nausea.

Communicating

Eardrops (usually oil) are usually prescribed for a few days prior to syringing to soften hard cerumen (wax). It is important to explain to the patient that feelings of slight dizziness may be experienced when this procedure is being carried out. If it is being performed to wash away wax which has been impairing the patient's hearing, there should be a marked improvement in hearing afterwards. If the patient wears a hearing aid, the nurse should check that it is working satisfactorily following the practice.

Mobilising

The patient's cooperation in remaining still while the procedure is being carried out is important, as the equipment could damage the tissue of the ear.

If there is any evidence of dizziness, the patient may have to rest for a time following the procedure.

Working and playing

Hearing difficulties may prevent the patient carrying out his job efficiently and can also prohibit participation in or limit enjoyment of hobbies and interests.

Patient education: key points

It should be explained to the patient that nausea or dizziness may be experienced for a short time after the procedure.

If the syringing was carried out to relieve impacted wax and improve hearing, the possibility of the condition recurring must be explained.

Further reading

Ashley J 1973 Journey into silence. Bodley Head
Bond M, Arthur A, Avis M 1995 Distant voices: hospital care of a woman with sensory impairments highlights the importance of touch in communicating with patients. Nursing Times 19 July: 38–40
Denyer S 1990 Foreign bodies: where do children put them? Health Visitor 63: 5
Kanda Y, Shigena K, Kinoshita N 1994 Sudden hearing loss associated with interferon. Lancet 343(8906): 1134–1135
Newman D 1990 Assessment of hearing loss in elderly people— the feasibility of a nurse-administered screening test. Journal of Advanced Nursing 15: 400–409
Roper N, Logan W, Tierney A 1996 The elements of nursing, 4th edn. Churchill Livingstone, Edinburgh
Russell J 1995 Ear screening. Community Nurse, May: 14–16
Stanley C 1995 The healing touch: admission to hospital can be a particularly unsettling experience for patients with dual sensory impairment. Nursing Times 19 July: 36–38
Surkitt-Par D 1989 The removal of foreign bodies. Nursing 3(35): 11–14
Thurgood K, Thurgood G 1995 Ear syringing: a clinical skill. British Journal of Nursing 4(12): 682–688
Verney A 1989 The patient with hearing impairment. Nursing 3(35): 17–20

18 Enema

Learning outcomes

By the end of this section you should know how to:

- prepare the patient for this nursing practice
- collect and prepare the equipment
- administer an enema
- describe the various enema preparations and their modes of action.

Background knowledge required

Revision of the anatomy and physiology of the colon, rectum and anus.
Revision of drug administration, particularly checking the drug with the prescription (see p. 1).

Indications and rationale for administering an enema

An enema is the introduction of liquid into the rectum by means of a tube. It is used:

- *to evacuate the bowel prior to surgery or investigations*
- *to administer medication.*

Equipment

Tray

Prescribed enema

Protective covering for the bed

Water-soluble lubricant

Disposable gloves

Apron

Medical wipes/tissues

Commode or bedpan if required

Receptacle for soiled disposables.

Types of enema (Fig. 18.1)

There are three main kinds:

- enemas containing medication, which should be retained as long as possible and should be inserted very slowly over half an hour
- stimulant enemas which are usually returned, with faecal matter and flatus, within a few minutes; a solution containing phosphates or sodium citrate is commonly used
- enemas which soften and lubricate faeces and should be retained for a

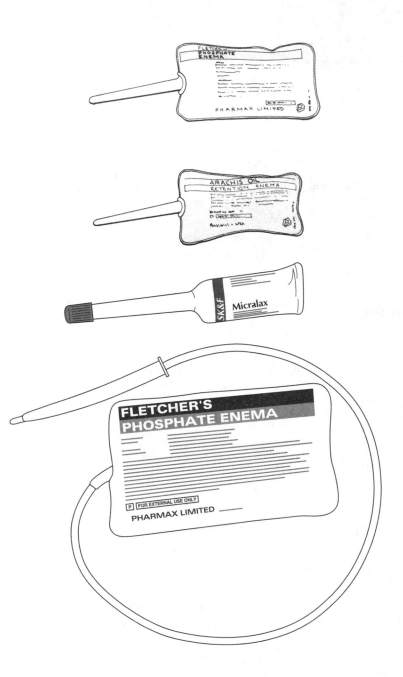

Figure 18.1 *Examples of disposable enemas*

specified time; they usually contain arachis or olive oil. They may be inserted, for example, at bedtime to be retained overnight for maximum efficiency of action.

Microenemas are being increasingly used in the community as they cause less discomfort to patients when administered. The other pre-prepared enemas can be obtained with long delivery tubes to facilitate self-insertion by patients.

At one time, a solution containing green soap was prescribed as an evacuant enema but it has been demonstrated that it can severely damage the mucosa of the bowel, and is no longer in use.

Guidelines and rationale for this nursing practice

- explain the nursing practice to the patient *to gain consent and cooperation. Patients should be encouraged to be active partners in care*
- assemble and prepare the equipment *for efficiency of practice*
- ensure the patient's privacy and help the patient into the left lateral position *to allow ease of access to the anal sphincter*
- observe the patient throughout this activity *to detect any signs of discomfort or distress*
- place the protective covering under the patient's buttocks *to contain any soiling or leakage*
- put on disposable gloves and apron
- lubricate the end of the enema tube *to ease entry into the rectum*
- squeeze a small amount of fluid down the tube to expel the air, *as air in the rectum will cause discomfort*
- insert the tube into the rectum in an upward and slightly backward direction for about 7.5 cm *following the natural line of the rectum*
- administer the solution gently and slowly *to minimise any discomfort*
- remove the tube when the prescribed amount has been administered
- dry the anal area *to prevent any irritation*
- the protective covering may be left in place *to help prevent soiling of bed linen by leaking faecal matter*
- provide a bedpan or commode when this is required although access to a toilet is preferable *as it reduces the patient's embarrassment*
- ensure that the patient is left feeling as comfortable as possible, *maintaining the quality of this nursing practice*
- dispose of the equipment safely *for the protection of others*
- document this nursing practice appropriately, monitor after-effects and report any abnormal findings immediately *to provide a written record and assist in the implementation of any action should an abnormality or adverse reaction to the practice be noted.*

Relevance to the activities of living

Maintaining a safe environment

Although aseptic technique is not required all the equipment used should be clean or disposable and the nurse should wash her hands before and on completion of the practice. Gloves and aprons are worn for protection.

Care should be taken to avoid damaging the rectal mucosa when inserting the tube of the enema into the rectum. If the tube meets with resistance it should be withdrawn slightly and no force used.

Communicating

It is important to explain clearly to the patient the reason for the enema being prescribed so that he knows whether it has to be retained for a time or returned quickly.

Eating and drinking

If the enema is being administered to relieve constipation, advice should be given on how to help avoid this problem in the future. An increased intake of dietary fibre and fluids may be of benefit.

Eliminating

Ensure that the patient has ready access to a bedpan, commode or toilet, and that assistance is given where necessary.

Mobilising

Research has shown that bedfast or immobile patients have a greater tendency to suffer from constipation.

Expressing sexuality

This can be an embarrassing and distasteful practice for the patient, so maximum privacy must be given, together with a clear explanation of the necessity for the practice.

Patient education: key points

If the enema is administered to treat constipation, a planned programme of increased dietary fibre, fluids and exercise should be explained to the patient to help relieve the problem. A self-completed bowel chart may be helpful in resolving the problem of constipation.

Tell the patient how long the enema requires to be retained for maximum effectiveness.

It may be appropriate to teach the patient to administer an enema to himself.

Further reading

Brown M, Everett I 1990 Gentler bowel fitness with fibre. Geriatric Nursing 1: 26–27
Chertow G, Brady H 1994 Hyponatraemia from tap water enema. Lancet 344(8924): 748
Clarke B 1989 Bowel preparation for operative procedures. Nursing Times 85(5): 46–47
Laming E 1994 A preventable problem. Journal of Community Nursing 8(7): 28–35
Lawler J 1991 Behind the screens. Churchill Livingstone, Edinburgh
Roper N, Logan W, Tierney A 1996 The elements of nursing, 4th edn. Churchill Livingstone, Edinburgh
Royle J, Walsh M 1992 Watson's Medical-surgical nursing. Bailliere Tindall, London, ch 16
Sadler C 1989 Elderly people with constipation. Nursing Times 3(44): 33
White T 1995 Dealing with constipation. Nursing Times 91(14): 57

19 Exercises: Active and Passive

Learning outcomes

By the end of this section you should know how to:
- prepare the patient for this nursing practice
- carry out active and passive exercises.

Background knowledge required

Revision of the anatomy and physiology of the musculoskeletal system.

Indications and rationale for active and passive exercises

Active and passive exercises (Fig. 19.1) are muscle and joint movements carried out *to assist circulation, maintain muscle tone and prevent the development of joint contracture*. These exercises can be performed by the patient (active) or by the nurse/carer helping the patient (passive) and are indicated:
- following an anaesthetic and surgery
- during reduced mobility such as bedrest
- during prolonged inactivity due to the effects of disease or trauma.

Guidelines and rationale for this nursing practice

These guidelines could be used by the nurse to teach a patient's carer(s) to become involved in this practice.
- explain the nursing practice to the patient *to gain consent and cooperation*
- ensure the patient's privacy *to reduce anxiety and/or embarrassment*
- observe the patient throughout this activity *to note any signs of distress or discomfort*
- wash the hands *to reduce the risk of cross-infection*
- help the patient into a comfortable position. The patient's position may require to be altered during the nursing practice *to permit easy comfortable access to each limb during the exercise programme*
- assist the patient to move the cervical spine and trunk through their normal range of movement *preventing damage and strain to any joint or muscle*
- taking each limb separately, assist the patient to move all the joints of the limb through their normal range of movement *allowing the patient and nurse to concentrate fully on the limb's movement, thus preventing damage to any tissue*
- ensure that the patient is left feeling as comfortable as possible *to ensure quality of patient care*
- document the nursing practice appropriately, monitor after-effects and report abnormal findings immediately *providing a written record and assisting in the implementation of any action should an abnormality or adverse reaction to the practice be noted.*

Figure 19.1
Passive (assisted) exercises for the bedfast patient (Reproduced with permission from Roper N, Logan W, Tierney A 1985 The elements of nursing, 2nd edn. Churchill Livingstone, Edinburgh)

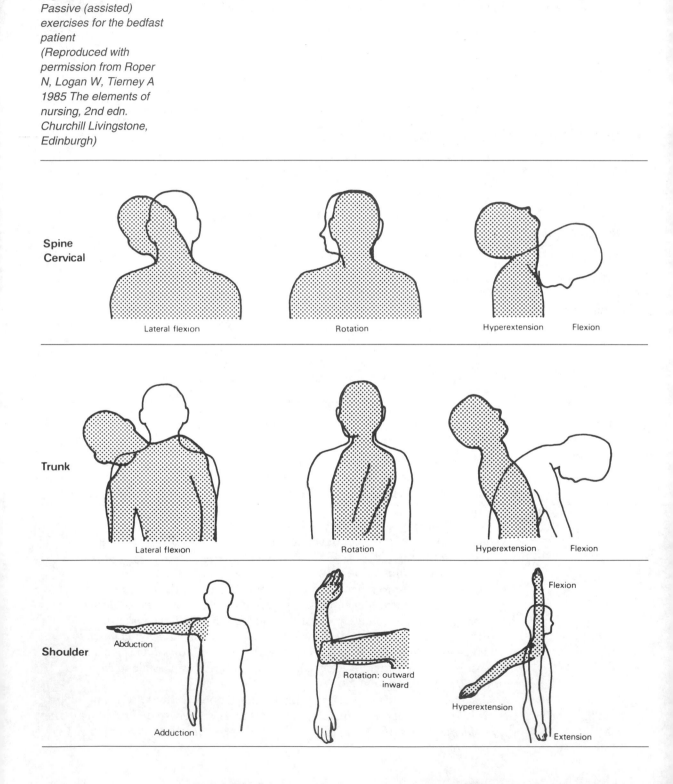

Spine Cervical

Lateral flexion   Rotation   Hyperextension   Flexion

Trunk

Lateral flexion   Rotation   Hyperextension   Flexion

Shoulder

Abduction

Adduction

Rotation: outward
inward

Flexion

Hyperextension

Extension

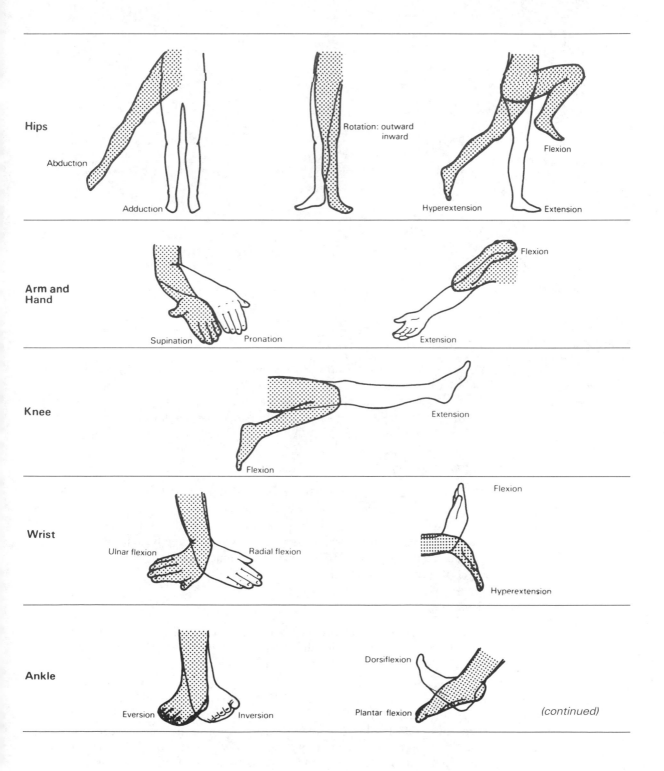

(continued)

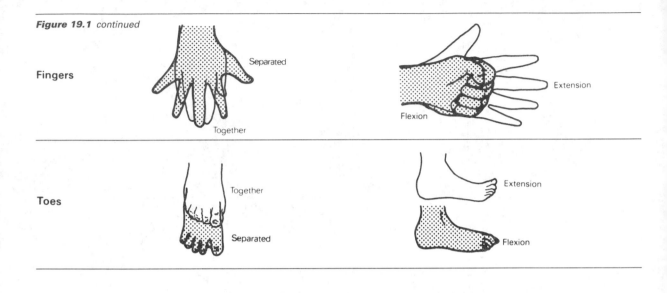

Figure 19.1 continued

Fingers

Separated

Extension

Flexion

Together

Toes

Together

Separated

Extension

Flexion

Relevance to the activities of living

Maintaining a safe environment

To prevent cross-infection the nurse should wash her hands before commencing and on completion of the nursing practice. The patient should not suffer any discomfort when regularly performing active or passive exercises unless there is an underlying disease such as rheumatoid arthritis or a developing complication such as deep vein thrombosis.

Communicating

The nurse should give to the patient an easily understood explanation of the importance of performing the active and/or passive exercises. When appropriate, the nurse should help to teach the patient to perform the exercises independently. Relatives or informal carers could be involved in the implementation of a regular exercise programme which can result in psychological benefits to all.

Breathing

Active and passive exercises have the benefit of increasing the patient's depth and rate of respiration, which may help to prevent the development of a chest infection during his period of reduced mobility.

The exercises can assist venous circulation, preventing venous stasis which can cause deep vein thrombosis (Jones 1992). Pulmonary embolism is a serious complication, occasionally fatal, following the development of a deep vein thrombosis (DVT), therefore the exercise pattern should be performed regularly. The benefit of exercise in the prevention of DVT may also be enhanced by the use of anti-embolic stockings and/or administration of subcutaneous heparin (Drinkwater 1989, Rodgers 1994).

Mobilising

In institutional settings, assisting the patient with active and passive exercises is usually the dual responsibility of the physiotherapist and the nurse; at home, the carer may be responsible for the implementation of the exercise programme.

Exercise helps to maintain muscle tone and movement so that when the patient's normal range of mobility can be resumed no joint stiffness or muscle weakness will hinder mobilisation (Jamieson & McFarlane 1994). Joints or muscle tissue should never be forced through any movement, as this could cause injury, with a resultant effect on the range of mobility.

When the nurse performs passive exercises, the joints and muscles not being exercised must be well supported otherwise injury will occur.

Exercising a paralysed limb may help to prevent joint and/or muscle contracture which would interfere with the patient's limited mobility and create a problem in positioning the limb.

Patient education: key points

Discuss with the patient and relatives the necessity and benefit of implementing this practice on a regular basis.

Should an abnormality or adverse reaction be noted, inform the patient of the action taken and any subsequent treatment.

References

Drinkwater K 1989 Management of deep vein thrombosis. Surgical Nurse 2(1): 24–26
Jamieson L, McFarlane C 1994 The musculoskeletal system. In: Alexander M, Fawcett J, Runciman P (eds) Nursing practice — hospital and home: the adult. Churchill Livingstone, Edinburgh
Jones D 1992 Caring for the patient undergoing surgery. In: Royle J, Walsh M (eds) Watson's Medical-surgical nursing and related physiology, 4th edn. Bailliere Tindall, London
Rodgers S 1994 The patient facing surgery. In: Alexander M, Fawcett J, Runciman P (eds) Nursing practice — hospital and home: the adult. Churchill Livingstone, Edinburgh

Further reading

Love C 1990 Deep vein thrombosis.
1. Threat to recovery. Nursing Times 86(5): 40–43
2. Methods of prevention. Nursing Times 86(6): 52–55
Roper N, Logan W, Tierney A 1996 The elements of nursing, 4th edn. Churchill Livingstone, Edinburgh

20 Eye Care

There are four parts to this section:

1 Eye swabbing
2 Eye irrigation
3 Instillation of eyedrops
4 Instillation of eye ointment

The concluding subsection, 'Relevance to the activities of living' refers to the four practices collectively.

Learning outcomes

By the end of this section you should know how to:

- prepare the patient for these four nursing practices
- collect and prepare the equipment
- carry out eye swabbing, eye irrigation, instillation of eyedrops and instillation of eye ointment.

Background knowledge required

Revision of the anatomy and physiology of the eye.
Revision of Administration of medicines (*see* p. 1) and Aseptic technique (*see* p. 383).

1 Eye swabbing

Indications and rationale for eye swabbing

- *to soothe the eye when a patient is suffering from an insensitive or diseased eye*
- *to precede the instillation of an eyedrop or the application of an eye ointment*
- *to remove eye discharge and/or crusts.*

Equipment

Sterile eye dressings pack containing a gallipot, small cotton wool balls and a disposable towel

Sterile swabbing solution, e.g. normal saline solution, to soften any crusted discharge

Good light source

Trolley or tray for equipment

Receptacle for soiled disposables.

Guidelines and rationale for this nursing practice

- explain the practice to the patient *to gain consent and cooperation*
- wash the hands *to reduce cross-infection* (Horton 1995)
- collect and prepare the equipment *to ensure that all equipment is available and ready for use*
- ensure the patient's privacy *to reduce anxiety*
- prepare the patient by helping him into a comfortable position either lying down or seated with his head inclined backwards *to allow the patient to maintain the position during the practice and permit easy access to the patient's eyes*
- observe the patient throughout this activity *to note any signs of distress*
- position the light source *to allow maximum observation of the patient's eyes without the beam shining directly into his eyes*
- open and arrange the equipment *in preparation for the practice*
- wash and dry the hands *to reduce the risk of cross-infection* (Horton 1995)
- place the disposable towel around the patient's neck *to catch any spillages and protect the patient's clothing*
- lightly moisten a cotton wool swab in the prescribed solution. *Excess moisture will cause the patient's face to be soaked with the cleansing solution*
- gently swab from the inner canthus to the outer canthus of the eye using each swab only once. *This decreases the risk of cross-infection of one eye to the other or infection of the lacrimal punctum (if both eyes are being swabbed, the healthy eye should be treated first as this again reduces the risk of cross-infection)*
- gently dry the patient's eyelids *to remove excess moisture*
- ensure that the patient is left feeling as comfortable as possible *maintaining the quality of this nursing practice*
- dispose of the equipment safely *to reduce any health hazard*
- document the nursing practice appropriately, monitor after-effects and report any abnormal findings immediately *providing a written record and assisting in the implementation of any action should an abnormality or adverse reaction to the practice be noted.*

2   Eye irrigation

Indications and rationale for eye irrigation

Irrigation involves the continuous washing of the eye surface with fluid:

- *to aid removal of a corrosive substance from the eye.*

Equipment

Waterproof sheet

Cotton towel

Sterile eye dressings pack containing a gallipot, small cotton wool balls and a disposable towel

Irrigation fluid, e.g. sterile water, sterile normal saline or universal buffer solution

Lotion thermometer

Irrigating utensil, e.g. undine or intravenous giving set

Receiver for the irrigating fluid

Trolley or adequate surface for equipment

Receptacle for soiled disposables.

Guidelines and rationale for this nursing practice	<ul><li>explain the nursing practice to the patient *to gain consent and cooperation*</li><li>wash the hands *to reduce cross-infection* (Horton 1995)</li><li>collect and prepare the equipment *to ensure that all equipment is available and ready for use*</li><li>ensure the patient's privacy *to reduce anxiety*</li><li>observe the patient throughout this activity *to note any signs of distress*</li><li>warm the irrigating fluid to 37.8°C *ensuring comfort of the patient when the irrigating fluid is applied*</li><li>help the patient into a suitable position either sitting or lying with his head and neck well supported *to allow the patient to maintain the position throughout the practice and permit easy access to the eyes*</li><li>apply the waterproof sheet and towel around the patient's neck *to absorb any spillage*</li><li>help the patient to turn his head to the side of the affected eye *to prevent any (or further) damage to the other eye by the corrosive substance when irrigation is commenced*</li><li>wash and dry the hands *to reduce cross-infection* (Horton 1995)</li><li>position the receiver below the affected eye against the patient's cheek *to collect the used irrigating fluid*</li><li>remove any discharge from the eye with a cotton wool ball *to prevent contamination of the eye when the irrigation commences*</li><li>explain to the patient that the flow of fluid is about to begin *permitting the patient to prepare for the introduction of the fluid*</li><li>hold the eyelids apart with the first and second fingers *as the natural defence mechanism of closing the eyes when an object closely approaches would interfere with the practice*</li><li>direct the flow from the irrigator onto the patient's cheek *to check that the temperature is comfortable for the patient*</li><li>hold the irrigator at a height 2.5 cm above the eye *to allow easy direction of the flow of fluid over the eye and prevent further damage to the eye*</li><li>direct a steady flow of irrigating fluid from the inner canthus to the outer canthus of the eye *allowing the fluid to cover the whole of the eye surface*</li><li>ask the patient to move his eye up, down and all around *to ensure the whole eye is irrigated*</li><li>remove the equipment from the patient and ensure that the patient is left feeling as comfortable as possible *maintaining the quality of this practice*</li><li>dispose of the equipment safely *to reduce any health hazard*</li><li>document the nursing practice appropriately, monitor after-effects and report any abnormal findings immediately *providing a written record and assisting in the implementation of any action should an abnormality or adverse reaction to the practice be noted.*</li></ul>

3   Instillation of eyedrops

Indications and rationale for instillation of eyedrops

Instillation involves the introduction of a liquid into a cavity drop by drop. In certain disease conditions and following injury eyedrops are prescribed:

- *to apply topically a local anaesthetic prior to diagnostic investigations, e.g. tonometry, removal of a foreign body or minor surgery*
- *to apply topically an antibiotic or anti-inflammatory medicine*
- *to apply topically a muscle constrictor or dilator to the eye*
- *to apply topically an artificial lubricant for the eye.*

Equipment

Sterile eye dressings pack containing a gallipot, small cotton wool balls and a disposable towel
Sterile solution for swabbing

} institutional settings

Eyedrops to be administered

Automatic dropper for self administration

Light source

Trolley or tray for equipment

Receptacle for soiled disposables.

Guidelines and rationale for this nursing practice

- explain the nursing practice to the patient *to gain consent and cooperation*
- wash the hands *to reduce cross-infection* (Horton 1995)
- collect and prepare the equipment *to ensure that all equipment is available and ready for use*
- ensure the patient's privacy *to reduce anxiety*
- observe the patient throughout this activity *to note any signs of distress*
- help the patient into a comfortable position *to allow easy access to the patient's eye and permit the patient to maintain the position throughout the practice*
- position the light source *giving good visualisation of the eye*
- check the medicine prescription with the eyedrops label *to ensure the correct medication will be administered*
- check the expiry date of the bottle of drops *ensuring administration of stable medication*
- verify which eye should receive the drops *to ensure the correct eye receives the medication*
- wash and dry the hands *to reduce cross-infection* (Horton 1995)
- swab the eye clean if a discharge is present *to remove contaminated debris*
- hold a swab in the non-dominant hand under the lower lid margin *to remove excess moisture after the drop instillation*
- ask the patient to look up and evert the lower lid *preventing the patient being aware of the approaching dropper*
- hold the dropper in the dominant hand *to provide controlled application*, about 2 cm above the eye, and allow one drop to fall into the lower conjunctival sac (Fig. 20.1)

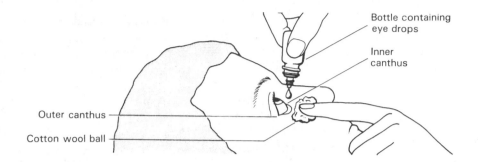

Figure 20.1 *Instillation of eyedrops: the lower lid is pulled gently downwards to create a pouch into which the drop is placed*

- ask the patient to close his eye *to remove axcess moisture*
- ensure that the patient is left feeling as comfortable as possible *maintaining the quality of this practice*
- dispose of the equipment safely *to reduce any health hazard*
- document the nursing practice appropriately, monitor after-effects and report any abnormal findings immediately *providing a written record and assisting in the implementation of any action should an abnormality or adverse reaction to the practice be noted.*

4   Instillation of eye ointment

Indications and rationale for instillation of eye ointment

In certain disease conditions, and following injury, eye ointment is prescribed:

- *to instil a medicine topically in place of eyedrops when a prolonged action of the medicine is required*
- *to form a protective film over the corneal surface of an eye*
- *to act as a soothing agent for the patient suffering from an inflamed eye or lid margin.*

Equipment

Sterile eye dressings pack containing a gallipot, small cotton wool balls and a disposable towel

Sterile solution for swabbing

} institutional setting

Eye ointment to be administered

Trolley or tray for equipment

Light source

Receptacle for soiled disposables.

Guidelines and rationale for this nursing practice

- explain the nursing practice to the patient *to gain consent and cooperation*
- wash the hands *to reduce cross-infection* (Horton 1995)
- collect and prepare the equipment *to ensure that all equipment is available and ready for use*
- ensure the patient's privacy *to reduce anxiety*
- observe the patient throughout this activity *to note any signs of distress*

- help the patient into a comfortable position *to allow easy access to the patient's eye and permit the patient to maintain the position throughout the practice*
- position the light source *giving good visualisation of the eye*
- check the medicine prescription with the label on the tube of eye ointment *to ensure the correct medication will be administered*
- check the expiry date of the tube of ointment *to ensure administration of stable medication*
- verify which eye should receive the ointment *ensuring the ointment is inserted into the correct eye*
- wash and dry the hands *to reduce cross-infection* (Horton 1995)
- swab the eye clean *to remove all traces of the previously instilled ointment and/or discharge*
- hold a swab in the non-dominant hand under the lower lid margin *to remove excess ointment after instillation*
- ask the patient to look up and evert the lower lid *to prevent the patient seeing the approaching nozzle which may cause the eyelid to close*
- hold the tube of ointment in the dominant hand *to permit good control of the insertion of the ointment*
- with the nozzle of the tube 2.5 cm above the lower lid, squeeze the tube *to allow a ribbon of ointment to run into the lower conjunctival sac from the inner canthus to the outer canthus* (Fig. 20.2)
- ask the patient to close his eye *to remove excess ointment*
- inform the patient that he may experience blurred vision for a few minutes following the instillation of the ointment *until the oily/greasy base disperses over the eye*
- ensure that the patient is left feeling as comfortable as possible *maintaining the quality of this practice*
- dispose of the equipment safely *to reduce any health hazard*
- document the nursing practice appropriately, monitor after-effects and report any abnormal findings immediately *providing a written record and assisting in the implementation of any action should an abnormality or adverse reaction to the practice be noted.*

Relevance to the activities of living

Maintaining a safe environment

To reduce the potential risk of cross-infection when caring for a patient's eye,

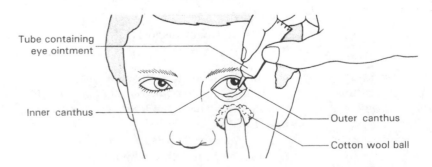

Figure 20.2 *Instillation of eye ointment: the lower lid is pulled gently downwards to create a pouch into which the ointment is placed*

the nurse must wash her hands thoroughly (Horton 1995). Only swab the eyes if debris/discharge is present; to reduce cross-infection swab the cleaner eye first from the inner canthus to the outer canthus. Use sterile swabbing solutions where possible or, at home, boiled cooled water; in an emergency, tap water may be used. To reduce the risk of cross-infection multiple-dose containers of eye medication should be changed regularly and each patient should have eyedrops or a tube of ointment reserved for his use alone (Heywood-Jones 1994).

When an eyedrop or ointment is to be instilled, care must be taken not to touch the eye surface with the applicator as this could cause injury to the eye and contamination of the applicator (Gardner & Studley 1994). If an eyedrop and eye ointment are to be instilled at the same time, the eyedrop should be instilled first. The greasy/oily base of an ointment once applied would prevent the absorption of the medicine within the eyedrop. The nurse is responsible for instilling the correct medicine into the correct eye. Any discrepancy must be reported immediately.

If the patient's vision is impaired, the nurse should assist the patient in maintaining a safe environment during his stay in hospital, and help to identify problems which may occur at home.

Should a patient need to continue eye medication following discharge, the nurse will assess and teach him or a relative to become competent in the practice. Self administration of eyedrops can be assisted with the use of an automatic dropper which clips onto the bottle of eyedrop solution (Heywood-Jones 1994).

Communicating

The nurse should explain the procedure simply to the patient and inform him of her intended actions. When an emergency eye irrigation is to be performed the nurse must be quick and precise with the explanation, so that the time the corrosive substance remains in the patient's eye is minimised. When a patient is extremely anxious or in severe pain the medical practitioner may prescribe local anaesthetic drops.

Should a patient complain of skin irritation, pain or a burning sensation following instillation of an eye medication this should be reported as it may indicate a drug allergy. Following the instillation of an eye ointment the nurse must warn the patient that his vision will be blurred for 5–6 minutes due to the greasy/oily base of the ointment.

As a result of the injury, disease or the effect of the topical medicine, the patient's previous range of vision may be temporarily or permanently impaired. The nurse will need to assist the patient to adapt to this change.

When a patient wears spectacles the nurse should assist the patient in the application and care of the spectacles according to his wishes.

Expressing sexuality

The visual appearance of some eye diseases or the effect of trauma to the eye may lead a patient to develop a negative body image, with resultant effects on his self esteem. He should be helped to come to terms with this altered body image, whether short-lived or permanent.

If vision in both eyes is suddenly impaired for any reason, many other Activities of Living will be affected and the patient will require help to adapt to this sudden loss of independence.

Patient education: key points

The patient/carer may require to be taught one or all parts of this nursing practice.

The nurse should ensure that the patient at home maintains safe and correct storage conditions of the medication.

A patient who requires to use the automatic dropper will need adequate information and practice to ensure skilled use of the equipment.

The nurse has a responsibility to provide and encourage education of the general population in the first aid measures needed following contamination of the eye by a corrosive substance.

References

Gardner R, Studley M 1994 Disorders of the eye. In: Alexander M, Fawcett J, Runciman P (eds) Nursing practice — hospital and home: the adult. Churcill Livingstone, Edinburgh
Heywood-Jones I 1994 Eye care. Community Outlook 4(1): 18–19
Horton R 1995 Handwashing: the fundamental infection control principle. British Journal of Nursing 4(16): 926–933

Further reading

Bocking H, Sercombe A, Kenny M et al 1990 Making sense of artificial eyes. Nursing Times 86(18): 40–41
Brooks J 1989 The red eye.
1. Practice Nurse 2(2): 73–75
2. Practice Nurse 2(5): 226–230
Josse E 1984 Corneal abscess from soft contact lenses. Nursing Times Journal of Infection Control Nursing 80(37): 3–4
Kelly J 1994 Nursing intervention in the treatment of cataracts. British Journal of Nursing 3(12): 602–606
Lloyd F 1990 Making sense of eye care. Nursing Times 86(1): 36–37
Murdoch A 1994 The unconscious patient. In: Alexander M, Fawcett J, Runciman P (eds) Nursing practice — hospital and home: the adult. Churchill Livingstone, Edinburgh, p 853
Roper N, Logan W, Tierney A 1996 The elements of nursing, 4th edn. Churchill Livingstone, Edinburgh, p 117
Smith J 1983 Ophthalmic problems in general nursing. Nursing 2(17): 507–508
Smith S 1987 Drugs and the eye. Nursing Times 83(25): 48–50
West G 1995 Picking up glaucoma. Community Nurse 1(4): 13–14

21 Gastric Aspiration

Learning outcomes

By the end of this section you should know how to:

- prepare the patient for this nursing practice
- collect and prepare the equipment
- pass a nasogastric tube
- aspirate the stomach contents.

Background knowledge required

Revision of the anatomy and physiology of the nose, pharynx, oesophagus and stomach.

Indications and rationale for gastric aspiration

Gastric aspiration is used *to keep the stomach empty of contents* by passing a tube into it and applying some form of suction. It is usually performed in the following circumstances:

- *obstruction of the bowel*
- *paralytic ileus*
- *preoperatively for gastric or some abdominal surgery, e.g. perforated gastric ulcer, oesophageal and gastric varices*
- *postoperatively, e.g. partial gastrectomy, cholecystectomy.*

Equipment

Trolley

Disposable gloves

Protective covering for the patient

Denture dish

Equipment for cleaning nostrils, if required

Nasogastric tube

Lubricant, e.g. iced water, water-soluble jelly

Catheter-tipped syringe

Litmus paper

Receiver for aspirated fluid

Receptacle for soiled disposables

Hypoallergenic tape

Stethoscope

Suction pump.

The size of tube selected depends on the size and age of the patient. The most commonly used sizes for the average adult are 14 and 16 FG

Guidelines and rationale for this nursing practice

- explain the nursing practice to the patient *to gain consent and cooperation. Patients should be encouraged to be active partners in care*
- collect and prepare the equipment *for efficiency of practice*
- ensure the patient's privacy *to maintain dignity and sense of 'self'*
- help the patient into as comfortable and relaxed a position as possible, sitting upright either in bed or on a chair *for ease of insertion of the tube*
- observe the patient throughout this activity *to detect any signs of discomfort or distress*
- measure approximately the distance from the patient's nose to stomach and mark it on the nasogastric tube *so that you will have an indication of when the tube is in the region of the stomach*
- put on gloves
- remove the patient's dentures, if present, and place in a labelled container
- ask the patient to blow the nose and sniff each nostril in turn, or clean the nostrils if necessary *to facilitate the passage of the tube*
- ascertain if the patient has any nasal defect or tenderness and change to the other nostril if the first nostril appears blocked. *Do not use great force as this may damage the nasal mucosa*
- ask the patient to relax as much as possible while the tube is being passed. *This eases the passing of the tube.*
- insert the tube and slide it gently but firmly inwards and backwards along the floor of the nose to the nasopharynx
- encourage the patient to swallow and breathe through his mouth when the tube reaches the pharynx, keeping the chin down and the head forward in order to assist the passage of the tube. *This is to try and overcome the gagging reflex which is present in the pharynx. Swallowing helps the tube to pass down by peristalsis*
- when the tube has reached the measured distance, carry out a test to confirm that it is in the stomach (see below)
- secure the tube with tape when there is confirmation that it is in the stomach (Fig. 21.1)
- aspirate the stomach contents. Either continuous or intermittent aspiration will be ordered by the medical practitioner
- ensure that the patient is left feeling as comfortable as possible *to maintain the quality of this practice*
- dispose of the equipment safely *for the protection of others*
- document this nursing practice appropriately, monitor after-effects and report abnormal findings immediately *to provide a written record and assist in the implementation of any action should an abnormality or adverse reaction to the procedure be noted*

The recommended test to confirm the presence of the tube in the stomach is to aspirate some of the stomach contents using a catheter-tipped syringe and test them for acidity with litmus paper. If the aspirate is from the stomach the acidity

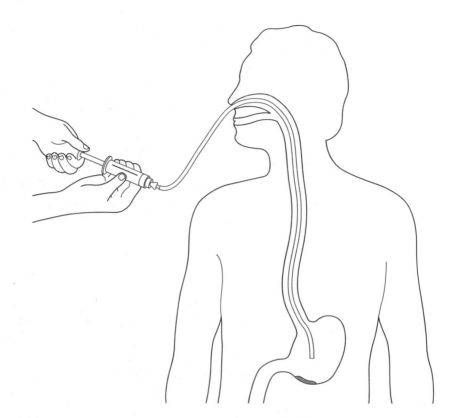

Figure 21.1 *Gastric aspiration: position of the nasogastric tube and the syringe attached to aspirate gastric contents*

will turn blue litmus paper pink. If it is not possible to aspirate sufficient stomach contents for testing, some air can be blown into the stomach through the syringe, while a second nurse listens with a stethoscope for the noise of the bubbles of air entering the stomach.

Continuous aspiration can be carried out by some form of pump; the recommended suction pressure is 20–25 mmHg. Lower pressure is ineffective and greater pressure can damage the lining of the stomach. Sometimes, usually postoperatively, a drainage bag and tubing may be attached to the end of the nasogastric tube. If the drainage bag is placed lower than the patient's stomach, the stomach contents will siphon into the bag.

Intermittent aspiration can be performed by pump or catheter-tipped syringe. Between aspirations, a clean spigot should be inserted in the end of the tube.

Relevance to the activities of living

Maintaining a safe environment

Although aseptic technique is not required, all the equipment should be clean or disposable and the nurse should wash her hands before commencing and on completion of this practice. Disposable gloves should be worn for the nurse's protection.

In order to prevent damage to the relevant respiratory and alimentary mucosa it is the nurse's duty to ensure that the tube is in the correct position and that the correct pressure of suction is applied.

Communicating

Communication, especially verbal, may be restricted. A pad of paper and pen may be helpful to the patient.

Breathing

The presence of a nasogastric tube may affect the rate and quality of respiration. It may also cause dryness and irritation in the patient's nose; a lubricant at, and just beyond, the nasal orifice may reduce discomfort.

Mouth breathing often occurs because of the size of the tube, so oral hygiene should be maintained.

Eating and drinking

When nasogastric aspiration is in progress the patient will not be permitted any solid food by mouth, but restricted fluids may be allowed.

Personal cleansing and dressing

The presence of the tube may predispose to dry mucous membranes in the nose and mouth, so frequent oral and nasal hygiene will be necessary.

Mobilising

Mobility may be limited because of the presence of the nasogastric tube and possible connection to suction apparatus.

Expressing sexuality

When a nasogastric tube is in position, the patient may be concerned about his appearance; if it remains in position for a length of time body image may be affected.

Sleeping

Sleep may be affected by the presence of the tube. The patient's sleeping pattern may also be interrupted if intermittent suction is being performed.

Patient education: key points

It will help the patient cope with the discomfort of the tube if the reason for it is explained.

The importance of not interfering with the tube should be explained to the patient, but if pain or extreme discomfort is experienced, he should tell someone.

It should also be explained that because the patient is unable to eat or drink he may experience a dry mouth, but that staff will help by giving mouthwashes, ice to suck, etc.

Further reading

Creach T 1988 Nasogastric warnings. Nursing Times 84(7): 46–47
Eaves D 1988 Making sense of gastric lavage. Nursing Times 84(20): 52–53
Price B 1989 Making sense of nasogastric intubation. Nursing Times 85(13): 50–52
Royle J, Walsh M 1992 Watson's Medical-surgical nursing. Bailliere Tindall, London

22 Gastric Lavage

Learning outcomes

By the end of this section you should know how to:
- prepare the patient for this procedure
- collect and prepare the equipment
- assist with the procedure of gastric lavage

Background knowledge required

Revision of the anatomy and physiology of the upper alimentary tract.

Review of health authority policy on gastric lavage.

Indications and rationale for gastric lavage

Gastric lavage involves introducing a wide-bore tube into the stomach and washing out the contents by pouring in and siphoning off a prescribed solution. It is sometimes necessary:
- *to obtain a specimen of gastric contents*
- *to remove harmful substances swallowed accidentally or deliberately*

There are various schools of thought about the efficacy of gastric lavage; advice on its use is conflicting following the results of research by Stoddart (1975), Goth & Vesell (1984) and others.

Outline of the procedure

Health authority policies vary on who is qualified to perform a gastric lavage. As a general rule, medical practitioners carry it out on unconscious patients, and specially trained nursing staff in accident and emergency units can carry it out on conscious patients.

The tube will be passed through the patient's mouth; if he is conscious he will be asked to swallow it. Once the marked length on the tube has been reached, one of the tests to check that the tube is in the stomach, described in the section on Gastric aspiration, will be performed (*see* pp. 144–145). Some of the stomach contents may then be aspirated to obtain specimens for analysis. The tubing and funnel are attached to the stomach tube and 150–300 ml of solution are poured into the stomach. If the stomach is overfilled some of the contents may be forced through the pylorus. The funnel is then lowered and the gastric contents siphoned into the bucket. The lavage will be repeated until the return flow is relatively clear. The tube is pinched when it is being withdrawn to maintain suction and prevent stimulation of the vomiting reflex.

Equipment	As for Gastric aspiration (*see* p. 143), but the tube should have a much larger lumen (e.g. 30 gauge Jacques stomach tube)

and

Apron

Funnel and connecting tubing

Bucket for aspirate

Tap water or prescribed solution at body temperature

Sterile containers appropriately labelled for specimens of aspirate

Laboratory form

Plastic specimen bag for transportation

Airway

Lubricating gel.

Guidelines and rationale for this nursing practice

- collect and prepare the required equipment *for efficiency of practice*
- explain the procedure to the patient if possible *to gain consent and cooperation*
- ensure the patient's privacy *to maintain dignity and sense of 'self'*
- remove dentures if appropriate and place in a labelled container
- insert an airway if it is usual practice. *This helps to prevent airway obstruction. On some occasions an anaesthetist will be standing by in case it is necessary to insert an endotracheal tube to maintain the patient's airway*
- measure the approximate distance between mouth and stomach and mark the tube. *This is helpful in indicating when the end of the tube has reached the stomach*
- help the patient into the position requested by the person passing the tube. Often the patient is requested to lie on his side
- observe the patient throughout this activity *to detect any signs of discomfort or distress*
- lubricate the end of the tube *to ease its passing down to the stomach*
- assist the person passing the tube as requested
- ensure the patient is left feeling as comfortable as possible *to maintain the quality of this practice*
- dispose of the equipment safely *for the safety of others*
- document this procedure appropriately, monitor after-effects, and report abnormal findings immediately *to provide a written record and assist in the implementation of any action should an abnormality or adverse reaction to the procedure be noted*
- dispatch labelled specimens and completed forms to the laboratory.

Relevance to the activities of living

Maintaining a safe environment

Although aseptic technique is not required all the equipment should be clean or disposable and the nurse should wash her hands before commencing and on completion of the procedure. Gloves should be worn.

The safety of the patient is a prime consideration; because of the obvious risks only a medical practitioner or a suitably qualified member of the nursing staff will carry out this procedure. If the patient is unconscious, a medical practitioner will carry out the procedure. For the safe transport of specimens see Specimen collection, page 297

Breathing

If the patient is unconscious a nasotracheal tube will be passed before the stomach tube to ensure the maintenance of a clear airway. The patient should be positioned in a way that will prevent aspiration of stomach contents.

Eating and drinking

The tube used for this procedure has a large lumen and cannot be left in position for a long period as it will cause tissue irritation and damage.

Sleeping

As mentioned already, this procedure may be carried out on an unconscious patient and so all reasonable precautions must be taken for the patient's safety. He should be placed in the recovery position and observed constantly. His vital signs should be monitored.

Patient education: key points	A clear explanation of the procedure and the reasons for performing it needs to be given to the patient to gain cooperation.

References

Goth A, Vesell 1984 Medical pharmacology: principles and concepts, 11 th edn. C V Mosby, St Louis
Stoddart J 1975 Intensive therapy. Blackwell Scientific Publications, Oxford

Further reading

Johnstone F 1987 Self poisoning. Nursing 3(16): 602–608

23 Hair Care

There are two parts to this section:

1 **Washing of the hair**
2 **Care of the infested head.**

The concluding subsection 'Relevance to the activities of living' refers to the two practices collectively.

Learning outcomes

By the end of this section you should know how to:

- prepare the patient for these nursing practices
- collect and prepare the equipment
- carry out washing of the hair and care of the infested head.

Background knowledge required

Revision of the anatomy and physiology of the skin with special reference to the hair follicles of the scalp.

Revision of the life cycle of the head louse (*Pediculus capitis*).

Review of the health authority policy on the use and type of insecticide.

1 Washing of the hair

Indications and rationale for washing of the hair

The hair covers the skin of the scalp, therefore sweat, sebum, dust and dead epithelial cells become trapped between the hair strands. The patient's hair, if left unwashed, may appear greasy and limp, and generally makes him feel unkempt. The patient may be unable to maintain his hair hygiene due to the effect of disease or injury or following surgery, or because of age (either a young child or a frail elderly person). The hair may therefore need to be washed:

- to maintain hygiene
- to improve the patient's self esteem.

Equipment

Basin

Large container of warm water ⎫

Container for used water ⎬ for a bedfast patient

Small jug or hair spray tap attachment ⎭

Cotton towels

Polythene sheeting

Patient's shampoo

Patient's own comb and/or brush

Disposable paper towel

Disposable plastic apron

Hair dryer

Trolley or adequate surface for equipment

Receptacle for soiled disposables.

Guidelines and rationale for this nursing practice

- explain the nursing practice to the patient *and gain consent and cooperation*
- collect and prepare the equipment *to ensure all equipment is available and ready for use*
- wash the hands *to reduce cross-infection*
- ensure the patient's privacy *to reduce anxiety*
- observe the patient throughout this activity *to note any signs of distress.*

Bedfast patient

- help the patient into a comfortable position, e.g. patient's head overhanging the edge of the bed, *to promote comfort and allow the patient to maintain the position during the practice*
- protect the patient's clothing, pillows and bedclothes using the polythene sheeting *to reduce water penetration*
- place a towel around the patient's shoulders *to absorb any water spillage*
- position the basin under the patient's head *to catch the water as it drains from the patient's head*
- protect the patient's eyes *preventing irritation from the shampoo*
- using the basin to catch the water, wet the hair and apply the shampoo *to commence washing the patient's hair*
- rinse off the lather *to remove the shampoo and leave the patient's hair clean.* Repeat if the patient wishes
- towel the hair dry *removing excess moisture*
- assist the patient to comb his hair into the usual style and dry using the hair dryer *to allow a positive body image to be reinstated*
- ensure that the patient is left feeling as comfortable as possible *confirming the quality of care delivered*
- dispose of the equipment safely *to reduce any health hazard*
- document the nursing appropriately, monitor after-effects and report abnormal findings immediately *providing a written record and assisting in the implementation of any action should an abnormality or adverse reaction to the practice be noted.*

Ambulant patient

- help the patient to the bathroom and ensure that he is sitting comfortably *to promote comfort and allow the patient to maintain the position during the practice*

- protect his clothing using the polythene sheeting *to reduce water penetration*
- drape a towel around his shoulders *to absorb any water spillage*
- protect the patient's eyes *preventing irritation from the shampoo*
- using the small jug or the hair spray tap attachment, wet the hair and apply the shampoo *to commence washing the patient's hair*
- rinse off the lather *to remove the shampoo and leave the patient's hair clean.* Repeat if the patient wishes
- towel the hair dry *removing excess moisture*
- assist the patient to comb his hair into his usual style and dry using the hair dryer *to allow a positive body image to be reinstated*
- ensure the patient is left feeling as *comfortable as possible, confirming the quality of care delivered*
- dispose of the equipment safely *to reduce any health hazard*
- document the nursing practice appropriately, monitor after-effects and report abnormal findings immediately *providing a written record and assisting in the implementation of any action should an abnormality or adverse reaction to the practice be noted.*

A patient can also have his hair washed during a shower or an immersion bath, using a hair spray tap attachment.

Patient education: key points	Emphasise the importance of adequate nutritional intake and daily grooming to maintain the health of the hair.
	Patients who are undergoing specialised treatment regimes involving the head and neck will require individualised information and education regarding care of their hair; for example, patients receiving radiotherapy to the scalp may not be permitted to wash their hair during and immediately following the course of treatment (Havard 1992).

2 Care of the infested head

Indications and rationale for care of the infested head	Scalp infestation is the parasitic infestation of the scalp by the head louse. The louse and its prelouse stage, the nit, cause irritation which may lead to scratching and potential infection of the abrasions. An insecticide is used:

- *to remove the parasite*
- *to prevent the infestation from spreading to family members, other patients and staff.*

Equipment	Insecticide can be used in shampoo or lotion form.

Medicated shampoo treatment

Shampoo containing phenothrin or permethrin

Disposable cap and gown

Fine-tooth comb

Equipment as for hair washing (*see* p. 153).

Medicated lotion treatment

Head lotion containing phenothrin or permethrin

Polythene sheeting

Disposable paper towel, cap and gown

Fine-tooth comb.

12 hours later, equipment for hair washing (*see* p. 153)

Trolley or tray for equipment

Receptacle for soiled disposables.

Guidelines and rationale for this nursing practice

- explain the nursing practice to the patient *to gain consent and cooperation*, and explain that you will wear a cap and gown *for your protection*
- collect and prepare the equipment *to ensure that the equipment is available and ready for use*
- wash the hands *to reduce cross-infection*
- apply a disposable cap and gown *for personal protection*
- ensure the patient's privacy *to reduce anxiety*
- observe the patient throughout this activity *to note any signs of distress*
- assist the patient into a comfortable position *to promote comfort and allow the patient to maintain the position during the practice.*

Medicated shampoo method

- follow the Guidelines for washing of the hair
- protect the patient's eyes *as the medication can be irritant to the eyes*
- use the medicated shampoo as recommended by the manufacturer. *Non-compliance may cause the medication to be ineffective*
- rinse the hair thoroughly *to remove all excess insecticide which could act as a skin irritant*
- comb the hair with the fine-tooth comb *to remove the nits and lice*, collecting them on a disposable paper towel with each stroke of the comb
- allow the patient's hair to dry *for the comfort and appearance of the patient*
- ensure the patient is left feeling as comfortable as possible *confirming the quality of care delivered*
- disinfect the patient's comb and/or hairbrush using the shampoo *to prevent re-infestation of the patient's hair*
- dispose of the equipment safely *to reduce any health hazard*
- remove the protective cap and gown and dispose of them safely *to prevent any cross-infestation*

- document the nursing practice appropriately, monitor after-effects and report abnormal findings immediately *providing a written record and assisting in the implementation of any action should an abnormality or adverse reaction to the practice be noted.*

Medicated head lotion method

- protect the patient's clothing using the polythene sheeting *to prevent staining by the medicated lotion*
- protect the patient's eyes *to prevent accidental spillage into the eyes*
- apply the head lotion as recommended by the manufacturer *to ensure effectiveness*, paying particular attention to the area above the ears and the nape of the neck *as the nits and lice tend to gather in these areas*
- leave the hair to dry naturally *as drying with a hair dryer could alter the effectiveness of the insecticide and cause a hazard*
- disinfect the patient's comb and/or hairbrush *to prevent re-infestation of the hair*
- 12 hours later, or as suggested by the manufacturer, wash the hair with a normal shampoo *to remove the insecticide*
- comb the hair with the fine-tooth comb *to remove the nits and lice*, collecting on a disposable paper towel with each stroke of the comb
- allow the patient's hair to dry naturally
- ensure the patient is left feeling as comfortable as possible *confirming the quality of care delivered*
- disinfect the fine-tooth comb with the head lotion *to prevent re-infestation of the hair*
- dispose of the equipment safely *to reduce any health hazard*
- remove the cap and gown and dispose of them safely *to prevent any cross-infestation*
- document the nursing practice appropriately, monitor after-effects and report abnormal findings immediately *providing a written record and assisting in the implementation of any action should an abnormality or adverse reaction to the practice be noted.*

Either of the two forms of treatment should be repeated as recommended by the manufacturer, and according to the success of the treatment.

Patient education: key points	The patient/carer/parents require to be given information and education regarding the care and future prevention of infestation of the head. At home, advice and information regarding the treatment of potentially infested bed linen should be given.
Relevance to the activities of living	### Maintaining a safe environment Although hair care does not require aseptic technique, all equipment should be clean or disposable and all precautions be taken to prevent cross-infection. The

nurse should wash her hands before commencing and on completion of hair care.

The nurse should test the temperature of the water prior to washing a patient's hair and be aware of any temperature change during the nursing practice, so that the patient's comfort is maintained. Protecting the patient's eyes reduces the potential problem of accidental introduction of shampoo or the medicated head lotion into the eyes; they would act as irritants to the eyes. Once the infestation is noted, treatment should start immediately as the condition spreads rapidly. Transmission of the louse is by direct physical contact or by contact with an infested comb, hairbrush, wig, hat or bedding. All family members and close contacts must be treated at the same time as the patient, otherwise re-infestation of the patient will occur. For her own safety, the nurse may wear a disposable cap and gown during the treatment of an infested scalp.

If left untreated, the sufferer may develop a variety of complications such as impetigo, dermatitis or undefined general malaise.

The louse can develop resistance to an insecticide. The insecticides suggested above are the two in common use at present, but advice from the pharmacy department should be sought about the current recommended insecticide. In the community the treatment regime is often the responsibility of the parent/carer with some input from the school nurse or community nurse. National guidelines in the treatment and use of insecticides for head lice are now available (Ibarra 1995a). Alternative methods of treatment without the use of insecticides are receiving positive recognition from children and parents (Ibarra 1995b).

Communicating

The patient with an infested scalp must be given a tactful, easily understood explanation about the reason for and the form of treatment. The patient's relatives and/or close contacts will also need to be informed about the infestation and given the necessary information about their own treatment. Some education of the patient and his family about the head louse may be necessary.

Personal cleansing and dressing

For normal hair cleanliness, the use of a dry shampoo can be of benefit to the patient who is unable to have his hair washed using shampoo and water. Wide-handled brushes or combs can assist the patient with hand grip or limited shoulder movement problems to remain independent in their hair care (Roper et al 1996).

A patient who experiences a chronic disease or a prolonged period of immobility will benefit both physically and psychologically from a visit by a hairdresser to cut and style their hair in hospital or at home.

As far as the infested head in concerned, the nits remain firmly attached to the hair even following insecticide treatment, therefore the fine-tooth comb must be used to remove them. The patient's hair should be left to dry naturally after insecticide application, as most of the lotions have an inflammable alcoholic base.

Expressing sexuality

A patient's hair should be kept in good condition as this helps to create a positive body image and maintain self esteem.

The nurse should style the patient's hair in the usual manner or as the patient wishes, as this helps to maintain his individuality.

Most people are embarrassed if it is discovered that the hair is infested with lice, and although the nurse should wear a disposable cap and gown while assisting the patient to remove the infestation, the explanation for doing so should be tactful and should not detract from the patient's dignity and self esteem.

References

Havard C 1992 Caring for the patient with cancer. In:Royle J, Walsh M(eds) Watson's Medical-surgical nursing and related physiology, 4th edn. Bailliere Tindall, London
Ibarra J 1995a A non-drug approach to treating head lice. Community Nurse 1(8): 25–27
Ibarra J 199b Commentary, originating data and references for the bug buster teaching pack. Community Hygiene Concern, London
Roper N, Logan W, Tierney A 1996 The elements of nursing, 4th edn. Churchill Livingstone, Edinburgh, pp 233, 236, 243

Further reading

Anonymous 1995 Bug buster teaching pack. Community Hygiene Concern, London (available from Community Hygiene Concern, 160 Inderwick Road, London N8 9JT, Tel: 0181 341 7167)
Cluroe S 1990 How to deal with head lice. Nursing 4(16): 9–12
Docherty C, Rose C 1994 Skin disorders. In: Alexander M, Fawcett J, Runciman P (eds) 1994 Nursing practice — hospital and home: the adult. Churchill Livingstone, Edinburgh
Roberts C 1989 Head lice. Practice Nurse 2(3): 108–111

24 Intrapleural Aspiration

Learning outcomes

By the end of this section you should know how to:
- prepare the patient for this nursing practice
- collect and prepare the equipment
- assist the medical practitioner during chest aspiration.

Background knowledge required

Revision of the anatomy and physiology of the respiratory system.
Revision of Aseptic technique (*see* p. 383).

Indications and rationale for aspirating the pleural cavity

The lungs are covered by the visceral pleura and the inner chest wall is lined by the parietal pleura. Between these pleura is a thin layer of serous fluid whose surface tension holds the two pleural linings together. As a result, the lung follows the movement of the chest wall, and lung volume is determined by the size of the thorax. An increase of fluid in the space upsets this mechanism. Chest aspiration involves the introduction of a needle into the pleural cavity between the visceral and parietal pleura. It may be performed for the following reasons:
- *to examine a specimen of the pleural fluid as an aid to the diagnosis of disease, e.g. tuberculosis, carcinoma*
- *to relieve dyspnoea, by removing excess pleural fluid*
- *to introduce medication, e.g. antibiotics, into the pleural cavity*

Outline of the procedure

Using aseptic technique, the medical practitioner washes and dries his hands, cleanses the patient's skin over the selected site of entry of the aspiration needle, injects a local anaesthetic and waits for it to take effect. He then inserts the aspiration needle into the cavity between the visceral and parietal layers of the pleura (Fig. 24.1). After withdrawing the stilette from the needle, specimens of fluid can be obtained from the cavity for laboratory investigation, and the remaining fluid may be allowed to drain out. If the fluid is purulent, it may have to be aspirated by attaching a large syringe to the needle. At the end of the procedure the aspirating needle is withdrawn, a sterile plastic spray applied to the wound puncture, and an adhesive dressing applied.

Equipment

Trolley
Sterile dressings pack
Sterile gloves

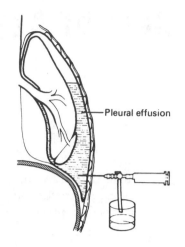

Pleural effusion

Figure 24.1 *Aspiration of pleural fluid (Reproduced with permission from Chilman A, Thomas M (eds) 1987 Understanding nursing care, 3rd edn. Churchill Livingstone, Edinburgh)*

Alcohol-based antiseptic for skin cleansing

Local anaesthetic, and equipment for its administration

50 ml sterile syringe

Sterile aspiration needles

Sterile two-way tap with length of sterile tubing

Sterile bowl for collecting fluid

Sterile specimen bottles, appropriately labelled laboratory form

Plastic specimen bag for transportation

Sterile plastic spray and adhesive dressing

Receptacle for soiled disposables.

Guidelines and rationale for this nursing practice

- help to explain the procedure to the patient, *ensuring that he has some understanding of the procedure, and obtain consent and cooperation*
- ensure the patient's privacy *to help maintain dignity and sense of 'self'*
- collect the equipment *for efficiency of practice*
- administer a sedative if prescribed by medical staff *to help relieve stress and anxiety in the patient*
- help the patient into a back-fastening gown *so that there is ease of access to the site for aspiration*
- assist the patient to sit up with arms extended over a bed table on which a pillow has been placed for the head to rest. If this is not comfortable for the patient, lying in bed on the unaffected side should still allow good access to the needle site. *The medical practitioner requires unobstructed access to the site of needle insertion*
- observe the patient throughout this activity *to detect any signs of discomfort or distress*
- open the sterile equipment as it is required by medical staff
- remain with the patient and help maintain the chosen position as required.

Continuing explanations and support will help the patient through this procedure

- observe the patient's respirations and attend to any complaints of pain during the procedure. *This may indicate that the needle has penetrated the pleura to the lung*
- ensure the patient is left feeling as comfortable as possible
- dispose of equipment safely *for the protection of others*
- dispatch the labelled specimen container in a plastic specimen bag immediately to the laboratory with the completed form. *Immediate dispatch ensures that the specimen arrives in optimal condition for the tests*
- document this nursing practice appropriately, monitor after-effects and report abnormal findings immediately *so that measures to overcome these can be instigated as soon as possible.*

Relevance to the activities of living

Maintaining a safe environment

This is an invasive procedure and all precautions for the prevention of infection must be taken. A meticulous technique should be used and thorough hand washing should be carried out using an antiseptic detergent and alcohol-based hand cleansing solution as appropriate.

For the safe transport of specimens *see* Specimen collection, page 297.

During and after this procedure there is some risk of a pneumothorax occurring, so the patient should be observed closely and a chest X-ray performed. A pneumothorax is collapse of the lung due to atmospheric air entering the pleural space and causing the loss of the normally negative intrathoracic pressure. The clinical features are chest pain, rapid respirations, and dyspnoea.

Breathing

By removing excess fluid from the pleural cavity and allowing the lungs to expand during inspiration, this procedure should help to relieve some of the patient's breathing problems and alleviate attendant pain.

Controlling body temperature

If infection is present in the pleural space the patient may have an elevated temperature. Tepid sponging may help to reduce the temperature to within normal range (*see* p. 319 for Tepid sponging).

Mobilising

Chest aspiration as such would not alter the patient's ability to mobilise, but rest is usually advised for 4–6 hours following the procedure.

Patient education: key points

A detailed explanation and step by step guidance through the procedure should help the patient to maintain cooperation.

If medication has been instilled into the cavity the patient should be helped to turn into different positions during the next couple of hours to facilitate its dispersal.

Further reading   Harvey J, Prescott R 1994 Simple aspiration vs intercostal tube drainage for spontaneous pneumothorax in patients with normal lungs British Medical Journal 309(6965): 1338–1339

25 Intravenous Therapy

There are four parts to this section:

1 **Commencing an intravenous infusion**
2 **Priming the equipment for intravenous infusion**
3 **Maintaining the infusion for a period of time**
4 **Care of a Hickman catheter for long-term intravenous therapy.**

The concluding subsection 'Relevance to the activities of living' refers to all four practices collectively.

Learning outcomes

By the end of this section you should know how to:

- prepare the patient for these nursing practices both at home and in an institutional setting
- collect and prepare the equipment
- assist the medical practitioner with the safe insertion of an intravenous cannula or catheter
- maintain an intravenous infusion as prescribed.

Background knowledge required

Revision of the anatomy and physiology of the cardiovascular system, with special reference to the circulation of the blood, and body fluids.

Revision of Aseptic technique (*see* p. 383).

Review of health authority policy in relation to intravenous therapy in both community and institutional care.

Indications and rationale for intravenous infusion

An intravenous infusion is the introduction of prescribed sterile fluid into the blood circulation; it may be indicated for the following reasons:

- *to maintain a normal fluid, nutrient and electrolyte balance when the patient is unable to maintain adequate intake by mouth, and nasogastric feeding is inappropriate,* e.g.:
  — a patient during the preoperative and postoperative period
  — a patient who has had surgery involving the alimentary system
  — a patient who has malabsorption problems
- *to replace severe fluid loss in emergency situations,* e.g.:
  — a patient who has severe haemorrhage and haemorrhagic shock
  — a patient who has severe burns or scalds
  — a patient dehydrated by vomiting or diarrhoea usually associated with enteric infection

- *to administer medication when other routes are not appropriate,* e.g.:
  — analgesic medication for effective pain relief
  — anticoagulant therapy for treatment of deep vein thrombosis
  — chemotherapy for treatment of patients with oncological problems.

1   Commencing an intravenous infusion

Outline of the procedure

Intravenous therapy is prescribed and initiated by the medical practitioner. The nurse may be required to help with the procedure, to maintain the infusion safely for a period of time, and to help with the removal of the cannula.

Using aseptic technique, the medical practitioner chooses a suitable vein site for access, the skin area being shaved as necessary and cleansed with antiseptic lotion. A local anaesthetic may be injected around the vein site if required. A sterile cannula is inserted into the vein so that the prescribed infusion fluid can enter the patient's blood circulation. The infusion fluid flows into the cannula through an administration set which will have been primed ready for use. The cannula is secured in position and covered by a sterile dressing. The flow of infusion fluid is maintained, and the containers of fluid replaced as prescribed, until the intravenous infusion is discontinued (Lamb 1995).

Sites chosen for intravenous cannulation

Short-term intravenous therapy   The veins at the back of the hand or the superficial veins of the wrist or lower arm are chosen for short-term infusions expected to last hours or a few days. Cannulation increases the risk of venous thrombosis in the veins used for access; if this occurs in the smaller branches of peripheral veins following an infusion, it is still possible to use the larger branches of the same vein at a later date if required. Veins of the lower limbs are rarely used because of the increased risk of thrombosis, due to a slower venous flow. The non-dominant limb should be used if possible to minimise the patient's discomfort.

Long-term intravenous therapy   For long-term intravenous infusions lasting several days or weeks, a long catheter is inserted into the subclavian vein or the internal jugular vein so that the tip of the catheter lies in the superior vena cava (see Hickman catheter, p. 175; Central venous pressure, p. 103) (Gabriel 1994).

Equipment

Trolley or tray

Sterile dressings pack, if required

Sterile cannula as required by the medical practitioner

Alcohol-based antiseptic for cleansing the skin

Gloves

Sterile administration set

Prescribed sterile infusion fluid

Sterile transparent dressing

Infusion stand

Tourniquet or sphygmomanometer

Hypoallergenic tape

Receptacle for soiled disposables.

Additional equipment if required

- Equipment for shaving the skin area
- Local anaesthetic and equipment for its administration
- Air inlet for glass containers
- Holder for glass containers (bottle holder)
- Splint and bandage to support the limb where the infusion is sited
- Continuous infusion pump and appropriate cassette (see Parenteral nutrition, p. 247).

Infusion fluids

The most commonly prescribed fluids are:
— normal saline (sodium chloride 0.9%)
— dextrose 5% in water
— Ringer's Lactate
— plasma or plasma expanders, e.g. Haemaccel, stable plasma protein solution (SPPS)
— blood (see Blood transfusion, p. 49)
— parenteral nutrients (see Parenteral nutrition, p. 247).

Most prescribed fluids are commercially prepared in sterile containers and they are labelled FOR INTRAVENOUS INFUSION. They may also be prepared by the hospital pharmacy. The containers used for these preparations are frequently soft plastic bags protected by an outer covering (see manufacturer's instructions), although glass bottles or semi-rigid plastic containers (Polyfusors) continue to be used for some preparations.

Cannulae

Various cannulae (Fig. 25.1) are available, and are prepared commercially in sterile packs. Those chosen by the medical practitioner may have an inner needle surrounded by a plastic cannula. The needle is withdrawn once the vein is punctured, allowing blood to flow back. Once the cannula is safely in situ the infusion fluid is connected and the cannula is secured in position. Some cannula packs include an accompanying syringe, e.g. Medicut. Small winged needles are used for access to scalp veins in babies and young children.

Administration sets

Administration sets are commercially prepared in sterile packs. The set contains specialised sterile tubing; at one end there is a rigid trocar protected by a sterile

Figure 25.1
Intravenous infusion:
cannulae in common use
A Cannula used when
intravenous drugs are to
be administered with the
infusion or post infusion
B Cannula used
preoperatively for short-
term infusion

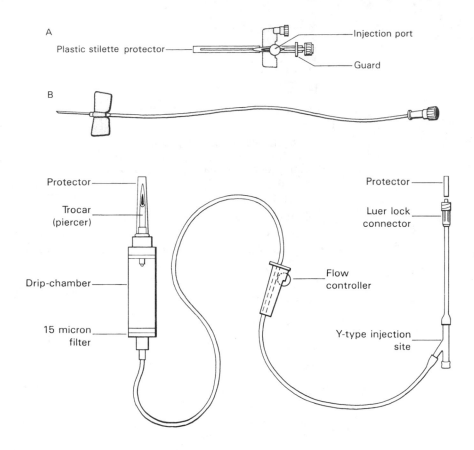

A

Plastic stilette protector

Injection port

Guard

B

Protector

Trocar
(piercer)

Drip-chamber

15 micron
filter

Protector

Luer lock
connector

Flow
controller

Y-type injection
site

Figure 25.2
Administration set for
intravenous infusion

sheath. At the other end is a similarly protected Luer connector nozzle. Towards the trocar end, the tubing widens into a drip chamber. An adjustable roller clamp surrounds the tubing below the drip chamber, which allows the flow of fluid to be regulated at the prescribed flow rate. Blood administration sets include a filter. Simple administration sets are available without filter, for infusion of clear fluids (Fig. 25.2).

Specialised administration sets (burette set)

A specialised administration set is used for infusions when a volumetric infusion pump is not available and a more accurate control of flow rate is needed. This is particularly important to reduce the risk of fluid overload when infusions are prescribed for babies or young children. The burette set has a calibrated drip chamber, with one roller clamp above and one roller clamp below. The drip chamber is filled with the amount of fluid prescribed in ml per hour; this amount of fluid is infused during one hour. The flow rate will depend on the drop factor and the amount prescribed (see manufacturer's instructions). In order for the infusion to continue, the drip chamber has to be refilled as prescribed each time it is emptied.

Volumetric infusion pumps

Some volumetric infusion pumps are used with specific sterile cassettes (e.g. Accuset) as well as a normal administration set so that an accurate flow of fluid can be maintained during the infusion. When primed and connected, these can be set to infuse fluid within a range of 1–999 ml per hour. Other volumetric infusion sets simply use a specifically adapted administration set. The infusion is controlled by a column of electronically controlled rollers which adjust the flow rate as required, e.g. Baxter Flo guard 6201 (see manufacturer's instructions). This equipment is expensive and is used extensively in intensive case areas and specialised units, e.g. oncology, but only occasionally in the general wards, mainly for the administration of intravenous medication or parenteral nutrition (Willis 1995) (*see* Parenteral nutrition, p. 247).

Syringe pumps may be used for a continuous infusion of prescribed intravenous medication of less than 10 ml per hour.

Guidelines and rationale for this nursing practice	<ul><li>help to explain the nursing practice to the patient *to gain consent and cooperation and encourage participation in care* (Corbett et al 1993)</li><li>ensure the patient's privacy, *respecting his individuality*</li><li>help to collect and prepare the equipment. Gloves should be worn *to prevent contamination with body fluid*</li><li>check the prescribed infusion fluid with a registered nurse or medical practitioner. *This is a legal requirement and part of professional practice*</li><li>prime the administration set with the infusion fluid, maintaining asepsis, *so that it is ready once the cannula is in position*</li><li>place the infusion fluid on the stand beside the patient, check that it is running freely and that all air is expelled from the system. *This prevents any danger of air embolus occuring.* If not connected immediately the end should be protected by replacing the sterile cap *to prevent contamination*</li><li>help the patient into as comfortable a position as possible *so that he will tolerate the intravenous therapy without distress*</li><li>observe the patient throughout this activity *to monitor any adverse affects as well as any improvement in his condition*</li><li>expose and support the area for cannulation *to facilitate access*</li><li>help to prepare the sterile equipment as required *to maintain a safe environment* (Recker 1992)</li><li>apply pressure around the limb above the cannulation site as directed using a sphygmomanometer cuff or tourniquet. *This will retain more blood in the veins and facilitate cannulation*</li><li>release the pressure as directed once the venous cannula is correctly positioned and the infusion lines are connected *to commence the flow of fluid to the veins*</li><li>regulate the flow rate as prescribed *to maintain the prescribed fluid intake*</li><li>help the medical practitioner to secure the dressing and tubing *to maintain asepsis and prevent disconnection of the tubing and cannula* (Thomas 1990) (Fig. 25.3)</li></ul>

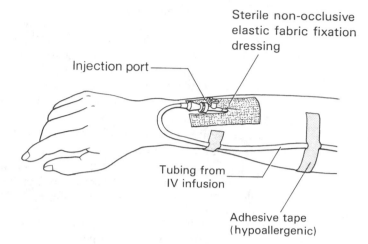

Figure 25.3 *Anchoring the tubing with adhesive tape*

- apply a splint to the limb *if the site of the infusion requires the limb to be immobilised*
- ensure that the patient is left feeling as comfortable as possible *so that he will continue to tolerate the intravenous therapy. Comfort helps to reduce stress levels and promotes healing*
- dispose of equipment safely *to prevent transmission of infection*
- document this nursing practice appropriately, monitor after-effects and report abnormal findings immediately, *ensuring safe practice and enabling prompt appropriate medical and nursing intervention to be initiated as soon as possible*
- maintain the infusion at the prescribed flow rate *for continuation of the treatment.*

2   Priming the equipment for intravenous infusion

This is the preparation of the prescribed infusion fluid by running it through the administration set. Asepsis should be maintained during this part of the practice *to prevent any internal or exposed areas being contaminated.*

Equipment

Prescribed intravenous infusion fluid

Sterile administration set

Sterile gallipot

Receptacle for soiled disposables

Infusion stand

Alcohol-saturated swab

Sterile air inlet

Bottle holder   } for use with glass container

Trolley or tray

Guidelines and rationale for this nursing practice

- check the infusion fluid, which is prescribed by the medical practitioner. Each container of fluid is checked by two people, one of whom must be a registered nurse or a medical practitioner (*see* Administration of medicines, p. 1) *for safe practice*
- check the following details against the patient's own documentation and the label on the infusion fluid *to make sure that the correct prescribed infusion is given:*
  - the patient's name and unit number
  - the date of the prescription
  - the type of infusion prescribed
  - the amount of infusion prescribed
  - the container labelled 'for intravenous infusion'
  - the expiry date of the infusion fluid
  - the time prescribed for commencement of the infusion
  - the time to be taken for completion of the infusion
  - the signature of the medical practitioner
- check the fluid for cloudiness, sediment or discoloration. The container should be checked for flaws, leaks or evidence of contamination. Any suspect fluid or containers must be discarded immediately according to health authority policies *to prevent any introduction of infection or contamination and to maintain a safe environment*
- include the serial number of the fluid as well as the signature of the nurse or medical practitioner checking the infusion prescription in the documentation. *If the patient suffers any adverse effects, the particular infusion can then be identified* (UKCC 1992)
- establish the identity of the patient by appropriate means, e.g. identification bracelet, *maintaining safe practice.*

When using a soft plastic container (bag):

- perform appropriate hand washing technique *to prevent infection*
- remove the outer plastic covering of the container *in preparation for use*
- remove the sheath covering the entry channel, without contaminating the inside, *maintaining asepsis*
- remove the administration set from its package *in preparation for use*
- close the flow control clamp *to prevent any uncontrolled flow of fluid*
- remove the protective sheath from the trocar of the administration set, maintaining asepsis *in preparation for insertion*
- insert the trocar firmly through the seal of the container's entry channel *so that fluid flows into the first part of the administration set*
- invert the container and hang it on the infusion pole *so that gravity will help the flow*
- gently squeeze the chamber of the administration set *to allow it to fill partly*
- temporarily remove the protective sheath covering the Luer connector at the end of the administration set and hold it over a sterile container (e.g. gallipot) *to prevent any contamination*

- slowly release the flow control clamp *to allow the fluid to fill the rest of the tubing*
- eliminate any air bubbles from the fluid in the tubing by running some fluid into a sterile container if necessary *to prevent any danger of air embolus*
- close the flow control clamp *to stop the flow of fluid*
- replace the protective cover on the Luer connector nozzle *to prevent any infection occurring*
- place the free end of the tubing in the notch provided on the flow control clamp, *to keep the Luer connector nozzle protected from contamination*
- place the primed equipment on the infusion stand beside the patient's bed *ready for connection to the intravenous cannula*

The equipment should only be primed immediately prior to the infusion *to minimise the risk of infection*

If contamination occurs or the container is punctured while priming the equipment, the infusion and the administration set are discarded and the procedure recommenced.

When using a glass container (bottle):

- maintain aseptic technique as before
- remove the seal from the top of the checked infusion fluid bottle *to expose the rubber bung*
- clean the rubber bung with alcohol solution *to prevent transmission of infection*
- prepare the administration set as before
- push the trocar firmly through the rubber bung *to access the fluid*
- remove the sterile air inlet from its outer package and remove the protective sheath from the needle
- insert the needle of the air inlet through the rubber bung *to equalise the pressure in the bottle and so facilitate the flow of fluid*
- hang the inverted bottle on the infusion stand using a bottle holder if required and support the end of the air inlet above the level of the fluid in the bottle if necessary *to allow the fluid to flow freely*
- proceed to prime the equipment as before.

When using a semi-rigid plastic container (Polyfusor):

- maintain aseptic technique as before
- remove the outer package of the checked infusion fluid
- cut off the end of the entry channel with sterile scissors *to maintain asepsis*
- prepare the administration set as before
- insert the trocar into the entry channel and twist it for a firm fit *to gain access*
- invert the container and hang it on the infusion stand *for gravity to help the flow*
- proceed to prime the equipment as before (no air inlet is required for this container)

3 Maintaining the infusion for a period of time

The number of drops per minute required for each particular infusion has to be accurately calculated *in order to maintain the flow of infusion at the prescribed rate.*

Guidelines and rationale for this nursing practice

Calculating the flow rate of infusion fluids

All administration sets include details of the number of drops per ml for that particular set. This is known as the drop factor. Some sets include a scale of drops per minute for a given time within the pack. *Using this information, an accurate assessment of the flow rate needed can be calculated.*

Formula used for calculation

$$\frac{\text{Total volume of infusion fluid x Drop factor (see administration set)}}{\text{Total time of infusion in minutes}}$$

Example

Total volume of fluid = 500 ml

Time for completion = 4 hours, i.e. 240 minutes (4 × 60)

Drop factor = 15

$$\frac{500 \times 15}{240} = 31.2 = 30 \text{ drops (approx)}$$

Thus the number of drops required to maintain the infusion at the required rate = 30 per minute when drop factor is 15 drops per ml.

The position of the cannula in the vein and the movement of the patient's limbs may have an effect on the flow rate. It is important to assess visually the rate of fall of fluid in the infusion container as well as to regulate the required drops per minute, e.g. when the time for completion is 4 hours, one quarter of the fluid should have been infused after 1 hour, and half the fluid after 2 hours.

Changing the infusion container

Within 24 hours the empty container can be replaced with a full container of prescribed infusion fluid without changing the administration set. The containers should be exchanged before the level of fluid drops below the point of the trocar in the neck of the container. Preparation for changing a container should begin while a small amount of fluid remains in the infusion container; *this prevents the formation of air bubbles in the system and the danger of air embolus.*

Guidelines and rationale for this nursing practice

- explain the nursing practice to the patient *to gain consent and cooperation*
- perform hand washing *and maintain asepsis during this practice as before*
- check the prescribed infusion fluid *continuing professional practice*
- prepare the new container of infusion fluid as for priming the equipment
- turn off the infusion temporarily, by closing the roller clamp
- remove the trocar of the administration set from the empty container and insert it into the new infusion fluid, *maintaining asepsis* (a new air inlet should be used when changing glass bottles)
- recommence the infusion as soon as possible at the prescribed flow rate
- maintain observations as before
- dispose of the used container safely *to prevent transmission of infection*
- document the nursing practice appropriately, monitor after-effects and report abnormal findings immediately *to ensure safe practice and enable prompt appropriate medical and nursing intervention to be initiated as soon as possible* (Locher 1992).

Removal of the intravenous cannula

This is performed using aseptic technique *when an intravenous infusion is discontinued or when a new site for access is needed to continue an infusion.*

- explain the procedure to the patient *to obtain consent and cooperation*
- ensure the patient's privacy *respecting his individuality*
- close the flow clamp *to discontinue infusion of fluid*
- prepare a trolley and sterile dressings as required *to maintain a safe environment*
- don sterile gloves *to prevent blood-borne infection*
- expose the site of insertion of the cannula, *maintaining asepsis*
- remove retaining sutures if present (*see* p. 391) *to release the cannula*
- apply pressure with a sterile swab using the non-dominant hand, and withdraw the cannula slowly with the dominant hand, maintaining pressure *to reduce any bleeding*
- retain pressure on the puncture site as required *until bleeding stops, maintaining asepsis*
- cover the site with a small sterile dressing, e.g. Airstrip, *to prevent infection*
- dispose of equipment safely *to prevent transmission of infection*
- resume observation of the site as appropriate *to monitor the healing process*
- document the nursing practice appropriately, monitor after-effects and report abnormal findings immediately *ensuring safe practice*

Occasionally the tip of the cannula is sent to the laboratory for microbiological investigation. If this is ordered the tip is cut off with sterile scissors, put into an appropriately labelled sterile specimen container, maintaining asepsis, and sent to the appropriate laboratory with the completed laboratory form (*see* Specimen collection, (p. 297).

4 Care of a Hickman catheter for long-term intravenous therapy

General indications and rationale for useof a Hickman catheter

As for Intravenous therapy (*see* p. 165)

Specific indications and rationale for use of a Hickman catheter

The use of a Hickman catheter may be chosen by the medical practitioner for continuous or intermittent intravenous therapy for a period of weeks or even as long as 2 years.

The patient may be at home or in an institutional setting (Stillwell 1992). *This method is chosen because the radio-opaque silastic catheter, which is usually 'tunnelled', can safely remain in situ for long periods if efficient care of the catheter is maintained.*

Patient education should help the patient to become independent in his own care *so that he can be discharged home with a long-term catheter in place, under the supervision of the community team* (Sheldon & Bender 1994).

Use of a Hickman catheter may be required for:

- administration of medicines, for example chemotherapy to give repeated doses of cytotoxic medication for treatment of malignant disease, e.g. leukaemia, over a period of weeks. *Cytotoxic medication can cause damage to peripheral vessels, but central venous access allows the irritant medication to be diluted rapidly in the circulating fluid of the large veins and transported round the body safely*
- long-term parenteral nutrition (*see* Parenteral nutrition, p. 247). *Nutrients in the parenteral feeding regime may also irritate the lining of the peripheral blood vessels; access via a central line prevents this occurring as the nutrients are infused directly into the central veins*
- taking blood samples over a period of time *to monitor the progress of treatment,* for example in children with malignant disease *to prevent repeated venepuncture.*

Skin-tunnelled catheters

A Hickman catheter will remain in situ for a period of time. The distal end of the catheter is usually tunnelled subcutaneously so that the entry site to the vein is separated from the skin exit site, *thus reducing the risk of infection entering the circulation from the catheter insertion site.* This is particularly important for patients having chemotherapy as both the disease and the treatment may cause immunosuppression, further reducing resistance to infection (RCN 1992).

A Hickman catheter has a Dacron cuff at the distal end, around which fibrous tissue will form, *anchoring the catheter in position and ensuring safer long-term use* (Fig. 25.4).

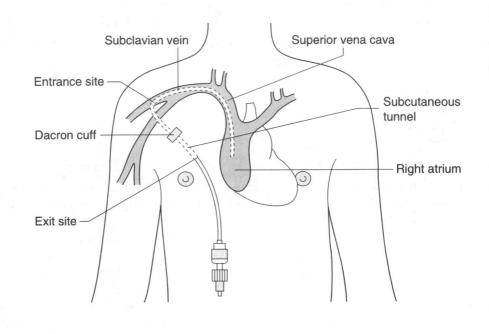

Figure 25.4 *Hickman catheter in situ*

Outline of the procedure	*See* Insertion of a central venous catheter, page 103, Parenteral nutrition, page 247.

Equipment	***Equipment for insertion of a Hickman catheter*** As for Intravenous therapy, page 166, Insertion of a central venous catheter, page 103. In addition: - Hickman catheter — a flexible, radio-opaque, silicone tube, 90 cm long (approx), incorporating a Dacron cuff at the distal end - injectable cap with a Luer lock for access to the line. ***Equipment for care at home*** - equipment for dressing entry site if required — *see* Wound care, page 383 - instruction sheet or booklet to reinforce the patient education commenced prior to discharge - suitable container for storing equipment - spare Luer lock cap with injection port — this usually includes a one-way valve so that no extra needle is needed (see manufacturer's instructions) - sterile 5 ml syringe - sterile 19 G needle for drawing up the heparin - prepared heparinised saline, 50 iu in 5 ml - alcohol-impregnated swabs, e.g. Mediswab - approved container for disposal of 'sharps'.

All the above should be available in the patient's home and continuously replaced as required for as long as the treatment continues. It is helpful if all the equipment is stored in a suitable container and used only for the care of the catheter, *to maintain a safe environment.*

<table>
<tr>
<td>

Guidelines and rationale for this nursing practice

</td>
<td>

These guidelines are applicable to the nurse and also to the patient or carer as the patient develops confidence in his own care.

- help to explain the procedure to the patient *to obtain consent and cooperation and encourage participation in care*
- ensure the patient's privacy *respecting his individuality*
- collect and prepare the equipment *so that everything is easily available*
- help the patient into as comfortable a position as possible *ensuring that there is easy access to the Hickman line and entry port*
- don gloves after efficient hand washing *to reduce any risk of infection and contamination with body fluids.* If the patient himself performs this procedure, he will not need to use gloves, but good hand washing technique should be part of patient education prior to discharge and continually reinforced afterwards (Cochrane 1994)
- draw up 5 ml of heparinised saline solution into the 5 ml syringe, *maintaining asepsis in preparation for flushing the line*
- observe the catheter site for redness, swelling or exudate *which may indicate infection.* The patient should inform the medical practitioner and the community nurse of any change in condition of the site
- observe the catheter for any damage or cracks *which may cause infection or an air embolus to occur.* Report any problems immediately and clamp the line above the damage until repaired or replaced
- clamp the line above the Luer lock cap if the cap needs changing. *This will ensure that air does not enter the line to cause an air embolus*
- maintaining asepsis, change the cap, *This may be necessary to ensure the continued efficiency of the valve, and also to reduce any risk of infection or contamination.* Refer to the health authority policy and manufacturer's instructions
- release the clamp from the line once the cap is safely in position *to ensure that the line is safely patent again*
- swab the end of the entry port of the cap with alcohol *to prevent transmission of infection*
- flush the line with 5 ml heparinised saline, maintaining asepsis, *to prevent a clot forming which would block the patency of the central line and prevent its continued use* (Fig. 25.5). Health authority policy will dictate the frequency of flushing with heparin. If resistance is felt, flushing should not be continued, *as a clot may be dislodged.* Resistance to flushing should be reported immediately, *as it may indicate a clot blocking the line*
- dress the catheter site as appropriate — *see* Wound care, page 383. Initially the site may be covered by a semi-permeable dressing (Keenlyside 1993). There is no need for a dressing once the site is clean and healed after the stitches have been removed — usually after the first 10 days

</td>
</tr>
</table>

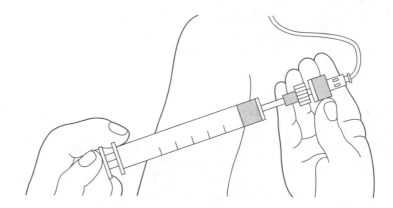

Figure 25.5 *Care of a Hickman catheter: flushing the line with heparinised saline*

- wash the site with clean water and dry thoroughly with low linting swabs *to keep the site clean and to prevent any risk of infection*. Catheter care can be timed to follow a shower or bath *to further prevent any risk of infection*, but the site itself should still be cleaned separately *to prevent contamination*
- ensure the patient is left feeling as comfortable as possible, *so that he can resume his normal activities of living*
- dispose of equipment safely *to prevent transmission of infection*
- document this nursing practice appropriately, monitor the effects and report abnormal findings immediately *to ensure safe practice and enable prompt appropriate medical or nursing intervention to be initiated.*

Relevance to the activities of living

Observations and further rationale for intravenous therapy will be included within each activity of living as appropriate.

Maintaining a safe environment

Intravenous infusion is an invasive practice so all precautions must be maintained to prevent any infection occurring at the venous access site, or infection entering the blood circulation via the infusion itself (Fig. 25.6). Efficient hand washing technique should be employed when handling equipment.

The drip rate and flow rate should be monitored to check that there is no occlusion in the system, and that the prescribed flow is maintained. Spasm of the vein or movement of the limb may cause slowing or stopping of the infusion; repositioning the limb may help to relieve the occlusion. If the stoppage is associated with soreness or swelling of the vein site this may indicate that the cannula is no longer in the vein and fluid is seeping into the surrounding tissues, or it may be evidence of developing thrombophlebitis. If this occurs the medical practitioner should be informed and the infusion discontinued and resumed at another site.

All the equipment connections should be inspected for disconnections, flaws or leakage, to prevent contamination or the possibility of an air embolus. The tubing should be inspected to check that there are no air bubbles.

Careful, considerate explanation of what the practice involves will help the

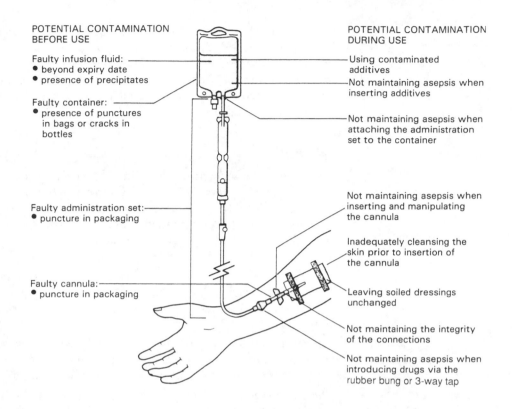

POTENTIAL CONTAMINATION
BEFORE USE

Faulty infusion fluid:
• beyond expiry date
• presence of precipitates

Faulty container:
• presence of punctures
  in bags or cracks in
  bottles

Faulty administration set:
• puncture in packaging

Faulty cannula:
• puncture in packaging

POTENTIAL CONTAMINATION
DURING USE

Using contaminated
additives

Not maintaining asepsis when
inserting additives

Not maintaining asepsis when
attaching the administration
set to the container

Not maintaining asepsis when
inserting and manipulating
the cannula

Inadequately cleansing the
skin prior to insertion of
the cannula

Leaving soiled dressings
unchanged

Not maintaining the integrity
of the connections

Not maintaining asepsis when
introducing drugs via the
rubber bung or 3-way tap

Figure 25.6 *Potential
routes for contamination
associated with
intravenous infusion*

patient to cooperate in maintaining a safe environment. He should understand the reasons why the lines must not be pulled or the dressing touched.

Patients who are confused or disorientated may require the appropriate use of splints and bandages to maintain the infusion safely in position.

The administration set should be changed every 24 hours, maintaining asepsis to minimise the risk of infection, unless long-term (96 hour) filters are used (Johnson 1994).

The dressing should be changed according to local practice. A transparent sterile occlusive dressing enables the site and the cannula to be observed without disturbing the dressing; this minimises the risk of infection. Gloves should be worn to prevent the risk of blood-borne infection.

Any abnormalities should be reported immediately, and the infusion discontinued or the rate of infusion reduced to a minimum until further instructions are given. Maintaining minimum flow will prevent clotting in the vein and also reduce the risk of further complications developing until the problem has been dealt with.

Communicating

The patient may find this practice very stressful; the nurse should give appropriate support, and simple explanations at each stage of the procedure.

It may be difficult for the patient to position spectacles or a hearing aid if one hand is immobilised. By anticipating his needs the nurse can greatly enhance the patient's ability to communicate. He should be reassured that a nurse is always nearby and constantly observant. When leaving the patient the nurse should ensure that articles he is likely to need are easily acessible and that a bell or other means of communication is available.

Breathing

Intravenous therapy in itself should not affect the patient's breathing but vital signs should be monitored hourly, 2-hourly or 4-hourly according to circumstances so that complications can be identified as soon as possible. For patients undergoing long-term intravenous therapy, e.g. with a Hickman line in situ at home, monitoring may only be necessary if the site is infected or any associated problems are identified.

The pulse rate   Tachycardia may indicate infusion reaction or infection. It may also indicate circulatory overload if the rate of infusion is too rapid and the patient's cardiac output has difficulty in responding to the extra fluid in the circulation.

The respiration rate   A rise in respiration rate may indicate infection or circulatory overload. Dyspnoea accompanied by a cough and frothy sputum may indicate pulmonary oedema and should be reported immediately.

The blood pressure   Changes in blood pressure will depend on the reason for infusion. If the infusion is given to replace fluid loss, the patient may be hypotensive initially and a gradual rise in blood pressure will be expected. Recordings outside the normal range should be reported.

The prescribed rate of the infusion will depend on the individual patient's requirements and condition. Patients who have congestive cardiac failure and elderly patients will have a lower infusion rate prescribed by the medical practitioner.

The prescribed rate of infusion for babies and young children will be adjusted for their age, weight and height ratio. A volumetric infusion pump or a burette set should be used to maintain an accurate flow rate, and observations monitored frequently.

For seriously ill patients a catheter may be inserted to record the central venous pressure, which can accurately monitor changes in circulating fluid volume during the period of intravenous infusion (*see* Central venous pressure, p. 103).

Disconnection of the infusion lines may cause a backflow of blood, increasing the risk of haemorrhage. Pressure over the venous site will prevent further blood loss, while appropriate action is taken by qualified staff.

An air embolus may occur if a bubble of air enters the blood circulation. The bubble may remain unnoticed until it reaches the heart. A large air embolus may cause a cardiac arrest; a small one may enter the pulmonary circulation and cause some respiratory distress. Every effort should be made to eliminate air from the tubing when priming the infusion equipment, and observations maintained to prevent any risk of air embolus occurring (*see* Central venous pressure, p. 103).

Eating and drinking

Fluid intake should be recorded and fluid balance charts accurately maintained (Daffurn et al 1994).

Normally the amount of infusion fluid is documented after the completion of each unit. However, with seriously ill patients both intake and output are recorded hourly. In this case the infusion fluid is usually given via continuous infusion pump or a burette set.

The patient may be unable to eat or drink normally during this procedure. Oral hygiene should be performed as appropriate to maintain a healthy oral and oropharyngeal mucosa (*see* Mouth care, p. 209).

The infusion may continue during the period of time when the patient recommences oral feeding. The food should be prepared so that the patient can comfortably use his available hand, and the nurse should ensure that prescribed oral fluids are readily accessible if one arm is partly immobilised by the infusion equipment.

Eliminating

Accurate documentation of fluid output should be maintained. This will help to monitor the patient's renal function during the infusion.

When using a commode the patient may need help to support the administration lines and prevent disconnection of tubing.

Personal cleansing and dressing

The condition of the skin should be noted. Local redness or heat may indicate infection, and swelling may indicate fluid leakage into the surrounding tissues; sweating, shivering, rigor, pallor or a rash may indicate an adverse systemic reaction (see pharmaceutical literature).

The patient may need appropriate help with personal cleansing and dressing. Clothing may have to be adapted to maintain access to the infusion site. The need for this and appropriate light clothing should be explained to the patient.

Controlling body temperature

Body temperature should be monitored hourly, 2-hourly or 4-hourly according to circumstances. A sudden rise in body temperature, or shivering and signs of rigor, may indicate infusion reaction or the onset of infection and should be reported immediately (*see* Blood transfusion, p. 49). For long-term intravenous therapy, the temperature should be monitored at the discretion of the community team if any infection is suspected.

It may be necessary for the area of the infusion site to be exposed for observation. The patient may need help to adjust his own clothing, or the bedcovers, for any perceived change in temperature.

Mobilising

Increasingly, patients are encouraged to move around and even to take a shower as their condition allows while an intravenous infusion is still in progress, especially during the postoperative period. The nurse should ensure that the lines are supported and that all precautions for prevention of infection and disconnection are maintained, with the patient's cooperation, during the period of mobilising.

Working and playing

The nurse should ensure that the patient maintains his interests, as his condition allows, while this practice is in progress. Access to newspapers, radio and television should be available if required.

Family and friends should be encouraged to visit the patient if there are no other contraindications.

Sleeping

The patient's general condition should be noted, e.g. restlessness, drowsiness and level of consciousness.

Tbe patient may find it difficult to lie in his normal sleeping position due to the infusion. Help in adjusting to a suitably comfortable position may induce sleep.

Necessary observations may waken the patient. Explanation of the need for these and reassurance may reduce the waking period. The observations which cause most disturbance are the recording of temperature and blood pressure; these observations may be reduced in frequency as the patient's condition allows, while maintaining the frequency of the pulse rate recording and observations of the lines and infusion rate.

Patient education: key points

The reason for the particular intravenous therapy should be explained to the patient.

The importance of maintaining the cannula/catheter in situ should be emphasised and the danger of disconnection explained, so that the patient does not pull the lines or dislodge the dressing.

Specific education for care of the site and lines should be given to the patient discharged home with an intravenous infusion. This may include:

- care of the infusion site and cannula/catheter port
- changing the infusion fluid as prescribed
- flushing the line to maintain patency for intermittent intravenous therapy
- observing the site for any adverse effects.

The patient at home should know what to do if the lines become disconnected. He and his carers should be familiar with the use of a simple clamp and be able to apply a dressing with firm pressure and a tight bandage while waiting for help from the community team.

All patients should understand the importance of reporting immediately any redness, swelling or pain at the infusion site, as well as any disconnection or blockage of the lines and any other adverse symptoms. A telephone 'help line' gives the patient at home added confidence to be self-caring.

References

Cochrane S 1994 A mask of approval: patient satisfaction with self infusion teaching programme. Professional Nurse 10(2): 106–111

Corbett K, Meehan L, Sackey V 1993 A strategy to enhance skills. Developing intravenous therapy skills for community nursing. Professional Nurse 9(1): 60–63

Daffurn K, Hillman K, Baumn A et al 1994 Fluid balance charts: do they measure up. British Journal of Nursing 3(16): 816–820

Gabriel J 1994 An intravenous alternative. Nursing Times 90(31): 39–41

Johnson S 1994 A time and money saver. Cost comparison of I.V. therapy with and without Pale 96 filters. Professional Nurse 10(2): 94–96

Keenlyside D 1993 Avoiding an unnecessary outcome. A comparative trial between I.V. 3000 and conventional film dressing to access rates of catheter related sepsis. Professional Nurse 8(5): 288–291

Lamb J 1995 I.V. therapy. Nursing Standard 9(30): 31–35

Locher C 1992 How to make the best of your charting. Journal of Practical Nursing 42(2): 35–43

RCN 1992 Skin tunnelled catheters. Guidelines for care. Royal College of Nursing, London

Recker D 1992 Catheter related sepsis: an analysis of research (I.V. catheters). Dimension of Critical Care Nursing 11(5): 249–262

Sheldon P, Bender M 1994 High technology in home care. An overview of intravenous therapy. Nursing Clinics of North America 29(3): 507–519

Stillwell B 1992 Skills update. Central venous lines (using Hickman lines). Community Outlook 2(5): 22–23

Thomas S 1990 Making sense of . . . . . semi permeable film dressings. Nursing Times 86(10): 49–51

UKCC 1992 Code of professional conduct. United Kingdom Central Council for Nursing — Midwifery and Health Visiting, London

Willis J 1995 Infusion devices: volumetric and peristaltic pumps. Professional Nurse 10(7): 433–435

Further reading

Cooper C, Hodgson J 1992 A learning experience. (District nurses extended role in administering I.V. therapy to an aids patient.) Journal of Community Nursing 6(2): 18–20

Goodson M 1990 Keeping the flora out. Professional Nurse 5(11): 572–575

Hagland M, Wilkinson B 1993 A flexible path to permanent change implementing standard setting in an intensive therapy unit. Professional Nurse 8(9): 578–582

Leighton H 1994 Maintaining patency of transduced arterial and venous lines using 0.9% sodium chloride. Intensive and Critical Care Nursing 10(1): 23–25

Pike S 1989 Family participation in the care of central venous lines. Nursing 3(47): 30–31

Sadler C 1989 How nurses help children cope with a Hickman catheter. Nursing 3(47): 30–31

Speechley V et al 1989 Managing an implantable drug delivery system (port-a-cath). Professional Nurse 4(6): 284–285, 287–288

26 Isolation Nursing

There are three parts to this section:

1 Source isolation
2 Protective isolation
3 Radioactive hazard isolation

The concluding subsection 'Relevance to the activities of living' refers to the three practices collectively.

Learning outcomes

By the end of this section you should know how to:

- prevent the spread of infection while nursing a patient with a specific communicable disease (source isolation)
- protect a patient from infection when he may be at a greater risk than normal (protective isolation)
- prevent hazard to carers and visitors when radioactive substances are used.

Background knowledge required

Revision of the modes of transmission of infection and related microbiology.

Review of health authority policy in relation to control of infection in both institutional and community settings.

Knowledge of the role of the infection control officer/nurse in your area.

Review of health authority policy in relation to the handling of radioactive substances.

Indications and rationale for isolation nursing

The aim of this nursing practice is to create an effective barrier between an infected area and a non-infected area, *to prevent occurrence of cross-infection*, or to use appropriate measures *to prevent contamination from radioactive substances*.

1   Source isolation (barrier nursing)

In this instance the infected area is the isolation area where the infected patient is nursed, and the non-infected area is outside the isolation area.

Indications and rationale for source isolation	This is carried out *to prevent the spread of infection from patients who have or are suspected of having a specific communicable infection*, for example: • a wound infection caused by *Staphylococcus aureus* • general infection caused by Methicillin Resistant *Staphylococcus Aureus* (MRSA) which may have few symptoms (Taylor 1990) • a respiratory infection caused by tuberculosis • an enteric infection caused by salmonella.
Equipment	The equipment required will depend on the infection, the patient's condition and health authority policies. It may include the following: Single room with toilet facilities Hand washing facilities for personnel inside and outside the isolation area Alcohol solution for rinsing hands Protective clothing, which may include: • cap • filter-type mask • gown • plastic apron • gloves • overshoes • goggles. These items should be disposable and a supply kept just outside the isolation area Disposable or individual crockery and cutlery Facilities for treatment of, or disposal of, infected linen and rubbish All equipment needed for appropriate nursing care should remain within the isolation area *to prevent transmission of infection.* The area should be equipped with a thermometer, sphygmomanometer, stethoscope and watch or clock with a seconds hand as required for recording vital signs. The patient's documentation should remain outside the isolation area and details of recordings and care be completed by 'uncontaminated' personnel *to maintain a safe environment.*
Guidelines and rationale for this nursing practice	• consult appropriate personnel *to obtain advice and guidance.* Most health authorities and hospitals have a member of staff designated to be responsible for the control of infection in that area e.g. infection control nurse (Alderman 1992) • plan the nursing so that everything required is carried out during one period of time in the isolation area. *Personnel continually entering and leaving the area greatly increase the risk of cross-infection*

- choose personnel with known immunity to care for patients with specific infections if possible *as they will be resistant to the infection*
- explain the importance of the precautions to the patient *to gain consent and cooperation and encourage participation in care*
- wash hands and apply alcohol solution before entering the isolation area *to maintain a safe environment*
- don protective clothing as required *to create an effective barrier against the infection* (Ayton 1984)
- enter the isolation area
- perform all necessary nursing care. Two nurses may be needed for certain nursing practices (Bowell 1990), e.g. to pass in equipment, the patient's meals, or prescribed medication from outside the isolation area. One nurse should remain in protective clothing within the area. The second nurse should remain at the entrance of the area and transfer articles to the nurse within the area without allowing any contamination to occur. *This prevents transmission of infection*
- observe the patient throughout this activity *to monitor any change in condition*
- ensure that the patient is left feeling as comfortable as possible *to help promote the healing process*
- ensure that the patient has a means of communication, e.g. bell, two-way radio, *as patients can feel very isolated in this situation* (Denton 1986)
- safely dispose of any infected material according to health authority policies *to prevent cross-infection*
- wash hands within the isolation area *to prevent transferral of infection out of the area*
- remove protective clothing without touching the outside of the garments and dispose of it safely *to prevent any cross-infection and maintain a safe environment for all*
- leave the isolation area once all nursing care is complete
- repeat hand washing outside the isolation area and apply alcohol solution *to further ensure no contamination occurs* (Elliot 1992)
- document the nursing practices appropriately, monitor after-effects and report abnormal findings immediately *so that care can be evaluated and any nursing or medical interventions can be altered as required*
- explain the precautions to visitors, who should be restricted to close relatives and friends, *to obtain their cooperation in maintaining isolation for the patient by wearing protective clothing.*

Disposal of infected material

Local guidelines should be followed by community nurses regarding the disposal of contaminated waste.

In an institutional setting two nurses are required: one to remain in her protective clothing within the isolation area, the second nurse to remain free from contamination outside the isolation area.

Disposal of waste   This should be put in a clinical waste disposal bag and closed as appropriate inside the isolation area by the isolation nurse. The second nurse outside the area remains at the entrance with an open clinical waste bag into which the isolation nurse places the infected bag without touching the outside of the second bag. The second bag is closed without contaminating the outside and treated as normal clinical waste. This procedure is known as 'double bagging' (Fig. 26.1).

Disposal of linen   Infected linen should be 'double bagged' in clear plastic bags and sent to the laundry in carriers designated for infected linen; sometimes disposable linen is used.

Disposal of sharps   The infected sharps container should be safely closed by the isolation nurse and placed in a clear plastic bag held by the second nurse, keeping the outside uncontaminated; it should then be sealed and disposed of in accordance with health authority policy *to prevent any transmission of infection.*

Domestic cleaning

The domestic manager should be informed whenever isolation procedures are required. Arrangements for cleaning the isolation area will be made in cooperation with the hospital infection control personnel, *maintaining a safe environment.*

Decontamination of the isolation area

When a patient leaves an isolation area, the nursing staff should dispose of all the infected equipment. The room or cubicle and associated furniture should be decontaminated as health authority policy dictates before being used again *to ensure that it is free of any infection.*

Specific precautions

Different precautions may be needed for specific infections.

Respiratory infections   The patient should be nursed in a single room or cubicle with the door kept closed *to reduce airborne and/or droplet infection.*

Masks which act as an efficient barrier may be worn by all personnel entering the area *to protect staff from infection.*

Gloves should be worn when handling sputum or contaminated linen, and when assisting the patient with oral hygiene. *This prevents contamination with body*

Figure 26.1 *Isolation nursing: removal of a disposal bag from the infected area to the 'clean' area. Infected bag already tied up is placed inside clean bag held by another nurse outside the area and tied up without contaminating the outside*

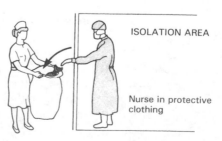

'Clean' nurse

ISOLATION AREA

Nurse in protective clothing

fluids. Good hand washing technique should give adequate protection otherwise. *This also prevents contamination with body fluids.*

Individual or disposable crockery and cutlery should be used as required *to maintain a safe environment.*

Urine and faeces do not require special treatment, but *the use of a separate toilet or commode helps to reduce cross-infection.*

Wound infections   The patient should be nursed in a single room or cubicle.

Gloves should be worn, especially when performing dressings or handling potentially infected bed linen or clothing *to prevent contamination with body fluids as well as preventing transmission of infection* (Thomas 1994).

A mask may only be necessary when performing dressings, depending on the infection.

A plastic apron may be adequate protective clothing depending on the organism causing the infection.

Good hand washing technique is essential *to ensure there is no transmission of infection.*

Enteric infections   The patient should be nursed in a single room or cubicle with adequate individual toilet facilities *as enteric infections are readily transmitted* (Epton 1990). Gowns, plastic aprons and gloves should be worn, but a mask is not necessary. Individual or disposable crockery and cutlery should be used as required *to prevent infection.* Vomitus and faeces will be infected and should be disposed of according to local policies. This may include covering the infected matter with disinfectant for a period of time *to destroy the causal organisms.*

Toilet utensils should be disposable and treated as infected waste *to maintain a safe environment.*

Before removing protective clothing, the gloved hands should be washed *to reduce contamination* and further hand washing performed as in the Guidelines above.

Viral infections   Special precautions are applicable when a patient has a viral infection caused by:

- hepatitis B virus
- human immunodeficiency virus (HIV) which may develop into acquired immune deficiency syndrome (AIDS) (Pratt 1994)

These patients may be suffering from the disease or carry the virus in their blood and should be treated as having infected blood and body fluids. The caring personnel are most at risk of infection in this situation. Precautions should be maintained for all patients suspected of being 'carriers' until investigations prove negative. According to current knowledge, the people most likely to be infected are:

- addicts who take drugs by the intravenous route and use contaminated needles *as the infection is blood-borne*
- male homosexuals, especially those with numerous partners, *as HIV can be*

transmitted during sexual intercourse. Recent figures show an increase among heterosexuals
- babies born to mothers who are infected *because the virus crosses the placenta barrier*
- people who have been transfused with contaminated blood or blood products
- patients from, or who have recently visited, tropical or subtropical countries *where there is a relatively higher incidence of the disease.*

Every precaution should be taken to prevent personnel in contact with the patient from being infected by the virus; it would have to enter the blood circulation through a break in the skin or through the mucosa of the non-infected individual. The degree of risk is assessed by the medical practitioner and precautions prescribed accordingly.

Low risk situations   Precautions should be taken when handling blood and body secretions. Gloves should be worn at all times. Special care should be taken when handling and disposing of syringes and needles. Sharps containers should be treated as infected and labelled with special stickers. Blood and other specimens for investigation should be labelled with special stickers and placed in 2 bags before being sent to the laboratory.

High risk situations   Additional precautions may be prescribed, for example when carrying out an invasive procedure for patients known to be infected by HIV or hepatitis B. Strict isolation nursing should be maintained and protective clothing should include goggles worn by attending personnel, as well as efficient masks *to prevent any infected secretion or blood splashing the eyes or mouth of the carer.* In some areas where such patients are known to be admitted, a protective 'pack' is available for immediate use. The infection control personnel should be the resource centre for any special requirements.

Health care personnel should be vaccinated against hepatitis B (refer to health authority policies).

2   Protective isolation (reverse barrier nursing)

In this situation the infected area is the environment of the ward and the non-infected area is the isolation area. Pathogens are prevented from entering the isolation area by protective isolation for the patient. The principles and the guidelines are the same but the procedure is reversed.

Indications and rationale for protective isolation

This is carried out *to prevent the spread of infection to patients who have a reduced resistance to infection due to their disease condition or to prescribed treatment,* for example:
- patients who have leukaemia *which causes immature and defective white blood cells and decreases resistance to infection*
- patients who have reduced autoimmunity due to cytotoxic medication for treatment of malignant disease, *and may have a reduced white blood cell count*

- patients who are receiving immunosuppressive medication following transplant surgery *which also reduces the level of white blood cells.*

The following precautions are emphasised:

A filter-type mask must be used by all personnel *to protect the patient from droplet infection.*

The form of protective clothing depends on the patient's condition. Gowns should be worn when nursing children, or patients who are at particular risk of infection, but in some instances a plastic apron will be sufficient *to prevent cross-infection from the nurse's uniform.*

A cap and overshoes may be worn *as a further precaution.*

All personnel must be meticulous in their hand washing technique *to maintain a safe environment* (Gould 1994).

Alcohol hand rub should be applied frequently to the nurse's hands *to further reduce the risk of cross-infection.*

Special air flow facilities, e.g. a laminar flow system, may be used *to prevent a flow of air from the ward area to the isolation area. This decreases the risk of infection from the ward environment.*

The precautions should be explained to visitors, who should be limited to close relatives and friends *reducing the risk of infection.* Appropriate protective clothing should be worn *to maintain a safe environment for the patient* (Curran 1994).

Visitors and other personnel should not be in contact with the patient if they have a cold, sore throat or other infection, however mild, *which might infect the immunosuppressed patient.* The reason for this precaution should be explained.

Nursing should be planned so that only one or two of the staff are caring for the patient during a span of duty *to reduce the risk of infection from ward personnel.*

3   Radioactive hazard isolation

Patients receiving large doses of radioactive isotopes, either systemically or by implant, are normally nursed in specially equipped units which have barriers against radioactivity built in to the environment and are equipped with specialised screens. However, radioactive isotopes are being used more frequently for diagnostic purposes, and nurses may care for patients undergoing such investigations in general wards.

Indications and rationale for radioactive hazard isolation

This is carried out *to prevent radioactive contamination to carers and others when radioactive substances are used*:

- to treat patients who have malignant tumours with radioactive implants or radioactive isotopes
- for diagnostic investigations using radioactive isotopes.

The isolation technique is aimed at *reducing the risk of radiation for other patients and caring personnel by limiting the time spent near the patient having radioactive treatment, and keeping a safe distance away at other times.* The patient should be nursed in a single room, or confined to one particular area of the ward. Lead screens should be used *as a shield from radiation when radioactive implants are inserted,* according to individual requirements. Radioactive material should be transported in lead containers *to prevent any escape of radioactivity.*

Guidelines and rationale for this nursing practice	<ul><li>consult the radiation protection officer and health authority policy *to ascertain appropriate precautions for particular radioactive substances used for treatment or investigations*</li><li>explain the precautions and their implications to the patient *and gain consent and cooperation*</li><li>ensure that all staff wear radiation detection badges. *This will monitor individual doses of radiation and ensure that no one is exposed to dangerous levels*</li><li>plan nursing so that no nurse is in an area of radiation for longer than necessary, and share care *so that each nurse has a reduced exposure time*</li><li>don protective lead aprons if appropriate *to block the passage of radiation*</li><li>wear gloves for all nursing practices and when handling any bed clothes or linen which may be contaminated by radioactive excreta and body fluid *to prevent contamination* (Thomas 1994)</li><li>dispose of linen and waste according to health authority policy, labelling materials with special radioactive warning stickers *to maintain a safe environment*</li><li>wear gloves to wipe up any spillage of suspected radioactive material immediately with paper tissues and rinse the area with water *to reduce radioactivity.* The tissues should be treated as radioactive waste</li><li>dilute urine and faeces with water and flush as soon as possible *to reduce radioactivity.*</li></ul>

Radioactive materials have a reducing 'half life' *so that precautions will only need to be carried out for a specific, prescribed period of time.* Once the danger of radioactivity is considered negligible, precautions may be discontinued.

It is advisable that staff who have had close contact with radioactive materials should have a shower and a change of clothing when coming off duty, as *an extra precaution.*

In radiotherapy units, special guidelines may apply and a Geiger counter may be used to assess radioactivity levels before disposing of radioactive material.

Relevance to the activities of living	Observations and further rationale for this nursing practice will be included within each activity of living as appropriate.

Maintaining a safe environment

The whole concept of isolation nursing is related to maintaining a safe environment for the patient or those who come into contact with him or his fomites.

With infected patients the emphasis is on maintaining a safe environment for other people by preventing the spread of the infection. The nursing and medical personnel are the key figures in this.

The safe environment of other hospital staff, e.g. porters and laundry staff, as well as the general public, is maintained by safe disposal of infected waste and linen. Bagging and labelling infected blood products for investigation ensures a safe environment for transportation and laboratory staff.

Protective isolation is aimed at maintaining a safe environment for the patient at risk of infection while the treatment for the disease is continued. Once the patient's immune system is able to maintain his own safe environment, isolation procedures can be reduced gradually; initially he may be allowed to eat unsterile food, while staff still wear masks and practise reverse barrier nursing. The patient is then re-introduced to a normal environment over a period of days. During the isolation period it is important that he is not exposed to any known infection. Staff and visitors with colds or sore throats should be excluded at all times, and the reason for this explained.

Radiation isolation is aimed at maintaining a safe environment for those in the vicinity of the radiation, while giving nursing care to the patient.

Appropriate hand washing technique is a most important means of maintaining a safe environment.

Communicating

This activity of living is most influenced by isolation nursing. Isolation immediately affects the normal person-to-person communication process. The patient often becomes depressed and bored because the number of people in contact with him is greatly reduced; visitors are limited and staff limit the number of times they enter and leave the area. The isolation increases when the door to a room is required to be shut and when the door and corridor wall are not made of glass.

The nurses need to be perceptive to the needs of the patient and should discuss with him and his visitors the best way of coping with the isolation problem.

An individual television is a great help, and should be considered essential equipment. A two-way radio or voice link system will enable staff to chat to the patient, and the patient to call the staff, thus reducing the feeling of isolation, but still maintaining the safe environment. A bell must be available so that the patient can summon assistance.

Interests such as reading, crafts, letter writing and jigsaw puzzles should be encouraged as the patient's condition allows. Most articles can be decontaminated, or sterilised as required. Isolation areas should ideally be glass cubicles where the patient can see the outside environment and have a window with an interesting view.

Blood-borne infection such as HIV has a high media profile. Nurses should be responsible communicators to promote health education on the subject, and should also help to minimise intolerant attitudes by using appropriate verbal and non-verbal communication skills.

Eating and drinking

Some patients are prescribed sterile food and drinks whilst in protective isolation, and these are available in cans, although the patient may find them boring after a while. It is important that the patient maintains an adequate diet while treatment continues. Microwave ovens can sterilise normal food and utensils, so food can be safely prepared in this way. The dietician should be asked for help as appropriate.

Patients with enteric infections may have an intravenous infusion in situ. When they are able to eat and drink, individualised or disposable crockery and cutlery should be used.

Eliminating

Ideally, all isolation patients should be nursed in a single room with individual toilet and washing facilities. Special precautions are needed for patients who have diarrhoea due to enteric infection.

Personal cleansing and dressing

Patients undergoing source isolation may have to wear hospital garments, or disposable clothes, which may add to the problems of isolation and stigma.

Patients in protective isolation should be encouraged to wear their own freshly laundered day and night clothes. (Arrangements for sterilisation may be necessary.) This will help to encourage individuality and self esteem.

Controlling body temperature

Patients isolated because of a specific infection should have their temperature recorded 2-hourly or 4-hourly as appropriate, to monitor the course of the infection and associated fever. All necessary equipment for recording should remain within the isolation area. Documentation should remain uncontaminated outside the area.

Expressing sexuality

The whole procedure of isolation may give the patient an impression of having an altered body image, due to the stigma felt by the patient who has an infection.

Perceptive and supportive nursing care and good communication skills will help to alleviate the feeling of rejection.

Patient education: key points

- The reason for the specific precautions should be explained to the patient and his relatives.

- Detailed patient education about the specific precautions for each individual infection will be needed throughout this nursing practice
- For immunosuppressed patients, specific teaching of skills in self care, i.e. mouth care, will be needed and the importance of these reinforced
- Patients with MRSA should understand the importance of reporting that they have had this infection when visiting outpatients or on re-admission, as recurrence may be a problem
- Patients with HIV and AIDS should have a good knowledge of precautions for the prevention of cross-infection to maintain a safe environment. Good communication skills, both verbal and non-verbal, are required to reinforce the nurse's non-judgmental attitude and to reduce any feeling of stigma on the part of the patient and his family
- Patients being discharged following recent investigations using radioactive isotopes should be given information sheets concerning the disposal of body fluids. Liaison with the community team will help to reinforce any precautions needed.

References

Alderman C 1992 Never a dull moment. Role of the infection control nurse. Nursing Standard 6(2): 18–19
Ayton M 1984 Protective clothing. What do we use and when? Nursing Times 80(20): 68–69
Bowell E 1990 Assessing infection risks. Nursing 4(12): 19–23
Curran E 1994 Taking down the barriers. Professional Nurse 9(7): 472–478
Denton F 1986 Psychological and physiological effects of isolation. Nursing 3(3): 88–91
Elliot P 1992 Hand washing, a process of judgement and effective decision making. Professional Nurse 7(5): 292, 294–296
Epton V 1990 Salmonella. What risk? Nursing 4(20): 14–16
Gould D 1994 Making sense of hand hygiene. Nursing Times 90(30): 63–64
Pratt R 1994 Safe practice (HIV and AIDS). Nursing Times 90(27): 64–68
Taylor L 1990 Infection control at your fingertips, procedures for preventing and controlling MRSA. Professional Nurse, July: 547–551
Thomas L 1994 Glove story: cost benefit analysis. Nursing Times 90(36): 31–35

Further reading

Akinsanya J, Rouse P 1992 Who will care. A survey of knowledge and attitudes of hospital nurses to people with HIV and AIDS. Journal of Advanced Nursing 17: 400–401
Clulow H 1994 A closer look at disposable gloves. An assessment of the value of vinyl, latex and plastic gloves. Professional Nurse 9(5): 324–329
Farnsworth B 1994 Managing health and safety in hospitals. British Journal of Nursing 3(16): 831–836
Gould D, Chamberlain A 1994 Infection control as a topic for ward based nursing education. Journal of Advanced Nursing 20(2): 275–285
Horton R 1995 Infection control and the bedside nurse. British Journal of Nursing 41(87): 428–430
Kingston J 1994 Same problems, different system. A UK perspective of infection control in an American hospital. Professional Nurse 9(12): 790–797
Oakley K 1994 Making sense of universal precautions. Nursing Times 90(27): 34–36
Siu A 1994 Methicillin-resistant staphylococcus aureus: do we just have to live with it? British Journal of Nursing 3(15): 753–759

27 Liver Biopsy

Learning outcomes

By the end of this section you should know how to:
- prepare the patient for this procedure
- collect and prepare the equipment
- assist the medical practitioner during the liver biopsy
- care for the patient prior to, during and following a liver biopsy.

Background knowledge required

Revision of the anatomy and physiology of the liver with special reference to the position and the functions of the liver.

Revision of Asceptic technique (*see* p. 383).

Indications and rationale for a liver biopsy

A liver biopsy is the removal of a small piece of liver tissue, using a specially designed needle, *to aid in the diagnosis of a liver disease.*

Outline of the procedure

Prior to this investigation the patient will have blood samples taken for estimation of bleeding, clotting and prothrombin times (Long et al 1995). A platelet count, grouping and cross-matching will also be requested by the medical practitioner (Topping 1992). A patient who requires a liver biopsy may be suffering from a blood clotting defect which may prevent or defer investigation. The patient may have some form of sedation prescribed prior to the procedure.

The biopsy will be carried out under local anaesthetic by a medical practitioner using an aseptic technique. It may be necessary for the biopsy to be obtained under ultrasound imaging if cells from a specific area of the liver are required by the medical practitioner (Miller et al 1994). The patient should lie in a supine position, using one pillow, with his right hand under his head. The biopsy needle will be inserted through a stab incision to rest above the surface of the liver. The patient is asked to hold his breath in full expiration as the medical practitioner advances the biopsy needle into the liver then withdraws the needle (Fig. 27.1). The patient can then resume his normal breathing pattern. Pressure should be applied to the biopsy site for 5 minutes using a sterile swab. Once the bleeding has ceased or is minimal the site can be covered with a sterile dry dressing.

Equipment

Sterile gloves
Sterile dressings pack

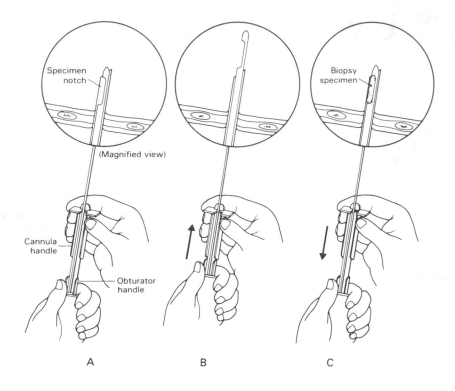

Figure 27.1 *Liver biopsy: method of securing a specimen of tissue*
A Introducing a biopsy needle: cannula (outer) and obturator (inner)
B Obtaining tissue specimen by advancing the obturator handle, and pushing the cutting edge of the obturator's specimen notch into the liver tissue
C Withdrawing the obturator handle to enclose the specimen within the cannula, then removing the entire biopsy needle

Alcohol-based antiseptic for skin cleansing

Local anaesthetic and equipment for its administration

Sterile disposable scalpel or similar equipment

Sterile liver biopsy needle, e.g. Trucut

Sterile adhesive dressing

Sterile specimen container with preservative appropriately labelled and with a completed laboratory form and plastic specimen bag for transportation

Trolley for equipment

Receptacle for soiled disposables.

Guidelines and rationale for this nursing practice

- help the medical practitioner to explain the procedure to the patient *to gain consent and cooperation*
- wash the hands *to reduce cross-infection*
- give the patient sedation if prescribed *as this may help to reduce excessive patient anxiety*
- ensure the patient's privacy *to further assist in the reduction of anxiety*
- collect and prepare the equipment and trolley as required *to ensure all equipment is available and ready for use*
- help the patient into the correct position *as this will assist in a positive outcome of the procedure*

- ensure that the patient is as comfortable as possible *as this position will require to be maintained throughout the procedure*
- observe the patient throughout this activity *to note any signs of distress*
- assist the medical practitioner as necessary during the procedure *to permit the procedure to be completed in a safe and competent manner*
- remain with the patient and help maintain his position as required during the biopsy *providing physical and psychological support during an unfamiliar experience*
- help the patient re-position himself onto his right side, with a small pillow under the costal margin, for 2 hours following the liver biopsy (Topping 1992) *to reduce the escape of blood and bile from the biopsy site*
- ensure that the patient is left feeling as comfortable as possible *maintaining the quality of this nursing practice*
- dispose of the equipment safely *to reduce any health hazard*
- dispatch the labelled specimen to the laboratory immediately with the completed laboratory form *to permit microscopic examination of the tissue of the correct patient*
- document the nursing practice appropriately, monitor after-effects, and report any abnormal findings immediately *providing a written record and assisting in the implementation of any action should an abnormality or adverse reaction to the practice be noted.*

Relevance to the activities of living

Maintaining a safe environment

As this is an invasive procedure all precautions against, and observations to detect, infection should be implemented. Unless a complication arises the adhesive dressing can be removed within 2–3 days following the biopsy.

For safe transportation of the specimen collection, *see* page 302.

Communicating

An easily understood explanation of the procedure and the aftercare should be given to the patient. This is primarily given by the medical practitioner but the nurse may be required to repeat the explanation.

Requesting the patient to turn his head to the left during the procedure could be helpful in the prevention of increased patient anxiety brought about by observing the medical practitioner's actions and the equipment used.

The patient may require a mild analgesic for pain at the biopsy site or referred pain, i.e. shoulder-tip pain. Should the patient complain of severe pain this must be reported immediately to the medical practitioner as it may be a sign of biliary peritonitis, which is known to be a potential complication following liver biopsy (Booth 1983).

Breathing

The patient should have frequent recordings of blood pressure, pulse and respiration rates for 24 hours following a liver biopsy while the biopsy site should be observed for continued bleeding or haematoma formation (Topping 1992).

A sudden change in the patient's cardiovascular or respiratory function, such as a drop in blood pressure or dyspnoea, must be reported. This may signify injury to other tissues during the biopsy leading to the development of the known complications of haemorrhage or a pneumothorax. The risk of tearing the liver and damaging the lung tissue is greatly reduced if the patient holds his breath in full expiration as the biopsy needle is advanced into the liver (Long et al 1995).

Mobilising

The patient may remain in bed for the 24 hours following the biopsy, the first 2 hours of the period spent quietly lying on his right side to compress the liver against the chest wall. This will help to reduce the possibility of haemorrhage.

Patient education: key points

The medical practitioner and the nurse should provide information regarding the necessity for this procedure. The patient and relatives will need time to ask questions and discuss any aspect of the planned procedure.

Before the procedure the nurse should give information and the rationale about the position the patient requires to adopt during and following the biopsy and the aftercare which will be delivered.

References

Booth J 1983 Handbook of investigations. Harper & Row, London, pp 25–27

Long B, Phipps W, Cassmeyer V (eds) 1995 Adult nursing: a nursing process approach. Mosby-Times Mirror International Publishers, London, ch 22

Miller R, Howie E, Murchie M 1994 The gastrointestinal system, liver and biliary tract. In: Alexander M, Fawcett J, Runciman P (eds) Nursing practice — hospital and home: the adult. Churchill Livingstone, Edinburgh

Topping A 1992 Caring for patient with disorders of the liver, biliary tract and exocrine pancreas. In: Royle J, Walsh M (eds) Watson's Medical-surgical nursing and related physiology, 4th edn. Bailliere Tindall, London

Further reading

Brunner I, Suddarth D 1992 The textbook of adult nursing. Chapman Hall, London, ch 16

28 Lumbar Puncture

Learning outcomes

By the end of this section you should know how to:
- prepare the patient for this nursing practice
- collect and prepare the equipment
- assist the medical practitioner to perform a lumbar puncture.

Background knowledge required

Revision of the anatomy and physiology of the brain and spinal cord, with special reference to the cerebrospinal fluid and the meninges.

Revision of the anatomy of the lumber vertebrae.

Revision of Aseptic technique (*see* p. 383).

Indications and rationale for lumbar puncture

Lumbar puncture is the insertion of a specialised needle into the lumbar subarachnoid space *to gain access to the cerebrospinal fluid (CSF)*. This may be required:
- *to obtain a sample of cerebrospinal fluid for investigative and diagnostic purposes* (Quigley et al 1989), e.g.:
  — bacteriological investigation for patients suspected of having meningitis or encephalitis
  — cytological investigation for patients suspected of having a malignant tumour
- *to identify the presence of blood in the cerebrospinal fluid following trauma or a suspected subarachnoid haemorrhage*
- *to introduce radio-opaque fluid into the subarachnoid space for radiographic investigation*
- *to identify raised intraspinal/intracranial pressure and provide relief if appropriate by removing some of the cerebrospinal fluid*
- *to introduce intrathecal medication such as cytotoxic agents or antibiotics.*

Outline of the procedure

A lumbar puncture is performed by a medical practitioner using aseptic technique. The patient is helped into the correct position. An area of skin above the 3rd, 4th and 5th lumbar vertebrae is prepared and cleansed with antiseptic solution prior to the administration of local anaesthesia. A special lumbar puncture needle is inserted between the 3rd and 4th lumbar vertebrae or 4th and 5th lumbar vertebrae in order to gain access to the subarachnoid space below the spinal cord in the region of the cauda equina (Fig. 28.1). Once in position the stilette of the needle is removed. A manometer is attached to the end of the

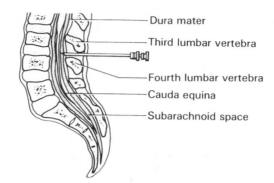

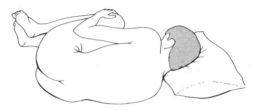

Figure 28.1   *Lumbar puncture: position of the needle in relation to the vertebrae*

Figure 28.2   *Lumbar punctre: position of the patient*

needle via a two-way tap and the cerebrospinal fluid is allowed to flow into the manometer to record intraspinal pressure. At this stage the medical practitioner may require Queckenstedt's test to be performed (*see* p. 204).

When pressure recordings are completed the manometer is occluded, and 2 or 3 ml of cerebrospinal fluid is allowed to flow into three separate sterile specimen containers as required while still maintaining asepsis. The medical practitioner will note the colour, consistency and opacity of the cerebrospinal fluid as well as observing the presence or absence of blood. On completion the needle is removed and the puncture site is covered by a small sterile dressing or plastic sealant spray. The patient remains lying flat in bed for 6–12 hours following this procedure and appropriate observations are maintained during this period (Allan 1989).

The position of the patient

The correct position is important for the success and safety of this procedure. The patient should lie on his side on a firm bed with one pillow. He should stretch his lumbar vertebrae by flexing his head and neck and drawing his knees up to his abdomen, holding them with his hands (Fig. 28.2). The nurse can assist by supporting the patient behind the knees and the neck, and helping to maintain the extension of the lumbar vertebrae, thus widening the intervertebral space. This will help to ensure that the insertion and correct placement of the lumbar puncture needle is safely achieved. Once the needle is in position the medical practitioner may ask the patient to slowly straighten his legs without moving the position of his back. This will reduce the intra-abdominal pressure which can cause an abnormal reading of intraspinal pressure.

Very occasionally this procedure is performed with a patient sitting straddled on a chair and facing the back of the chair with his head resting on folded arms. This position may be chosen by the medical practitioner when performing a lumbar puncture for an obese patient with dyspnoea who may be distressed when lying flat.

Equipment	Trolley

Trolley

Sterile dressings pack

Sterile drapes

Sterile surgical gloves for the medical practitioner

Sterile lumbar puncture set containing:
- lumbar puncture needle
- spinal manometer
- two-way tap

Alcohol-based antiseptic lotion for cleansing the skin

Local anaesthetic and equipment for its administration

Syringe and needles for local anaesthetic

Sterile dressing, e.g. Airstrip or plastic sealant spray

Three sterile specimen containers appropriately labelled, completed laboratory forms, and plastic specimen bag for transportation. These may be required for three separate samples of CSF for microbiological, biochemical and cytological investigation

Watch with seconds had for Queckenstedt's test

Receptacle for disposables.

Lumbar puncture needle

This is a rigid stainless steel needle 5 cm (approx) in length, complete with its own sharp-pointed stilette; this helps the entry of the needle into the correct position. Once the stilette is removed, the blunt end of the needle lies within the subarachnoid space, and should cause no damage to tissue during the procedure. Needles are usually supplied with their own metal two-way tap, but a Luer disposable tap may be used.

Guidelines and rationale for this nursing practice

- help to explain the procedure to the patient *to gain consent and cooperation to encourage participation in care*
- ensure the patient's privacy *to respect his individuality and maintain his self esteem*
- help to collect and prepare the equipment
- help to prepare the sterile field *to maintain asepsis*
- help the patient into the appropriate position, and remain with him *to maintain that position and maximise the safety of the procedure*
- observe the patient throughout this activity *to monitor any adverse effects*

- help to expose the lumbar region of the patient's back and assist the medical practitioner, as required, *to maintain asepsis and help to reassure the patient*
- encourage the patient to breathe quietly *in order to prevent hyperventilation which gives a false low pressure reading*
- assist the medical practitioner with the Queckenstedt's test if required by compressing the jugular vein, or veins, as directed (see below)
- hold the appropriate sterile containers *to receive the flow of CSF as directed, maintaining asepsis*
- ensure that the puncture site is covered with a sterile dressing or plastic sealant spray once the needle is removed *to prevent leakage of CSF and maintain asepsis*
- help the patient into a comfortable position, lying flat with only one pillow, once the procedure is completed, explaining the importance of maintaining this position for 6–12 hours following the procedure *as changes in pressure sometimes cause headache* (Bass & Vandervoort 1988)
- ensure the patient is left feeling as comfortable as possible with everything he requires at hand *to reassure him and help the healing process*. Ideally, a period of rest should be encouraged after any stressful experience
- dispose of the equipment safely *to maintain a safe environment and prevent transmission of infection*
- document the procedure appropriately, monitor after-effects, and report abnormal findings immediately, *ensuring safe practice and enabling prompt appropriate medical and nursing action to be initiated* (UKCC 1993)
- dispatch the labelled CSF specimens to the laboratory with their completed forms immediately *so that investigations may be initiated and decisions about appropriate treatment can be made as soon as possible* (Allan & Craig 1994)

Queckenstedt's test

This test is performed to determine whether or not there is an obstruction in the spinal subarachnoid pathway. Obstruction may be caused by a fractured or dislocated vertebra, or a tumour. Normally there is a rapid rise in intraspinal pressure when jugular compression is applied and an equally rapid return to normal when pressure is released. Any obstruction will cause a much slower rise and fall of the intraspinal pressure. The test is only performed to investigate a spinal lesion. It is never performed when an intracranial lesion is suspected, as raised intracranial pressure could increase the risk of brain damage.

The medical practitioner will ask for jugular compression to be applied for the maximum of 10 seconds and released for 10 seconds. Pressure readings are recorded for each 10-second interval. (Fig. 28.3)

Relevance to the activities of living   Observations and further rationale for this nursing practice will be included within each activity of living as appropriate.

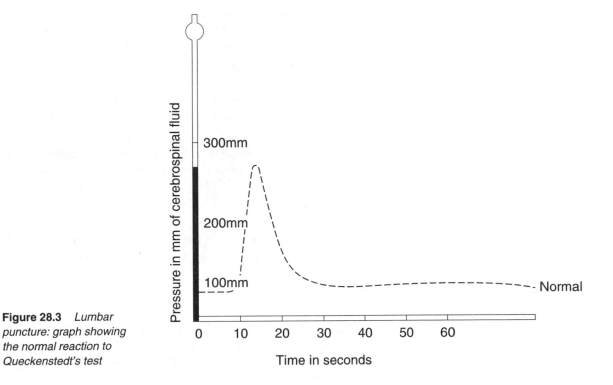

Figure 28.3 *Lumbar puncture: graph showing the normal reaction to Queckenstedt's test*

Maintaining a safe environment

This is an invasive procedure which involves direct access to the spinal and brain tissue via the cerebrospinal fluid. Asepsis should be maintained during and following the procedure, and adequate hand washing technique should be practised to prevent cross-infection. The puncture site should be observed for evidence of localised infection or leakage; accurate observations of the patient's condition will help to monitor any evidence of developing infection.

A lumbar puncture is performed as a neurological investigataion. A patient who is confused or disorientated may need cot sides on the bed to prevent falls and maintain the safety of his environment.

A lumbar puncture should not be performed if raised intracranial pressure is suspected. The raised pressure may cause the brain stem tissue to herniate through the foramen magnum. This is known as 'coning' and could be fatal.

Safety of staff transporting specimens should be maintained by enclosing containers in plastic specimen bags (*see* Specimen collection, p. 297).

Communicating

After the procedure, the patient should lie horizontally with only one pillow, either supine or on his side. This will minimise the effect of changes in intraspinal pressure caused by the removal of 1–3 ml of CSF during the procedure, and help to prevent headache or dizziness occurring. This position is usually maintained for 6–12 hours, depending on the patient's condition. There is, however, conflicting evidence about the length of time the patient needs to remain horizontal following this procedure (Carpaat & Vancrevel 1981).

The patient's general condition should be noted, e.g. orientation, restlessness, drowsiness, nausea.

Any evidence of cerebral irritability should be observed. Fitting, twitching, spasticity or weakness of limb movements should be reported immediately and recorded (Hart et al 1988).

The patient's level of consciousness should be recorded as prescribed, depending on his condition. Neurological observations should be maintained for 18–24 hours following this investigation (*see* care of the Unconscious patient, p. 347).

The patient may complain of a headache following this procedure. Analgesic medication should be administered as prescribed. The nurse should be observant for any non-verbal communication indicating pain, and anticipate the patient's needs as appropriate. The fact that the patient might experience discomfort should be explained to him.

Breathing

The pulse, respiration and blood pressure should be recorded 4-hourly, or as indicated by the patient's condition, Abnormalities may indicate developing infection or evidence of cerebral changes, and should be reported immediately.

Eating and drinking

A normal diet may be ordered as the patient's condition allows. However, while he is lying flat some adjustments and help may be needed. An adequate fluid intake should be maintained following the procedure. Drinks should be easily accessible to the patient, and specialised cups or straws used as appropriate.

Eliminating

It may be necessary for the patient to use a urinal/bedpan instead of a commode for a period following the procedure because of the 6–12 hours' bedrest; the reason for this should be explained to the patient.

Controlling body temperature

The temperature should be monitored for as long as necessary following the procedure. Four-hourly recordings should be maintained for 48 hours and any rise in temperature which might indicate a developing infection should be reported.

Mobilising

The patient should remain flat in bed for 6–12 hours following the procedure to prevent headache or dizziness. Mobilising should commence with the patient sitting up in bed for a period of time before progressing to further activity, as his condition allows. This will reduce any further risk of headaches or dizziness, which can occur if the patient changes his position too rapidly following this procedure.

Patient education: key points

The reason for the investigation and the importance of a lumbar puncture for diagnostic purposes should be explained. This should include the fact that the investigation itself should have no long-term effects.

The importance of retaining a correct position should be carefully explained and reinforced.

Following the lumbar puncture the patient should be told the importance of remaining flat for a period of time, and the reason for this.

The patient should understand the importance of reporting a headache or any other adverse effects to the nursing staff, who will be monitoring her condition following a lumbar puncture.

Any redness, swelling or soreness at the site should be reported. If the patient is discharged home, adverse effects should be reported to the medical practitioner or community nurse immediately.

References

Allan D 1989 Making sense of . . . lumbar puncture. Nursing Times 85(49) 39–42

Allan D, Craig E 1994 The nervous system. In: Alexander M, Fawcett J, Runciman P (eds) Nursing practice — hospital and home: the adult. Churchill Livingstone, Edinburgh, pp 363–364

Bass B, Vandervoort M K 1988 Post lumbar puncture headache. Canadian Nurse 84(4): 15–18

Carpaat P, Vancrevel H 1981 Lumbar puncture headache. Controlled study. Lancet 8256(11): 1133–1134

Hart I, Bone I, Hadley D 1988 Development of neurological problems after lumbar puncture. British Medical Journal 296(2): 51–52

Quigley J et al 1989 Neurological investigations. Nursing 3(33): 12–17

UKCC 1993 Standards for records and record keeping. United Kingdom Central Council for Nursing, Midwifery and Health Visiting, London

Further reading

Allan D (ed) 1988 Nursing and the neurosciences. Churchill Livingstone, Edinburgh, pp 54–56

Roper N, Logan W, Tierney A 1996 The elements of nursing, 4th edn. Churchill Livingstone, Edinburgh, pp 114–138

29 Mouth Care

Learning outcomes	By the end of this section you should know how to:

By the end of this section you should know how to:

- prepare the patient for this nursing practice
- collect and prepare the equipment
- carry out mouth care according to the individual needs of the patient in both a community and institutional setting.

Background knowledge required

Revision of the anatomy and physiology of the mouth and pharynx, with special reference to the teeth, the salivary glands and the oral mucosa.

Revision of pharmaceutical literature related to mouthwashes and mouth-cleaning preparations in current use.

Review of health authority policy related to mouth care in both community and institutional care.

Indications and rationale for mouth care

Mouth care is the use of a toothbrush and paste, a mouthwash or other mouth-cleaning preparation *to help the patient maintain the cleanliness of his teeth or dentures,* and *to encourage the flow of saliva to maintain a healthy oropharyngeal mucosa.* The condition of the teeth, gums and mouth is not only an indication of the general health of an individual but may also influence overall health status (WHO 1988).

This nursing practice is also known as oral hygiene and may be required:

- for any patient who has not eaten for a period of time or whose diet is restricted, *as reduction in mastication decreases the flow of saliva,* e.g. during the preoperative or postoperative period, and especially for patients who have undergone oral or abdominal surgery
- for patients who are dehydrated for any reason *as the normal flow of saliva will be reduced*
- for patients suffering from nausea or vomiting *as they will be reluctant to eat*
- for patients being treated with oxygen therapy *which has a drying effect on the oral mucosa*
- for patients who are having radiotherapy or cytotoxic medication for malignant diseases, *as this may adversely affect the cells of the oral mucosa* (Porter 1994)
- for patients with any form of facial paralysis or muscle weakness *as inability to masticate adequately reduces the flow of saliva and may cause food debris to be retained in the mouth.* This may include an unconcious patient or one in the terminal stages of illness.

The frequency of mouth care will vary for each individual. Intensive mouth care may be carried out every 2 hours, whereas mouthwashes may only be required 2 or 3 times a day.

Equipment

Suitable tray or trolley

Plastic gloves (non-sterile)

Pencil torch

Spatula

Toothbrush

Toothpaste

Container for dentures (for institutional care this should be appropriately labelled)

Beaker

Bowl or receiver

Towel or other protective covering

Mouthwash solution

Soft tissues for wiping the mouth

Receptacle for disposables.

Additional equipment for specialised mouth care as required

- Mouth-care pack or equivalent equipment
- Plastic gloves (non-sterile)
- Foam sticks
- Cotton buds
- Prescribed medication, e.g. antifungal agent, if thrush is diagnosed
- Solution for mouth cleaning
- Lubrication for lips, e.g. petroleum jelly
- Suction equipment.

Toothbrush and toothpaste

The patient's own equipment may be used if available, otherwise a soft small-headed nylon brush and toothpaste can be supplied. Usually this is the most appropriate equipment for this nursing practice.

Solutions for mouthwashes

Various solutions are available. Professional knowledge or individual prescription and patient preference will influence the choice of preparation used (Hatton-Smith 1994).

All solutions used should be clearly labelled and diluted according to instructions. The procedure for checking the preparation is as for Administration of medicines (p. 2).

Saline   This can be made up using common salt, one level teaspoon (4.5 g approx) in 500 ml water. It is also available in sterile sachets. This is an effective mouthwash for patients who have had oral surgery, especially dental extractions.

Thymol   This is prepared in solution and is the main component of most mouthwash tablets. It has a mild antiseptic effect and is well tolerated when diluted to suit the patient's taste.

Sodium bicarbonate   This may be made up immediately prior to use. One level teaspoon of powder in 500 ml of water is a useful mouthwash for dissolving mucus and debris. A stronger solution can be used for soaking dentures before cleaning them.

Corsodyl   This is a commercial preparation containing chlorhexidine which is thought to inhibit plaque formation. It may be prescribed for patients having cytotoxic therapy.

Cold water   This may be the most refreshing and appropriate mouthwash to use after brushing the teeth.

Other aids for mouth care (if permitted)

Soda water   This may be appreciated as an alternative mouthwash.

Ice cubes   These may be sucked, but the number should be limited if the patient has restricted oral intake.

Fresh fruit   This can be sucked and removed. Pineapple, if allowed, can be very refreshing and will stimulate saliva.

Solutions for mouth cleaning

Any mouthwash solution can be used for mouth cleaning, as well as solutions which actively stimulate the flow of saliva.

A mild toothpaste applied with a soft small-headed toothbrush remains the most efficient method of mouth cleaning.

The toothbrush may be dipped in any mouthwash/mouth cleaning solution acceptable to the patient.

Mouth-care pack

This prepared sterile pack is used when intensive mouth care is needed for patients for whom a mouthwash alone, or tooth-brushing, is not appropriate. The pack may contain:

- plastic tray divided into compartments to hold the mouth-cleaning solution
- plastic forceps
- dental rolls or cotton sticks
- foam sticks
- gauze swabs.

If the pack is not available a sterile mouth-care tray can be assembled using:

- foil tray
- gallipot
- plastic forceps
- gauze swabs
- foam sticks
- dental rolls or cotton sticks.

The mouth-care pack should be covered, labelled with the patient's name and the date, cleaned and replenished after use, and replaced every 24 hours or as required. In the patient's own home, equipment will be adapted appropriately, maintaining a safe environment.

Guidelines and rationale for this nursing practice

- explain the nursing practice to the patient *to gain consent and cooperation and encourage participation in care, ensuring that there is some understanding of this practice*
- collect and prepare the equipment *to ensure efficient use of time and resources.* Some solutions are more effective if prepared immediately before use
- ensure the patient's privacy *to respect her individuality and maintain her self esteem*
- help the patient into a comfortable sitting position, either in bed or on a chair *to help patient cooperation and promote as much independence as possible.* Sometimes it is possible for the patient to sit comfortably in front of the wash-hand basin either in his own home or in an institution
- place some protective material over the patient's chest and under his chin *to protect his clothes.* The patient's own towel could be used
- observe the patient throughout this activity *to monitor any adverse effects*
- don clean plastic gloves after efficient hand washing *to prevent contamination with body fluids and to maintain a safe environment*
- ask or help the patient to remove his dentures and place them in a bowl of clean water (labelled if necessary) *to gain access and a clear view of the oral cavity*
- examine the patient's mouth and tongue using the torch and spatula, *to observe the condition of the teeth, gums and mucosa. Note any food debris; any ulcers or sores and the condition of the lips* (Holmes & Mountain 1993)
- discuss with the patient, if possible, the most suitable and acceptable mouth care for his particular needs *to promote individualised care and help compliance*
- help the patient to clean his teeth or his dentures with his toothbrush and toothpaste
- offer a suitable mouthwash, explaining that it should not be swallowed, and help to hold the equipment as necessary *to rinse the mouth until all debris and cleaning paste are removed*
- offer tissues *for drying the mouth*
- help to apply lubrication to the lips as required *to maintain the skin integrity of the lips.* This can be done by placing the lubricant on a gloved finger and applying it directly, or using a dental roll or a gauze swab, or the patient may apply it himself *to encourage independence*

- return the patient's clean dentures to him in a bowl of clean water and encourage him to wear them *to maintain the shape of the oral cavity*
- ensure the patient is left feeling as comfortable as possible. Ideally, a period of rest should be encouraged after this nursing practice
- dispose of equipment safely *to maintain a safe environment*
- document the nursing practice appropriately and report immediately any deterioration or improvement in the condition of the mouth, as well as abnormal findings. *This enables changes in practice to be implemented to maintain optimum mouth care for each patient.*

Intensive mouth care for dependent patients

- explain the nursing practice *to again the patient's consent and cooperation if possible*
- ensure the patient's privacy *to respect his individuality*
- help the patient into a comfortable position *so that he tolerates the practice*
- collect and prepare the equipment including the mouth-cleaning pack or tray
- don clean plastic gloves *to prevent contamination with body fluids*
- remove dentures if present *to gain access and a clear view of the oral cavity*
- examine the patient's mouth as before
- clean all round the mouth, gums and tongue with the mouth-cleaning solution, using a soft toothbrush if possible. *This will help to dislodge debris and remove plaque* (Buglass 1995). A cotton wool stick dipped into the solution may be used. A gauze swab wrapped round a pair of plastic forceps, or a dental roll held lengthways in forceps may also be used. However, care is needed *to prevent damage to the oral mucosa* (Peate 1993). Proprietary foam or flavoured sticks are a convenient and acceptable tool for mouth care *if a toothbrush is not appropriate* (Fig. 29.1)
- help the patient to use a mouthwash if possible, or rinse the mouth with a gauze swab soaked in mouthwash solution, allowing the patient to suck it. For patients with a wired mandible following oral surgery, a syringe of mouthwash in conjunction with suction may be used. This will require good cooperation from a patient with an adequate swallowing reflex *to prevent inhalation of the rinsing fluid* (Kelly 1994).
- help the patient to clean his dentures or clean them for him using toothbrush and toothpaste, under a running tap if possible, *to retain a healthy oral mucosa*
- proceed with the nursing practice as before.

Mouth care for an unconscious patient

Mouth-care guidelines are as for a dependent patient, with the following exceptions:

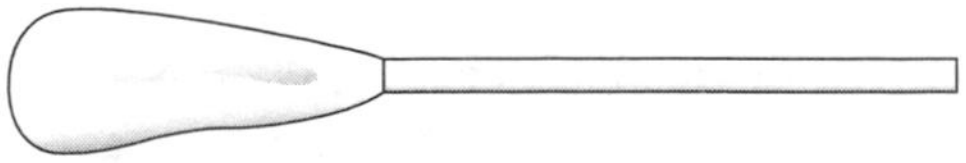

Figure 29.1 *Cotton wool or foam stick for mouth cleaning.*

- position the patient on his side, with no pillow, and his head supported *so that no secretion or mouth-cleaning solution can flow into the trachea and be inhaled* (Kite & Pearson 1995)
- place waterproof material on the bed before placing tissues under the lower side of the face *to absorb solution and saliva draining from the mouth*
- check that suction equipment is at hand and in working order and, if required, perform oral suction before commencing and during the nursing practice *to prevent any danger of fluid being inhaled*

The dentures should have been removed, cleaned, appropriately labelled and stored with the patient's belongings on admission (*see* care of the Unconscious patient, p. 347).

Relevance to the activities of living

Observations and further rationales for this nursing practice will be included within each activity of living as appropriate.

Maintaining a safe environment

The oral mucosa itself is part of the body's defence against infection. Mouth care, which helps to keep the teeth and oral mucosa in good condition, is important in maintaining a safe environment for the patient.

Although mouth care does not need aseptic technique, all the equipment should be clean or disposable, and all precautions should be taken to prevent cross-infection. The nurse should wash her hands before commencing and on completion of mouth care for each patient.

The nurse herself should be protected from any blood-borne viral infection which might be present in the saliva, e.g. hepatitis B or HIV. It is an advisable precaution to wear gloves for all mouth care as it may involve direct contact with the oral mucosa and oral secretions (Thomas 1994).

Patients who are receiving cytotoxic medication for malignant disease, e.g. leukaemia, may be at greater risk of infection than normal. The treatment itself may also affect the cells of the oral mucosa. A special mouth-care regimen using mouthwashes, suspensions or creams may be prescribed for these patients. If possible, the patient himself should apply these once the nurse has shown the procedure, to minimise the risk of cross-infection. The importance of this care in the prevention of infection should be explained to the patient, and the nurse may use this time as an opportunity for patient education.

Mouthwashes should only be given to patients who are alert and well oriented, with a good cough reflex, otherwise there is a danger of accidental inhalation of the solution. For patients with poor swallowing and cough reflex oral suction equipment should be used to prevent any danger of aspiration of excess fluid in the oral cavity during this nursing practice.

Communicating

A patient who has a dry or infected mouth will find it uncomfortable to talk, and dry lips can also be painful when speaking, so appropriate mouth care can help with communication. Having a mouth which feels fresh can help to raise the patient's morale and encourage him to take an interest in other people and his surroundings.

Breathing

Patients who have a cough and sputum may appreciate regular mouthwashes to clear mucus which may have lodged round the teeth and gums. A mouthwash should be given after chest physiotherapy to freshen the mouth and encourage a feeling of well-being, although an opportunity to clean the teeth may be even more welcome. Oxygen therapy dries the oral mucosa. Patients receiving this treatment either at home or in institutional care will appreciate regular mouth care.

Eating and drinking

The opportunity for mouth care should be provided for all patients after meals. They should be encouraged to clean teeth and/or dentures, as well as to rinse the mouth; the nurse may need to assemble the equipment and give appropriate help. This regular encouragement should form part of patient education in personal hygiene. The importance of a healthy mouth, teeth and gums should be emphasised (WHO 1988).

A dry or 'dirty' mouth may discourage a patient from eating. Good mouth care can be a help in promoting the appetite and an encouragement to eat when this is important to aid recovery.

Conversely, patients who are not allowed to eat by the oral route will need frequent mouth care as masticating food stimulates saliva which helps to maintain a healthy mucosa. Some patients go home with nasogastric feeding or parenteral nutrition and may need assistance with mouth care from the community nurse for some time until they can manage their own mouth care.

Adequate fluid intake is an additional help in maintaining a moist, healthy oral environment.

Personal cleansing and dressing

An important part of this activity of living is the patient's own oral hygiene. The nurse should be able to identify any associated problems during her assessment of the patient, and this may be an opportunity for patient education in relation to dental and oral hygiene. Giving a rationale for treatment and nursing care should enable the nurse to include the whole family in health promotion related to oral hygiene and dental care, e.g. using a toothbrush effectively (Trevelyan 1994).

Using a toothbrush effectively   Brushing the teeth loosens and removes debris trapped in the spaces and also prevents the growth of plaque which harbours bacteria and may be a precursor of dental caries. The brushing also stimulates the blood circulation in the gums and helps to keep the soft tissue healthy. The teeth should be brushed with the toothbrush held at an angle of 45°. Vibrating strokes of the brush at the gum level will help to dislodge plaque and debris. This is known as the 'Bass' method (Thurgood 1994). Inner aspects of the teeth should be brushed in the same way. Efficient tooth cleaning should not be hurried. The mouth should be well rinsed several times during and after tooth cleaning. Facilities for cleaning the teeth or dentures should be offered after meals to all patients who are not self-caring.

The correct use of dental floss can be included when discussing dental hygiene (Fig. 29.2).

The importance of regular visits to the dentist should also be emphasised when the opportunity arises. This is an opportunity for the community nurse to extend health education to the whole family (Levine 1993).

Expressing sexuality

Sexuality can be expressed positively in the form of non-verbal communication. For example, smiling is an important way of projecting self to other people; teeth and gums which are well cared for enhance the body image and the feeling of well-

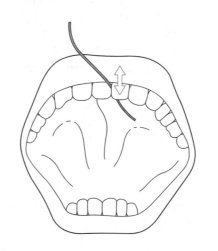
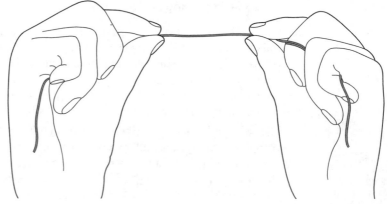

Figure 29.2 *Mouth care: use of dental floss*

being. If a patient is feeling depressed, appropriate mouth care and a fresh mouthwash may encourage a male patient to agree to having a shave in preparation for meeting his sensitive visitors, and a female patient may feel encouraged to put on make-up, lipstick and perfume. At home, an increase in self esteem will encourage the patient's interest in family events and aid rehabilitation.

Patient education: key points

Health education and health promotion for the care of the mouth should be multidisciplinary from childhood to old age: the health visitor, school nurse, practice nurse, district nurse as well as the dentist and the dental hygienist may be involved. Advice should include:

- the importance of good care of the mouth, teeth and gums related to general health
- good teeth cleaning technique and care of dentures
- nutritional advice about the relationship of the incidence of dental caries to food and drink with a high sugar content
- the importance of the removal of debris from the teeth and fornices of the mouth after meals
- the influence of fluoride in the development of teeth.

Patients with a suppressed immune system should be taught oral hygiene procedures to prevent mucosal infection.

References

Buglass E 1995 Oral hygiene. British Journal of Nursing 4(9): 516–519
Hatton-Smith C 1994 A last bastion of ritualised practice? A review of nurses knowledge of oral health care. Professional Nurse 9(5): 304–308
Holmes S, Mountain E 1993 Assessment of oral status. Evaluation of three oral assessment guides. Journal of Clinical Nursing 2(1): 35–40
Kelly R 1994 Disorders of the mouth. In: Alexander M, Fawcett J, Runciman P (eds) Nursing practice — hospital and home: the adult. Churchill Livingstone, Edinburgh, ch 15
Kite K, Pearson L 1995 A rationale for mouth care: the integration of theory with practice. Intensive and Critical Care Nursing 11(2): 71–76
Levine R 1993 The scientific basis of dental health education. Health Authority, London
Peate I 1993 Nurse administered oral hygiene in the hospitalised patient. British Journal of Nursing 2(9): 459–462
Porter H 1994 Mouth care in cancer. Nursing Times 90(14): 27–29
Thomas L 1994 Glove story. Gloves, cost benefit analysis. Nursing Times 90(36): 31–35
Thurgood G 1994 Nurse maintenance of oral hygiene. British Journal of Nursing 3(7): 332–334, 351–353
Trevelyan J 1994 Oral traditions. Nursing Times 90(14): 24–27
WHO 1988 Oral health: global indicators for health. WHO, Geneva

Further reading

Boyle S 1992 Assessing mouth care. Nursing Times 88(15): 44–46
Day R 1993 Mouth care in an intensive care unit: a review. Intensive and Critical Care Nursing 9(4): 246–252
Heywood Jones I 1994 Mouth care (skills update). Community Outlook: 26–27
Roper N, Logan W, Tierney A 1996 The elements of nursing, 4th edn. Churchill Livingstone, Edinburgh, pp 231–264
Walsh M, Ford P 1989 Nursing rituals — research and rational actions. Heinemann Nursing, Oxford, pp 112–114, 154–156
Watson R 1989 Care of the mouth. Nursing 3(46): 20–24

30 Moving and Handling

Learning outcomes

By the end of this section you should know how to:

- assess the requirements correctly
- plan the safest method of moving the patient
- adapt the principles of movement to suit each particular situation.

Background knowledge required

Revision of the anatomy and physiology of the spinal column and main joints and muscles of the body.

Revision of the current theories on safe and efficient moving and handling practices (particularly the articles on the neuromuscular approach by Vasey & Crozier 1982, in Suggested reading).

EC Guidelines on lifting and handling.

RCN Guidelines on lifting and handling.

Local policies on lifting and handling patients.

Indications and rationale for moving and handling a patient

It may be necessary for one, two or more staff, with the help of mechanical aids, to move a patient when he is unable to move himself because of:

- *severe injury*
- *major surgery*
- *paralysis*
- *acute illness*
- *weakness*
- *unconsciousness*
- *disability.*

Outline of the procedure

It is important to understand the theories of safe and efficient moving and handling practices. In normal adults the imaginary 'centre of gravity' point is near the base of the spine. If suspended from this point, in theory, the body would balance (Fig. 30.1). The feet form what is called the 'base' and if the centre of gravity moves beyond the area of the base, the body will become unbalanced and fall unless all the major muscles of the trunk and legs tense and hold the body upright. A prolonged period of imbalance or 'top heavy' action can lead to stress and strain of these muscles and ultimately injury and pain

Figure 30.1 *Centre of gravity*

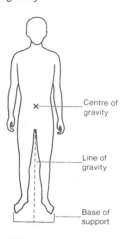

- Centre of gravity
- Line of gravity
- Base of support

(Fig. 30.2). Widening of the base to keep the centre of gravity within the baseline will help to avoid this. Most adults have developed bad movement habits and their movements involve many 'top heavy' actions. The re-education of the body to adopt safe movement habits is to be encouraged (McCall 1991).

When preparing to move a patient, soften the spine, relax the knees and widen the base appropriately. Approach the load to be moved with open palms and hold from underneath upwards to avoid pinching grips on the load and unnecessary stress on the muscles of the fingers, hands and arms. Hold the load as near to your body as possible. Just before the 'effort' phase of the move, re-soften the spine so that the move begins with the spine in a non-fixed position, then lead with the top of the head in the direction of the move and re-form the spine. The momentum caused by this action should allow the patient to come with you. If necessary, break the move into several stages, repositioning yourself after each move.

Equipment

Mechanical aids, e.g. lifting device (Fig. 30.3), patient sling.

Guidelines and rationale for this nursing practice

- assess the requirements with regard to the condition of the patient, weight, ability to help, the number of helpers, the most appropriate way of moving the patient, which may involve equipment as well as manpower and the immediate environment (RCN 1992) *as thoughtless actions can lead to back injury*
- clear the area, if possible, of any obstacles *for ease of movement*
- ensure appropriate bed height *to reduce the risk of back injury*
- collect any help or mechanical aids required *to reduce any risk involved* (Barker et al 1994)
- explain fully to the patient and any helpers what is going to happen and what is expected of them *so that they can cooperate as much as possible*

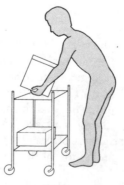
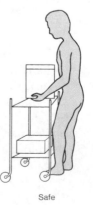

Figure 30.2 *Examples of safe and unsafe lifting*

Unsafe   Safe

- observe the patient throughout this activity *to detect any signs of distress*
- adopt a suitable position for the move or manoeuvre the mechanical aid into position for the move
- apply the recommended theories of safe and efficient moving and handling practices when performing the move, *to protect nursing staff from back injury*
- carry out the lift, with one nurse acting as the leader and giving instructions *so that everyone knows what is expected of them and can act together*
- ensure that the patient is left feeling as comfortable as possible

There should always be a minimum of two nurses to move a patient when the person being moved cannot fully bear weight, or a mechanical aid such as a hoist should be used.

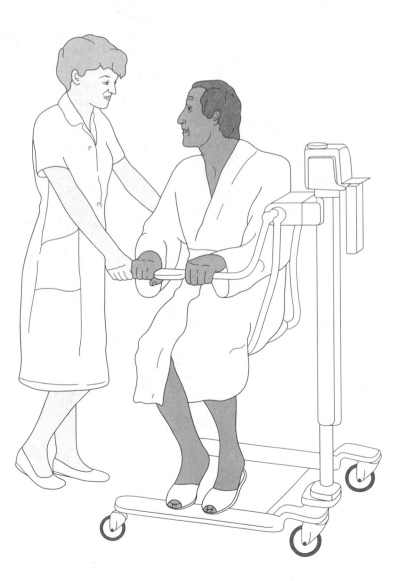

Figure 30.3 *Examples of mechanical aids*

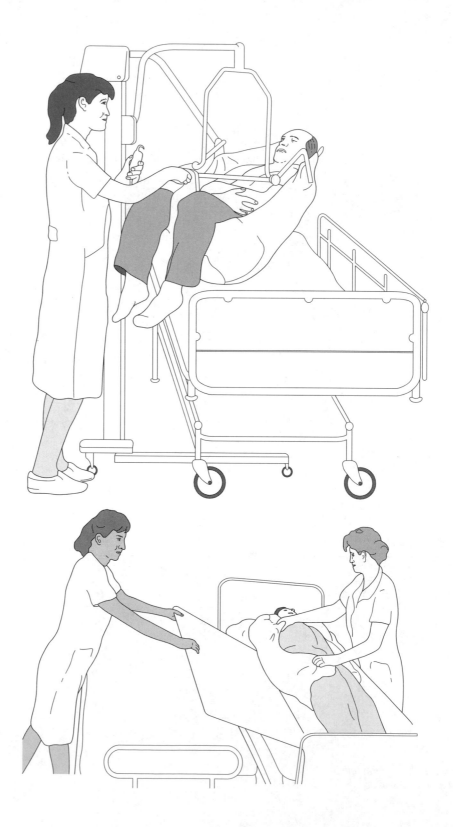

Figure 30.3 *Cont'd*

Australian or shoulder move

This method of moving is recommended if a mechanical aid is not appropriate and the patient cannot bear his own weight. Research has demonstrated that this move produces significantly lower intra-abdominal pressure in the lifter than any of the others (Pheasant & Stubbs 1991).

The patient is helped to sit upright in bed on a sliding sheet and both nurses stand level with the patient's hips. The nurses soften their spines and widen their base, pointing the foot nearest the top of the bed in the direction of the lift. It may allow closer access to the patient if the knee nearest the patient is placed on the bed, level with the patient's buttocks. The shoulder nearest the patient is placed firmly under his axilla so that his arms rest on the nurses' backs. The arms of the shoulders which are pressing into the patient's axilla are placed on the handles of the sliding sheet or across the front of the patient's chest and abdomen. The nurse's free hand can be placed on the bed above the patient but this is not necessary for the move. The leader gives the start signal and the nurses begin the 'effort phase' of the move by leading with the top of their heads, re-forming their spines and transferring their weight to their forward foot. They move the patient with them and soften their spines again to rest the patient back on the bed in the new position. The patient is left feeling as comfortable as possible (Fig. 30.4).

Through arm move

Two nurses help the patient to sit forwards and give support while they stand facing the foot of the bed. It will allow closer access to the patient if the nurse places her knee nearest the patient onto the bed. The patient crosses his arms and, using safe movement habits, the nurses ease the arm nearest the patient through, from the back, between the patient's arm and chest. The arm moves further than necessary and as it is withdrawn the open hand fixes on the patient's forearm. Using the movements described earlier, and on the instruction of the leader, the nurses move the patient up the bed. If the patient is unable to bend his knees and give some assistance to the move by digging his feet into the bed then a sliding aid or a rolling pillow may be placed under the patient's ankles to avoid them dragging on the bed (Fig. 30.5).

Relevance to the activities of living

Maintaining a safe environment

The safety of the patient and of nursing staff is of equal importance. To avoid the danger of back injury to staff, mechanical aids should be used on all possible occasions.

Know your own moving capacity and do not exceed it (RCN 1992). Do not move patients unnecessarily. If something goes wrong with the move do not be afraid to lower the patient gently to the floor. Make him comfortable and summon help.

A full assessment must be carried out prior to moving and handling patients. In

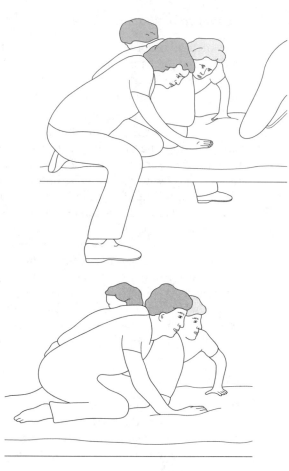

Figure 30.4 *Two nurses lifting a patient in bed: Australian move (Adapted from Roper N, Logan W, Tierney A 1990 The elements of nursing, 3rd edn. Churchill Livingstone, Edinburgh)*

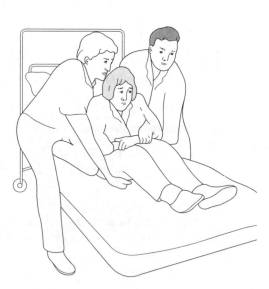

Figure 30.5 *Two nurses performing a through-arm move*

the community, liaison between the community nurse, occupational therapist and physiotherapist is essential in ensuring that equipment and appropriate moving/handling techniques are used. The physiotherapist will normally provide equipment for patients such as walking sticks or zimmers, while occupational therapists will offer items such as bathing equipment, seating and housing adaptations. The community nurse may provide nursing aids such as hoists, commodes, monkey poles and special beds.

Communicating

Good communication between the nurses, and between the nurses and the patient, is very important for successful movement which does no harm to the movers or the patient.

Successful communication will enable the patient to feel safer and more confident in the nurses' moving abilities.

Personal cleansing and dressing

Appropriate clothing and footwear for nurses and patient can help the success of a move.

Mobilising

Patients should be encouraged to help move themselves as much as possible. Sometimes nurses move patients unnecessarily because it is quicker than waiting for the patient to move himself.

Patient education: key points	Mechanical aids should be installed in the patient's home prior to transfer from hospital to community.
	Carers require to be taught safe moving and handling techniques.
	Patients should be encouraged to move themselves whenever possible.
	To gain the patient's cooperation and to ensure that he will not react to moves in an unexpected way it is important to provide a full explanation of what is going to happen.

References	Barker A, Cassars S, Gabbett J 1994 Handling people: equipment advice and information. Disabled Living Foundation, London
	McCall J 1991 Watch your back. Nursing Standard 5(24): 50–51
	RCN 1992 Code of practice for the lifting and handling of patients. RCN, London
	Pheasant S, Stubbs D 1991 Lifting and handling: an ergonomic approach. National Back Pain Association, London

Further reading	Brewer S 1993 The back injury battle. Nursing Standard 7(40): 20–21
	Hawkey B, Clarke M 1990 Dress sense or nonsense. Nursing Times 86(3): 28–31

Hempel S 1993 Home truths. Nursing Times 89(15): 40–41

Naish J 1996 Campaign aims to change the culture on manual lifting. Nursing Times 92(15): 27–29

Pilling S 1993 Calculating the risk. Nursing Standard 8(6): 18–20

Roper N, Logan W, Tierney A 1996 The elements of nursing, 4th edn. Churchill Livingstone, Edinburgh

Vasey J, Crozier L 1982 A neuromuscular approach.
1. A move in the right direction. Nursing Mirror 154(17): 42–47
2. Get into condition. Nursing Mirror 154(18): 22–28
3. At ease. Nursing Mirror 154(19): 28–31
4. Handle with care. Nursing Mirror 154(20): 30–32
5. Easy on the base. Nursing Mirror 154(21): 36–42
6. Safety first. Nursing Mirror 154(22): 44–48

31 Nebuliser Therapy

Learning outcomes

By the end of this section you should know how to:
- prepare the patient for this nursing practice
- collect and prepare the equipment
- administer medication via a nebuliser, either in the community or in an institutional setting

Background knowledge required

Revision of the respiratory system with special reference to respiratory diseases associated with bronchospasm.

Revision of Oxygen therapy (*see* p. 255).

Revision of Administration of medicines (*see* p. 1).

Indications and rationale for using nebuliser therapy

A nebuliser attached to a flow of air or oxygen converts a liquid into an aerosol mist which is used as a therapeutic inhalation (BNF 1995).

The use of a nebuliser may be indicated for the following reasons:
- to administer bronchodilators *for the relief of bronchospasm associated with respiratory disease*, e.g.:
  — asthma
  — chronic obstructive airways disease (COAD) (Flynn 1993)
- to administer mucolytic medication *to lower the viscosity of the secretions and aid expectoration*, e.g.:
  — chronic obstructive airways disease (COAD)
  — cystic fibrosis
  — bronchial carcinoma

The medication, as well as the administration by air or oxygen, is prescribed by a medical practitioner. It may require to be diluted with 2–3 ml normal saline, and is normally prescribed 3–4 times a day. The procedure may be coordinated with chest physiotherapy, and may be administered by a nurse or the physiotherapist. For the patient with asthma, an estimation of peak flow of tidal volume may be recorded before and after nebuliser therapy. If long-term treatment is needed the patient may become efficient in his own self care with nebuliser treatment at home, under the supervision of the community team (Tettersell 1993).

Equipment

Prescribed air supply: piped, in cylinders, or portable air compressor

Prescribed oxygen supply, either piped or in cylinders

Flow meter

Adapter

Oxygen tubing

Nebuliser (Fig. 31.1)

Mouthpiece or appropriate oxygen mask, e.g. Hudson mask (Fig. 31.1)

Prescribed medication

Sputum carton as required

'No Smoking' signs as appropriate (*see* Oxygen therapy, p. 255)

Receptacle for soiled disposables.

For peak flow measurement

- Peak flow meter (Fig. 31.2)
- Disposable mouthpiece
- Specific chart for documenting results.

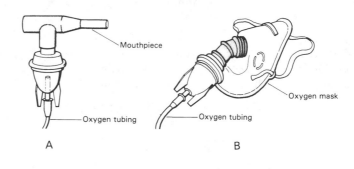

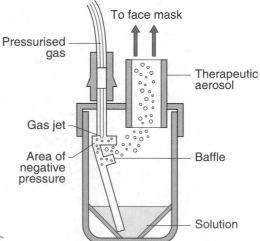

Figure 31.1 *Nebuliser*
A Attached to a mouthpiece
B Attached to an oxygen mask
C Cross section

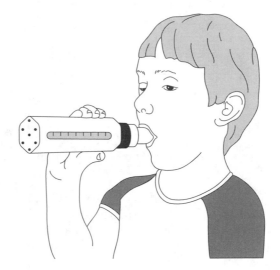

Figure 31.2 *Peak flow meter*

Guidelines and rationale for this nursing practice

- explain the nursing practice to the patient *to gain consent and cooperation and encourage participation in care*
- ensure the patient's privacy *to respect individuality and maintain self esteem*
- prepare and assemble the equipment *so that everything is ready*
- explain the dangers of smoking to the patient and his visitors and position 'No Smoking' signs as appropriate, *making sure they understand the increased risk of fire when oxygen is administered*
- help the patient to estimate the peak flow of his tidal volume by recording the best of three results on the peak flow meter before commencing nebuliser therapy. *This will help to evaluate the efficiency of the treatment* (Kendrick & Smith 1992)
- help the patient into a comfortable position *so that he will tolerate the therapy without distress*
- observe the patient throughout the activity *to monitor the effects of the nebuliser therapy*
- identify and check the medication prescription (*see* Administration of medicines, p. 2). *This is a professional requirement for prescribed medication* (McKenzie 1994)
- prepare the prescribed dose in a suitable sterile syringe *to maintain a safe environment*
- fill the nebuliser with prepared medication (Fig. 31.3)
- adjust the flow meter to 5 litres or turn on the air compressor *to ensure efficient vaporisation of the medication*
- observe the fine spray from the nebuliser *to ensure that the equipment is working*
- encourage the patient to breathe the nebulised vapour through the mouthpiece *for maximum effect; a mask may be used if a patient has difficulty with the mouthpiece*

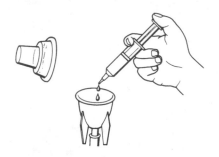

Figure 31.3 *Nebuliser taken apart to introduce a prepared medication*

- remain with the patient *until all the solution has been nebulised*
- encourage the patient to expectorate *as the medication may help to loosen the bronchial secretions* (Hough 1992)
- ensure that the patient is left feeling as comfortable as possible. *Bronchospasm is further reduced if the patient is relaxed and reassured*
- help the patient to estimate the peak flow of his tidal volume by recording the best of three results on the peak flow meter. This should preferably be recorded half an hour after the completion of nebuliser therapy *as some bronchodilators have their maximum effect during this period* (Brewin & Hughes 1995)
- wash and dry the nebuliser, tubing and mask or mouthpiece *to maintain a safe environment*
- retain the equipment in a polythene bag *for the patient's next administration. To prevent infection, the equipment should be changed every 24 hours*
- document the nursing practice appropriately, monitor after-effects and report abnormal findings immediately, *to ensure safe practice and enable prompt appropriate medical and nursing intervention to be initiated as soon as possible.*

Relevance to the activities of living

Observations and further rationale for this nursing practice will be included within each activity of living as appropriate.

Maintaining a safe environment

If oxygen is used, all precautions to prevent the risk of fire should be maintained, as with Oxygen therapy.

This is not a sterile procedure but adequate standards of cleanliness should be maintained. The nurse should wash her hands before commencing and on completion of this nursing practice.

The equipment for each patient should be kept clean and dry when not in use. It should be changed every 24 hours to prevent infection.

The prescription should be checked by a registered nurse or medical practitioner (*see* Administration of medicines, p. 1).

Communicating

During the nursing practice itself the patient will not be encouraged to speak.

Normally all of the solution is administered within 10 minutes, this can be explained to the patient.

Breathing

Monitor the respiration rate, the depth and type of respirations and maintain recordings as frequently as required. The patient should take deep regular breaths through the mouthpiece of the nebuliser to ensure that the medication reaches the mucosa of the bronchi and bronchioles and not just the oropharynx (Everard et al 1993).

Patients will often experience less dyspnoea following this procedure and there may be a dramatic relief of bronchospasm for patients with asthma. This can be monitored by peak flow recordings over a period of time.

Occasionally two drugs are prescribed via the nebuliser and, unless specifically stated, these should NOT be mixed. They should be administered in separate nebulisers, one after the other; prescribed bronchodilators should always be administered first. The nebulisers should be labelled appropriately and kept clean and dry for future use.

For efficient vaporisation a flow of oxygen 4–5 litres on the flow meter is required. However, for patients with chronic obstructive airways disease this will administer a dangerously high percentage of oxygen (*see* Oxygen therapy, p. 255), and air should be prescribed for administration instead. This can be in the form of a piped supply or from an air compressor (Dodd et al 1995).

For patients in intensive care areas a nebuliser can be introduced into the ventilator circuit and medication administered as prescribed.

Observe and record the amount, colour and type of any sputum.

Eating and drinking

A healthy mouth and oropharyngeal mucosa is essential for maximum absorption of the medication. Frequent oral hygiene should be performed as appropriate.

A mouthwash after expectorating may be appreciated and should be available if desired.

Patient education: key points

The reason for the nebuliser therapy should be carefully explained to the patient and his family so that compliance is continued.

If oxygen is used for nebulisation, information about fire risks and the precautions needed should be explained (*see* Oxygen therapy, p. 255).

If the patient is self caring, instructions about preparing the medication and using the equipment should be given and the nurse should ensure that these continue to be prepared and used correctly.

At home, the nurse should ensure that the patient and carers keep the equipment clean and separate from other household equipment to maintain a safe environment.

The patient should understand the importance of reporting immediately any changes in respiratory function such as increased dyspnoea, cough, sputum, or any general feeling of distress.

References

Brewin A, Hughes J 1995 Effect of patient education on asthma management. British Journal of Nursing 4(2): 81–82, 99–101

British National Formulary (BNF) 1995 Drugs used in the treatment of the respiratory system. BNF, March: 108–118

Dodd M, Hanley S, Johnson S, Webb A 1995 District nebuliser compressor service: reliability and costs. Thorax 50(1): 81–82

Everard M, Hardy J, Milner A 1993 Comparison of nebulised aerosol deposition in the lungs of healthy adults following oral and nasal inhalation. Thorax 48(10): 1045–1046

Flynn M 1993 Management of chronic obstructive airways disease. British Journal of Nursing 2(14): 717–723

Hough A 1992 Making sense of ---- sputum retention, Nursing Times 88(36): 33–35

Kendrick A, Smith E 1992 Respiratory measurements: 2. Simple measurement of lung function. Professional Nurse 7(1): 748–754

McKenzie S 1994 Drugs used to control asthma. British Journal of Nursing 3(17): 872–880

Tettersell M J 1993 Asthma patients' knowledge in relation to compliance with drug therapy. Journal of Advanced Nursing 18(1): 103–113

Further reading

Abbott J, Dodd M, Bilton D et al 1994 Treatment compliance in adults with cystic fibrosis. Thorax 49(2): 115–120

Barnes K, Rollo C, Holgate S et al 1987 Bacterial contamination of home nebulisers. British Medical Journal 295: 812

Cattell R, Jones S 1995 Nebulised therapy and nursing knowledge. British Journal of Nursing 4(16): 954–957

Heslop A, King M 1994 Let's treat body and mind: collaborative rehabilitation for chronic breathlessness. Professional Nurse 10(3): 188–192

Hurrell F 1995 Asthma and activity. Practice Nurse 6(6): 14–17

Nevin M, Nevin M 1992 Help the parent and you help the child: a parents' view of coping with the asthmatic child. Paediatric Nursing 4(1): 25–27

Steventon R, Wilson R 1986 A guide to apparatus for home nebuliser therapy. Allan & Hanbury, Greenford, pp 3–17

Stokesay J 1989 Breathless. Nursing Times 85(17): 28–31

32 Neurological Examination

Learning outcomes

By the end of this section you should know how to:

- prepare the patient for a neurological examination
- collect and prepare the equipment
- assist the medical practitioner during neurological examination if required.

Background knowledge required

Revision of the anatomy and physiology of the nervous system.

Revision of care of the Unconscious patient (*see* p. 347).

Indications and rationale for neurological examination

Neurological examination is a method of obtaining some objective data on the function of a patient's nervous system (Brunner & Suddarth 1992). This may be required:

- *to aid in the diagnosis of a neurological disease*
- *to monitor the effect of a neurological disease*
- *to aid in the assessment of treatment during the course of a neurological disease.*

Outline of the procedure

This procedure is carried out by a medical practitioner and is usually done in conjunction with an examination of the motor and sensory function of the patient's trunk and limbs. The ophthalmoscope and pencil torch are used to assess the function of the optic, the oculomotor, the trochlear and the ophthalmic branch of the trigeminal cranial nerves. The auriscope and tuning fork are used to examine the ears and assess the function of the vestibulocochlear cranial nerve, respectively. Assessment of the patient's sensation to pain, touch and temperature is made using a sterile needle, a cotton wool ball and the test tubes of hot and cold water. The olfactory cranial nerve is assessed when the patient is asked to identify the odours of the various strong-smelling substances. The tendon hammer is used by the medical practitioner when testing a spinal reflex such as the knee jerk. Assessment for an upper motor neurone lesion will also require the use of a tendon hammer for stroking the lateral aspect of the sole of the patient's foot. The function of the facial cranial nerve is assessed by asking the patient to identify various substances, i.e. salt, sugar, vinegar and lemon juice. The patient will be required to use the mouth rinse after each substance is tasted to prevent inaccurate results.

Equipment	Ophthalmoscope
	Pencil torch
	Auriscope
	Tuning fork
	Sterile injection needle
	Non-sterile cotton wool balls
	Test tubes filled with hot and cold water
	Small containers of various strong-smelling substances, e.g. peppermint, oil of cloves
	Tendon hammer
	Small samples of salt, sugar, lemon juice and vinegar
	Glass of water for rinsing the patient's mouth
	Trolley or tray for equipment
	Receptacle for used mouth rinse
	Receptacle for soiled disposables.

Guidelines and rationale for this nursing practice

- help to explain the procedure to the patient *to gain consent and cooperation*
- wash the hands *to reduce cross-infection* (Horton 1995)
- prepare the equipment *to ensure that all equipment is available and ready for use*
- ensure the patient's privacy *to reduce anxiety*
- observe the patient throughout this activity *to note any signs of distress*
- help the patient into a comfortable position *to allow the patient to maintain the position and provide easy access for the medical practitioner*
- assist the medical practitioner during the examination *to enhance the overall quality of the procedure* (Pemberton 1988)
- ensure the patient is left feeling as comfortable as possible *maintaining the quality of this nursing practice*
- dispose of the equipment safely *to reduce any health hazard*
- document the nursing practice appropriately, monitor after-effects and report any abnormal findings immediately *providing a written record and assisting in the implementation of any action should an abnormality or adverse reaction to the practice be noted.*

Relevance to the activities of living

Maintaining a safe environment

All equipment should be clean or disposable and all precautions taken to prevent cross-infection. The nurse should wash her hands before commencing and on completion of the nursing practice (Horton 1995).

A nurse is not always present during a neurological examination, but assistance may be required by the medical practitioner, for example with a paralysed patient.

Communicating

The medical practitioner who carries out the examination gives the patient an explanation of the procedure, but the nurse may be required to repeat the explanation (Brunner & Suddarth 1992).

Depending on the nature of the disease condition which requires the neurological examination (they are many and diverse), any of the patient's activities of living may be affected, but the examination itself does not have any adverse effects on the Activities of Living.

Patient education: key points

The patient should be given an initial explanation of the procedure by the medical practitioner which may need to be repeated by the nurse.

The patient should have the initial results of the examination explained and discussed (Pemberton 1988).

References

Brunner L, Suddarth D (eds) 1992 The textbook of adult nursing. Chapman & Hall, London, ch 31
Horton R 1995 Handwashing: the fundamental infection control principle. British Journal of Nursing 4(16): 926–933
Pemberton L 1988 Assessment of the nervous system. In: Allan D (ed) Nursing and the neurosciences. Churchill Livingstone, Edinburgh

Further reading

Roper N, Logan W, Tierney A 1996 The elements of nursing, 4th edn. Churchill Livingstone, Edinburgh, pp 103–140

33 Nutrition

There are three parts to this section:

1 Feeding a dependent patient
2 Enteral feeding
3 Parenteral nutrition.

1 Feeding a dependent patient

Learning outcomes

By the end of this section you should know how to:

- prepare the patient for this nursing practice
- collect and prepare the equipment
- carry out feeding a dependent patient.

Background knowledge required

Revision of the anatomy and physiology of the mouth and oesophagus with special reference to the physical acts of mastication and swallowing.

Indications and rationale for the feeding of a dependent patient

The nurse may be required to feed a dependent patient *to maintain adequate nutrition in:*

- *a patient who is unable to use his upper limbs due to paralysis or serious illness*
- *a patient who has lost upper limb coordination due to a physical or mental disease*
- *a patient who has recently lost his eyesight*
- *a patient who has an injury around the mouth.*

Equipment

Feeding utensils such as a fork, knife, spoon, drinking cup with a spout or cup with an angled straw

Disposable napkin or paper towel

Diet as ordered by the patient

Trolley or tray for equipment

Receptacle for soiled disposables.

Guidelines and rationale for this nursing practice

In hospital or at home this practice may be undertaken by the patient's relatives or carers.

- explain the nursing practice to the patient *to gain consent and cooperation*

- collect and prepare the equipment *to ensure that all equipment is available and ready for use*
- help the patient into a comfortable position *to allow easy access to the patient by the nurse and also allow the patient to maintain his position during the practice*
- observe the patient throughout this activity *to note any signs of distress*
- wash the hands *for general hygiene purposes and to reduce cross-infection*
- *for patient satisfaction and enjoyment* keep the food not being eaten at a suitable temperature
- remind the patient of his ordered menu *to permit psychological preparation for the food*
- where possible the nurse should sit down while feeding the patient *so that this is made an enjoyable social occasion* (Sanford 1987, Roper et al 1996)
- ask the patient which food he wishes to eat first *thereby giving the patient some control during the activity*
- offer the food to the patient at a rate set by the patient *as hurrying the patient while he eats may induce nausea or vomiting*
- *to prevent gagging or choking* place the spoon or fork accurately into the patient's mouth
- offer sips of fluid during the meal *to aid in the mastication and swallowing of the food*
- discontinue feeding when asked by the patient *to prevent a feeling of distension and excessive fullness*
- assist the patient with mouth care following the meal *as this will promote dental health and may reduce the incidence of dental caries* (Kelly 1994)
- ensure the patient is left feeling as comfortable as possible *maintaining the quality of this nursing practice*
- dispose of equipment safely *to reduce any health hazard*
- document the nursing practice appropriately, monitor after-effects and report abnormal findings immediately *providing a written record and assisting in the implementation of any action should an abnormality or adverse reaction to the practice be noted.*

Relevance to the activities of living	**Maintaining a safe environment**

All equipment should be clean and all precautions be taken to prevent cross-infection. The nurse should wash her hands before commencing and on completion of the nursing practice.

The nurse will require to check the temperature of the food with the patient to prevent a burn of the mouth, lips or tongue.

Communicating

The patient should be assisted to choose and order his own food from the hospital menu. Eating is a pleasant social occasion for most people, therefore the nurse must help to maintain the atmosphere (Sanford 1987).

The patient should be shown the food to be eaten as this will assist in the digestion of the food.

A blind patient should be told what food to expect, to avoid the shock of an unexpected taste.

Breathing

The nurse should observe the patient for difficulty in swallowing which may precede choking. Placing the spoon or fork too far back in the patient's mouth may produce gagging or choking.

A patient who may have temporarily lost the ability to swallow, such as a stroke victim, may be assisted by a skilled speech therapist to regain the swallowing reflex.

Eating and drinking

Sips of fluid will assist a patient to swallow food and also rid the mouth of the taste of one food prior to a different taste.

When appropriate the patient should be given the choice of feeding utensil to be used. Some patients do not like to use a feeding cup with spout, but prefer a straw used with a cup or glass.

A patient who has a motor or sensory loss of one side of the face will need to be fed on the unaffected side of the mouth. The nurse should check that food does not accumulate in the cheek of the affected side.

When possible the patient should be assisted to put the food into his own mouth as this may help him to feel less dependent on the nurse.

Drinks and other foods such as a piece of fruit should be offered at frequent intervals other than meal times.

Relatives of the patient may wish to assist the patient in taking food. This should be encouraged as it is of great psychological benefit both to the patient and the relatives.

Information and education regarding the constituents of a healthy diet should be discussed with the patient, relatives and carers. The National Advisory Committee on Nutrition Education (NACNE) produced dietary guidelines (1983) which reflect the current emphasis on prevention of major diseases such as heart disease and cancer. These guidelines and the dietary reference values (Department of Health 1991) should be the basis of any discussion pertaining to a healthy diet in the United Kingdom.

Personal cleansing and dressing

On ending the meal, the nurse should ask the patient if he wishes his face to be washed and if mouth hygiene is desired. The nurse/carer has a role in the prevention of dental caries by the provision and maintenance of good oral care (Kelly 1994).

Ensure that all visible traces of food debris, spillages and soiled napkin are removed from the patient's appearance, thereby maintaining a positive body image which may enhance the patient's self esteem.

Patient education: key points

Advice on a healthy dietary intake and the benefits of such a diet should be given by the nurse to both the patient and his carers.

The nurse should provide information and education on the constituents of a special diet which is required by the patient.

Information regarding the maintenance of oral health should be given by the nurse.

2   Enteral feeding

There are two parts to this section:

A **Enteral feeding via a nasogastric tube and intermittent bolus or a continuous drip system**

B **Enteral feeding via a gastrostomy/jejunostomy tube**

The concluding subsection 'Relevance to the activities of living' refers to the two practices collectively.

Learning outcomes

By the end of this section you should know how to:

- prepare the patient for this nursing practice
- collect and prepare the equipment
- describe the principles of enteral feeding
- outline some of the problems of enteral feeding.

Background knowledge required

Revision of the anatomy and physiology of the gastrointestinal tract.
Revision of the nutritional requirements of the human body.

Indications and rationale for enteral feeding

Enteral feeding is the introduction of the daily nutritional requirements, in liquid form, directly into a patient's stomach or small intestine by means of a tube. The tube may be inserted through the nostril and passed down into the stomach or it may be introduced directly into the stomach or small intestine by a surgical incision made in the abdominal wall.

It may be performed to maintain adequate nutrition in the following circumstances:

- obstruction of oesophagus, e.g. neoplasm
- loss of swallowing reflex
- oesophageal fistula
- preoperative preparation of malnourished patients
- during radiotherapy treatment
- postoperatively for patients who have had some types of oral surgery or oesophageal surgery

- some unconscious patients
- patients who have severe burns
- during radiotherapy treatment.

Enteral feeding can be administered in several ways. It may be administered through a fine tube, e.g. Clinifeed, with its own administration set and container for the feed, or it can be channelled through a pump. Enteral feeding may also be given through a self-retaining tube, e.g. Foley's catheter or Percutaneous Endoscopic Gastrostomy tube (PEG) via a surgical opening in the abdominal wall into the stomach, duodenum or jejunum.

2A Enteral feeding via a nasogastric tube and intermittent bolus or continuous enteral feeding

Equipment

Clinifeed tube and introducer

Lubricant, e.g. iced water or jelly

Hypoallergenic tape

Container with prepared feed

Clinifeed administration set (Fig. 33.1)

Intravenous infusion stand

Gravity or volumetric pump if required

Receptacle for soiled disposables.

Guidelines and rationale for this nursing practice

- help to explain the nursing practice to the patient *to gain consent and cooperation*
- collect and prepare the equipment *for efficiency of practice*
- observe the patient throughout this activity *to detect any signs of discomfort or distress*
- assist the qualified practitioner to insert the Clinifeed tube and then remove the introducer
- before commencing the feed an X-ray to confirm the position of the tube is necessary *as the lumen is too narrow to allow the usual tests to be carried out and it is necessary to ascertain that the tube has been correctly positioned*
- attach the prepared feed in the container to the infusion stand
- join the administration set to the container and allow the feed to run through to the end of the set before it is connected to the Clinifeed tube *so that as little air as possible is introduced to the patient's stomach*
- adjust the flow rate as required or connect to the appropriate pump *and ensure the rate of flow is as prescribed so that the patient's stomach does not become overdistended and produce feelings of nausea*
- when intermittent bolus feeding is the method of choice, run through some water at the end of the feed *to clear the tube*
- ensure that the patient is left feeling as comfortable as possible *maintaining the quality of this practice*

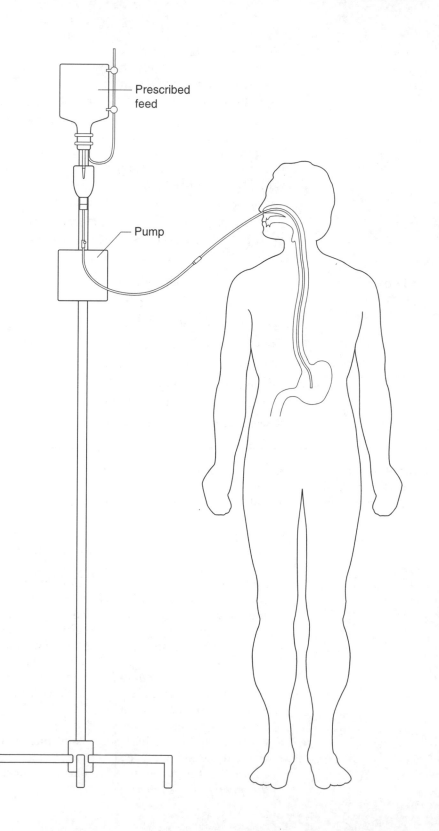

Prescribed
feed

Pump

Figure 33.1   *Enteral
feeding: nasogastric
continuous drip system*

- record appropriately the time of commencement of feeding, the amount and type of feed given, monitor after-effects and report abnormal findings immediately *providing a written record and assisting in the implementation of any action should an abnormality or adverse reaction to the practice be noted.*

Narrow-bore tubes for continuous enteral feeding are made of silicone or polyurethane, with diameters from 1–3 mm. They are more comfortable for the patient than the wide-bore tube and less likely to cause ulceration or erosion of the mucosa. They do, however, become blocked more easily and it is almost impossible to clear them by aspiration.

2B Enteral feeding via a gastrostomy/jejunostomy tube (Fig. 33.2)

Equipment	Water
	Prepared feed in container
	Sterile spigot
	Sterile dressings pack
	Water-based antiseptic
	Hypoallergenic tape
	Receptacle for soiled disposables.

Guidelines and rationale for this nursing practice

- explain the nursing practice to the patient *to gain consent and cooperation. Patients should be encouraged to be active partners in care*
- assist the patient into a suitable position such as semi-recumbent *to enable easy access to the gastrostomy site and to lessen the risk of a kink in the tube.* Ideally, the patient should not be lying flat as this increases the risk of reflux and aspiration (Fawcett, 1995)
- observe the patient throughout this activity *to detect any signs of discomfort or distress*
- collect and prepare the equipment *for efficiency of practice*
- connect the administration set to the gastrostomy tube after expelling all the air from the set *so that unnecessary air is not introduced into the stomach as this can cause pain and distension*
- pour a little water through the tube *to ensure it is clear*
- start the flow by adjusting the administration set or switching on the pump
- flush the tube through with water when all the prepared feed has been given *to clear the tube*
- disconnect the administration set and put a clean spigot in the end of the tube
- clean and re-dress the enterostomy site using an aseptic technique. *See* Wound care, page 383
- ensure that the patient is left feeling as comfortable as possible *maintaining the quality of this practice*

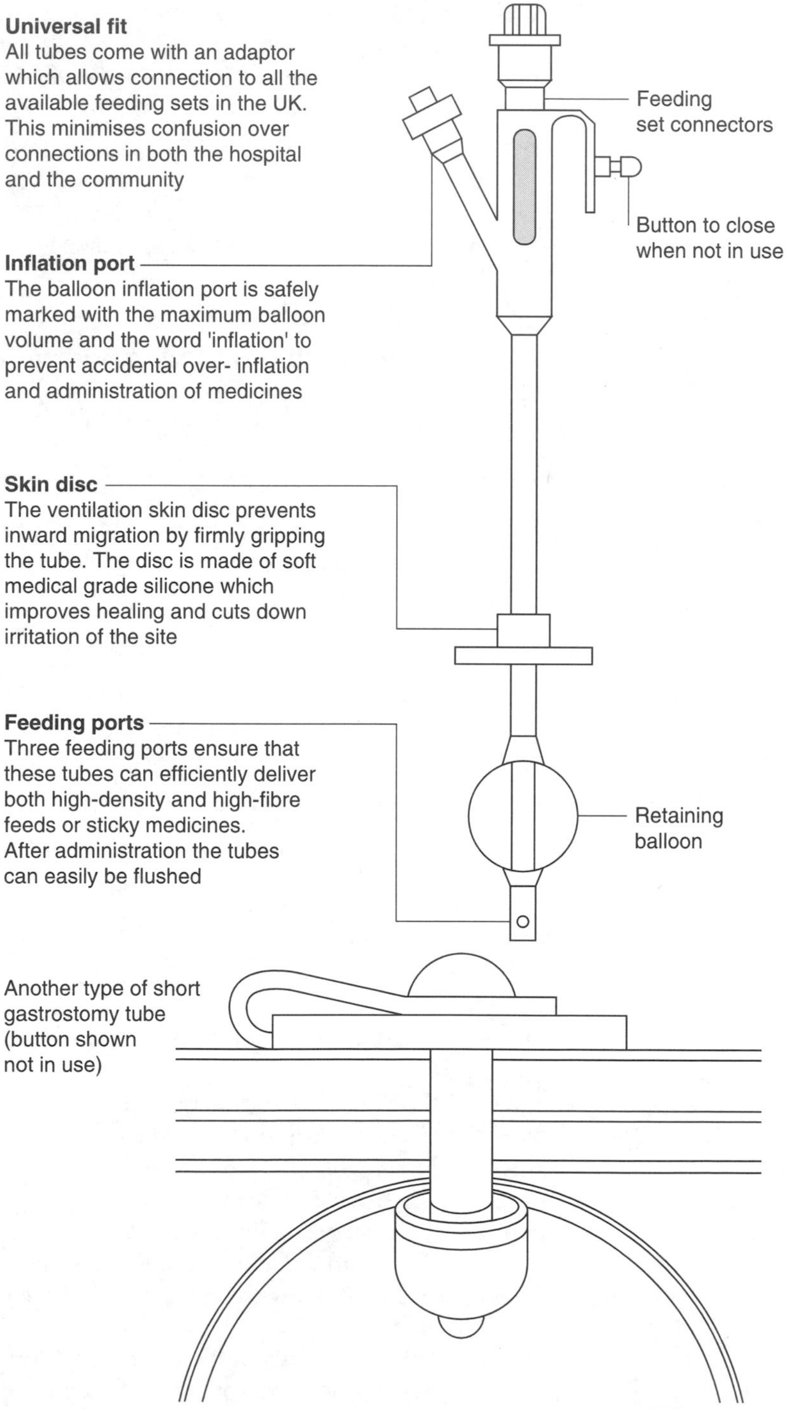

Universal fit
All tubes come with an adaptor which allows connection to all the available feeding sets in the UK. This minimises confusion over connections in both the hospital and the community

Feeding set connectors

Button to close when not in use

Inflation port
The balloon inflation port is safely marked with the maximum balloon volume and the word 'inflation' to prevent accidental over- inflation and administration of medicines

Skin disc
The ventilation skin disc prevents inward migration by firmly gripping the tube. The disc is made of soft medical grade silicone which improves healing and cuts down irritation of the site

Feeding ports
Three feeding ports ensure that these tubes can efficiently deliver both high-density and high-fibre feeds or sticky medicines. After administration the tubes can easily be flushed

Retaining balloon

Another type of short gastrostomy tube (button shown not in use)

Figure 33.2 *Enteral feeding via a gastrostomy tube*

- dispose of the equipment safely *to reduce any health hazard*
- record appropriately the time, amount and type of feed, monitor after-effects and report abnormal findings immediately *providing a written record and assisting in the implementation of any action should an abnormality or adverse reaction to the practice be noted.*

Relevance to the activities of living

Maintaining a safe environment

Although aseptic technique is not necessary when administering enteral feeding, a good standard of hygiene must be maintained to prevent the patient developing a gastrointestinal infection. A strict aseptic technique is necessary when re-dressing the gastrostomy site to help prevent the wound becoming infected.

No feed should be administered via nasogastric tube until the nurse has checked that it is in the correct position.

Eating and drinking

The patient may be allowed a small amount of liquid orally. This can help to stimulate secretion of some of the digestive juices. It is necessary to ensure that the patient receives an adequate amount of fluid in 24 hours and all the essential nutrients.

A formal dietetic assessment should be carried out and the patient's nutritional requirements discussed with a nutritionist.

Nausea, distension and diarrhoea can be a problem and is often caused by the feed being administered too rapidly. The continuous drip system helps to overcome this. Intermittent bolus feeding is waning in popularity for this reason although it is very convenient for community patients as it allows them to carry on their normal routine between feeds and also means they can conform to family meal times.

Eliminating

Diarrhoea can be a problem and is usually caused by too rapid feeding or administering a feed which is too concentrated. A feed contaminated by pathogens would also result in diarrhoea.

Personal cleansing and dressing

Frequent oral hygiene should be offered to the patient receiving enteral feeding because his lips, tongue and the mucosa of his mouth rapidly become dry and cracked if no fluid is passing over them.

Sleeping

Patients may prefer to receive their food by the continuous drip system while they are asleep at night. This allows them more freedom of movement during the day.

| **Patient education: key points** | A clear explanation of the necessity of this form of feeding will help gain the patient's cooperation. If the patient is self-administering feeds the importance of hygiene needs to be stressed. Patterns of feeding also need to be agreed with the patient. |

3 Parenteral nutrition

| **Learning outcomes** | By the end of this section you should know how to: |

- prepare the patient for this nursing practice
- collect and prepare the equipment
- assist the medical practitioner with the insertion of a central venous catheter
- maintain an infusion of parenteral nutrition for a period of time in an institutional or community setting.

| **Background knowledge required** | Revision of the anatomy and physiology of the cardiopulmonary system with special reference to the circulation of the blood, and the veins of the neck and upper thorax. |

Revision of the nutritional needs required to maintain health.

Revision of Intravenous therapy (*see* p. 165) and care of a Hickman catheter (*see* p. 175).

Revision of Aseptic technique (*see* p. 383).

Review of health authority policy regarding parenteral nutrition both in community and institutional care.

| **Indications and rationale for parenteral nutrition** | Parenteral nutrition is the intravenous infusion of essential nutrients for patients who are unable to maintain an adequate nutritional intake by the oral or nasogastric route. It may be indicated for anyone who is unable to ingest, digest or absorb sufficient oral or enteral feeding, e.g.: |

- patients who have had surgery involving major resection of the intestine *as they will have a reduced ability to digest food*
- patients who have extensive inflammatory disease of the alimentary system. *Inflammation of the gut reduces the efficiency of the digestive process*
- patients who have malabsorption problems *as, despite reasonable intake, there will be inadequate amounts of nutrients absorbed and available for tissue cells*
- patients who have severe nausea and vomiting, e.g. following chemotherapy for malignant disease. *The appetite is reduced and food will not remain in the stomach long enough for digestion to occur.*

Total Parenteral Nutrition (TPN) is the term used when all the patient's nutritional requirements are given by intravenous infusion. Parenteral nutrition may also be given as a supplement to nasogastric or oral feeding (Zainal 1994).

Outline of the procedure

Ideally this procedure should be performed in theatre. If the procedure is performed in the ward, it should take place in the treatment room.

The insertion of the intravenous catheter used for an infusion of parenteral nutrition is performed by a medical practitioner using aseptic technique. A cap and theatre mask are worn. Having washed his hands, the medical practitioner dons a theatre gown and gloves, and prepares the sterile equipment on the trolley, maintaining asepsis. When the patient is in the correct position, sterile drapes are placed round the area of the access site. A local anaesthetic may be administered. The skin area of the access site is cleansed prior to the insertion of an intravenous catheter through the subclavian or the internal jugular vein to allow the tip of the catheter to lie in the superior vena cava. A flow of prescribed infusion fluid is established, and the distal end of the catheter is stitched in position. The access site is covered with a sterile dressing (*see* Central venous pressure, p. 103).

Occasionally a catheter will be tunnelled subcutaneously so that the entry site to the vein is separated from the skin entry site to reduce the risk of infection. This is performed when long-term parenteral nutrition is envisaged (RCN 1992).

The concentration of the nutrients is irritant to peripheral vessels, and could cause damage to peripheral veins, so parenteral nutrition should always be infused through a central venous catheter. The infusion fluid enters the circulation at the superior vena cava, is rapidly diluted by the volume of blood entering the heart, and is quickly distributed by the circulation of the blood thus reducing any problems of irritation to the vessels involved (Springett & Murray 1994).

The position of the patient is important during this procedure, and is dependent on the choice of entry site for catheterisation. There are three main entry sites:

The subclavian vein   The patient lies supine with no pillow, and the neck is extended. The head of the bed is lowered by 10°.

The internal jugular vein   The patient lies supine with no pillow, and the neck is extended. The head is rotated away from the site of entry, and is well supported in position. The head of the bed is lowered by 10°. This position is important to prevent the development of an air embolus.

The median cephalic vein   The patient lies supine. The chosen arm is extended with the palm upwards and the elbow supported. Peripherally inserted central catheters (PICC) via the cephalic or basilic vein are being used increasingly as technology advances (Gabriel 1994).

Equipment

As for intravenous infusion (*see* p. 166)

Additional equipment

- Theatre cap and mask
- Sterile gown
- Sterile gloves

- Sterile minor operation pack or sterile drape and towels
- Waterproof protection for the bed
- Alcohol-based lotion for cleansing the skin
- Prescribed infusion fluid for parenteral nutrition
- Appropriate sterile catheter depending on the site of entry used, e.g. Hickman catheter, double or triple lumen catheter
- Sterile needles and black silk sutures
- ECG monitoring equipment if required
- Volumetric infusion pump, e.g. IMED infusion pumps, nos 922, 960, 965, Baxter Flo guard 6201
- Cassette for priming infusion pump or specialised infusion set
- Dark bag for excluding light from prepared infusion fluid.

Infusion fluid for parenteral nutrition

This will be prescribed by the medical practitioner for each 24-hour period, depending on the patient's nutritional needs and related blood chemistry. A combination of nutrients will be used to give a balanced intake, and vitamins and trace elements will be included in the prescription (Torrance & Gobbi 1994).

In areas where pharmacy services are available the intravenous feeding regimen is prepared as prescribed for each patient in 2 or 3 litre bags under laminar flow conditions every 24 hours. Everything for parenteral nutrition, including vitamins and trace elements, is added at one time. This reduces the risk of infection which might occur when an infusion of several different fluids in separate containers is prescribed and a series of taps, or Y connectors, are needed for the infusion.

A combination of the following intravenous fluids may be prescribed. All are available in 500 ml containers (see current pharmaceutical literature)(BNF 1995):

- carbohydrates, e.g. dextrose 20%
- fats, e.g. Intralipid 10%, Intralipid 20%
- proteins, e.g. Vamin 14 EF, Vamin 18 EF.

Many other products are available and the choice will depend on the patient's needs and the medical practitioner's preference.

In addition the following may be added:

- vitamins, e.g. Multibionta. *Note:* Some vitamins are destroyed by sunlight; if added to a 24-hour parenteral infusion the container must be covered by a dark bag to exclude light
- electrolytes, e.g. potassium, phosphates
- trace elements, e.g. zinc, magnesium.

Hickman catheter

This intravenous catheter may be chosen by the medical practitioner for a parenteral infusion which is needed over a period of weeks. This radio-opaque silastic catheter has a small sponge-like Dacron cuff at the distal end. The line is tunnelled subcutaneously and the cuff helps to retain the line in position as fibrous tissue forms round it. Patients may go home with this catheter in situ and become proficient in self care under the supervision of the primary health care team (*see* p. 175) (Corbett et al 1993).

The Hickman catheter is also used for infusions of intravenous cytotoxic medications which are prescribed over a long period and are not suitable for a peripheral infusion because of their irritant properties.

Volumetric infusion pumps

Parenteral nutrition should be infused by a continuous volumetric infusion pump. This ensures that a steady flow of prescribed nutrients is infused at a rate suitable for the patient's metabolism. If a pump is unavailable, a burette administration set should be used. Infusion pumps are primed with a special cassette and introduced into the infusion circuit between the administration set from the infusion fluid, and the infusion catheter (Fig. 33.3). There are clear manufacturer's instructions for all infusion pumps which should be followed when setting up infusions.

Infusion pumps can be set to give an hourly flow rate of 1–999 ml per hour. All pumps are fitted with alarm systems which will monitor any occlusion of the lines, air bubbles and completion of the available fluid. Recent equipment has a digital read-out of details of the infusion, and the alarm system. New equipment for controlled administration of intravenous infusion is being developed continually. There are different types of infusion pumps and gravity-feed infusion sets on the market, and the choice for use may depend on health authority policy.

Guidelines and rationale for this nursing practice

- help to explain the procedure to the patient *to gain consent and cooperation and encourage participation in care* (Hamilton 1993)
- ensure the patient's privacy, *respecting her individuality and maintaining her self esteem*
- collect and prepare the equipment *for efficiency of practice*

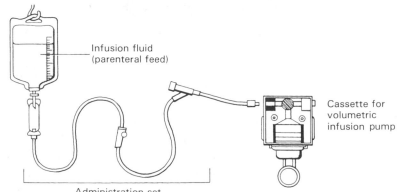

Infusion fluid (parenteral feed)

Cassette for volumetric infusion pump

Figure 33.3 *Parenteral nutrition: equipment for priming the volumetric infusion pump*

Administration set

- check the prescribed intravenous fluid for parenteral nutrition (*see* Administration of medicines, p. 1)
- prime the equipment (*see* Intravenous infusion, p. 165)
- help the patient into the appropriate position, depending on the site of entry used for the insertion of the central venous catheter, *so that optimum safety is maintained for the patient*
- observe the patient throughout this activity *to monitor any adverse effects*. The central line enters the large veins adjacent to the heart and occasionally may cause arrhythmias, so monitoring the patient's ECG may be helpful
- adjust the tilt of the bed to lower the patient's head if necessary *to minimise the risk of an air embolus*
- remain with the patient and *help maintain her position*. Reassurance will be needed *as the patient may find this part frightening*
- assist the medical practitioner as required *to ensure the safe outcome of this practice*
- commence the infusion of parenteral nutrition at the prescribed rate once the catheter is in position and the sterile dressing is applied to the access site (*see* Central venous pressure, p. 103)
- cover the infusion with a dark bag *to protect any vitamins from light, which may cause deterioration*
- ensure that the patient is left feeling as comfortable as possible. Ideally, the patient should have a period of rest after this nursing practice *to reduce anxiety and stress*
- Dial the required number of ml per hour on the infusion pump (see manufacturer's instructions) or fill the burette chamber hourly with the prescribed volume of fluid *to maintain the infusion as prescribed*
- dispose of the equipment safely *to maintain a safe environment*
- document the nursing practice appropriately, monitor after-effects and report abnormal findings immediately. *This ensures safe practice and enables prompt appropriate medical and nursing intervention to be initiated.*

Relevance to the activities of living

Observations and further rationale for this nursing practice will be included within each activity of living as appropriate.

Maintaining a safe environment

All precautions and observations for the prevention of infection should be maintained.

The whole infusion and the administration set should be changed every 24 hours, maintaining asepsis.

The lines should be observed for air bubbles and all the connections checked regularly and the lines supported to prevent any disconnection, in order to help prevent the development of an air embolus.

The alarm systems of the infusion pumps should be familiar to the staff using the equipment, and appropriate action taken when they are activated.

The nurse should ensure that dressing of the catheter site is performed using aseptic technique (*see* p. 383) and that interventions are conducted in the knowledge of recent research on this invasive procedure (Roberts 1994).

The nurse may help with patient education in maintaining a safe environment. Learning aseptic technique of wound cleaning and dressing will allow some independence for patients discharged home with long-term TPN (Stillwell 1992) (*see* Hickman catheter, p. 175).

Breathing

The respirations should be observed, and all the vital signs recorded 4-hourly or as frequently as necessary. Breathlessness accompanied by a moist cough and frothy sputum may indicate pulmonary oedema due to circulatory overload. Any abnormalities should be reported so that the rate of the prescribed infusion can be adjusted (*see* Intravenous therapy, p. 165).

A rare complication is the development of a pneumothorax; this is more likely to occur at the time of insertion of the catheter. Any sudden change in the patient's general condition or respiratory function should be reported immediately.

Eating and drinking

Accurate fluid balance recordings should be maintained. Fluid intake should be recorded as frequently as necessary, depending on the patient's condition — hourly, 2-hourly or 4-hourly.

Details of IV nutrients infused should be recorded accurately and any adverse effects reported.

Initially the patient's blood sugar levels may be monitored regularly while parenteral nutrition is in progress. The results will indicate the patient's ability to metabolise the nutrients infused. Blood sugar estimation using BM sticks or Dextrostix should be performed 4-hourly or as ordered. Ward urinalysis should be performed for sugar and acetone 4-hourly for the same reason, until the blood sugar has returned to normal.

Occasionally a continuous infusion of insulin is prescribed for patients who need a large calorie intake but whose metabolism is temporarily deficient. This may occur when a patient has severe trauma, burns or scalds.

A patient receiving parenteral nutrition has little or nothing to eat or drink by mouth. Frequent oral hygiene should be performed to maintain a healthy oral mucosa until a normal diet is resumed. With appropriate health education, patients with long-term TPN may be helped to become independent in keeping their oral mucosa healthy.

Eliminating

Fluid output should be recorded to maintain accurate fluid balance charts and help monitor renal function

The patient may need help when using a commode to support the infusion lines and prevent any disconnection.

Personal cleansing and dressing

Light comfortable clothing will allow access to the infusion site; the reason for this should be explained to the patient. Help may be needed with washing and showering. Some patients may be discharged home with TPN, and help given by carers and the district nurse.

Expressing sexuality

A continuous infusion and a long-term central line will result in an altered body image. Perceptive and supportive nursing care and good communication skills will help to alleviate the effects of this.

At home, adaptation of normal clothes, as well as counselling and help from the primary health care team, will enable normal activities to resume as far as possible, restoring the patient's self esteem.

Mobilising

In some instances parenteral nutrition may continue when the patient is up and about in the ward, and staff can help the patient to take his infusion with him. A light mobile pole and supportive explanations in relation to maintaining a safe environment will give the patient confidence to be more independent and visit other patients or the television room, as his condition allows. Occasionally patients may be discharged home while still receiving parenteral nutrition; with supervision and counselling from the primary health care team they can resume many normal activities.

Sleeping

The normal sleeping position may have to be adapted to accommodate the infusion lines, and the patient helped into a comfortable position.

Patients on long-term home TPN (HTPN) may choose the times of their nutritional infusion period. TPN may be given overnight, so that a more normal lifestyle may be resumed during the day.

Patient education: key points

Explanations given before, during and after the line is inserted, as well as the rationale for continuing parenteral nutrition, will help the patient to understand and interpret his condition and treatment.

The nurse should be sensitive to the timing and relevance of the information for each stage of this practice.

The community team will help to encourage the independence of the person having TPN at home. This will include teaching the relevant aspects of:

- aseptic technique
- care of the central venous catheter
- observation of the site
- preparation of the intravenous feed

- use of the volumetric infusion pump
- mouth care.

The patient requiring long-term care should understand the importance of reporting redness, swelling or pain at the catheter site or any feeling of being generally unwell. He may have increased independence if he is taught the principles of simple urinalysis to monitor glycosuria.

Patient education should be part of the discharge planning and should commence well before the patient goes home. It is helpful to have a liaison nurse working between the community and the institution. Written information in the form of an education leaflet will reinforce the patient's and carer's knowledge and confidence.

A contact telephone number to use as a 'help line' will give confidence to the patient for continuing independence.

References

Feeding a dependent patient

Department of Health 1991 Dietary reference values for food energy and nutrients for the United Kingdom (Report No. 41). HMSO, London

Kelly R 1994 Disorders of the mouth. In: Alexander M, Fawcett J, Runciman P (eds) Nursing practice — hospital and home: the adult. Churchill Livingstone, Edinburgh

National Advisory Committe on Nutrition Education 1983 A discussion paper on proposals of nutritional guidelines for health education in Britain. Health Education Council, London

Roper N, Logan W, Tierney A 1996 The elements of nursing, 4th edn. Churchill Livingstone, Edinburgh, pp 173–176, 181–188

Sanford J 1987 Making meals a pleasure. Nursing Times 83(6): 31–32

Further reading

Feeding a dependent patient

Baughen R 1989 Hospital food — a literature review. Surgical Nurse 2(3): 18–22

Bodey S, White G 1995 Working together for a nutritional balance. Community Nurse 1(7): 11–12

Cabell C 1990 Regaining a basic pleasure (describes care to regain the swallowing reflex). Nursing Times 86(47): 27–29

Committee on Medical Aspects of Food Policy 1984 Diet and cardiovascular disease. HMSO, London

Gregory J, Foster K, Tyler H, Wiseman M 1990 The dietary and nutritional survey of British adults. HMSO, London

Hempel S 1994 Alcohol consumption. Community Outlook 4(4): 35–36

Sadler C 1990 Sandwich course (discusses the axing of hot evening meals). Nursing Times 86(36): 19

Scott D 1986 Time and patience. Nursing Times 82(32): 36–37

Taylor M 1985 Care about food: 'Nurse I'm starving'. Nursing Times 81(23): 31

World Health Organisation 1990 Diet, nutrition and the prevention of chronic diseases. WHO, Geneva

Reference

Enteral feeding

Fawcett H 1995 Nutritional support for hospital patients. Nursing Standard 9(48): 25–28

Further reading

Enteral feeding

Anderton A 1995 Reducing bacterial contamination in enteral tube feeds. British Journal of Nursing 4(7): 368–376

Beadle L, Townsend S, Palmer D 1995 The management of dysphagia in stroke. Nursing Standard 9(15): 37–39

Fawcett H 1991 A tube to suit all nasogastric needs? Evaluation of finebore nasogastric tubes. Professional Nurse 6(6): 324–329

Delaney C 1991 Nasogastric intubation: use and abuse. Surgical Nurse 4(3): 4–9

Holmes S 1992 Enteral feeding. Community Outlook 2(10): 15–18

Langley P 1994 From tube to table. Nursing Times 90(48): 43–45

Liddle K 1995 Making sense of percutaneous endoscopic gastrostomy. Nursing Times 91(18): 32–33

Methaney N, McSweeney M, Wehole M 1990 Effectiveness of the auscultatory method of predicting feeding tube location. Nursing Research 39: 262–267

RCN Nursing Update 1994 Clinical enteral nutrition. Nursing Standard 8:32 (suppl)

Taylor S 1989 Preventing complications in enteral feeding. Professional Nurse 4(5): 247–249

Wakefield S, Mansell N, Baigrie R, Dowling B 1995 The use of a feeding jejunostomy after oesophogastric surgery. British Journal of Surgery 82(6): 811–813

Willow J 1995 Enteral feeding pumps. Professional Nurse 10(10): 635–640

References

Parenteral nutrition

British National Formulary 1995 British Medical Association and Royal Pharmaceutical Society of Great Britain, ch 9

Corbett K, Meehan L, Sackey V 1993 A strategy to enhance skills. Developing intravenous skills for community nursing. Professional Nurse 9(1): 60–63

Gabriel J 1994 An intravenous alternative. Nursing Times 90(31): 39–41

Hamilton H 1993 Care improves, while costs reduce. The clinical nurse specialist in total parenteral nutrition. Professional Nurse 8(9): 592–596

RCN 1992 Skin tunnelled catheters. Guidelines for care. RCN, London

Roberts P 1993 Simply a case of good practice. Professional Nurse 8(12): 775–779

Springett J, Murray C 1994 Direct input. Nursing Times 90(17): 48–52

Stillwell B 1992 Skills update: central venous lines (using Hickman lines). Community Outlook 2(5): 22–23

Torrance G, Gobbi M 1994 Nutrition. In: Alexander M, Fawcett J, Runciman P (eds) Nursing practice — hospital and home: the adult. Churchill Livingstone, Edinburgh, pp 672–676

Zainal G 1994 Nutrition of critically ill people. Intensive and Critical Care Nursing 10(3): 165–169

Further reading

Parenteral nutrition

Clarke R 1990 A cost effective system for TPN. Nursing Times 86(31): 65–68

Finnegan S 1989 Home parenteral nutrition. Professional Nurse 4(2): 79–81

Lee H, Venkat Raman G 1990 A handbook of parenteral nutrition. Chapman & Hall, London

Miller R, Howie E, Murchie M 1994 The gastrointestinal system, liver and biliary tract. In: Alexander M, Fawcett J, Runciman P (eds) Nursing practice — hospital and home: the adult. Churchill Livingstone, Edinburgh, pp 101–104

Raper S, Maynard N 1992 Feeding the critically ill patient. British Journal of Nursing 1(6): 273–280

Roper N, Logan W, Tierney A 1996 The elements of nursing, 4th edn. Churchill Livingstone, Edinburgh, pp 190–191

Thompson A et al 1989 Long term central venous access: the patient's view. Intensive Care and Clinical Monitoring 10(5): 142–145

34 Oxygen Therapy

Learning outcomes

By the end of this section you should know how to:

- prepare the patient for this nursing practice
- collect and prepare the equipment
- administer oxygen therapy at home or in an institutional setting.

Background knowledge required

Revision of the anatomy and physiology of the cardiopulmonary system, with special reference to the exchange of gases and the mechanism of respiration.

Revision of the dangers of the use of oxygen.

Review of health authority policies regarding fire precautions and oxygen therapy, both in institutional and community care.

Indications and rationale for oxygen therapy

Oxygen therapy is the introduction of increased oxygen to the air available for respiration *to prevent hypoxia, a condition where insufficient oxygen is available for the cells of the body, especially those in the brain and vital organs.*

Hypoxia may occur in the following circumstances:

- respiratory disease, *when the area available for respiration is reduced,* e.g. by:
  — infection
  — chronic obstructive airways disease (COAD)
  — pulmonary infarction/embolus
  — asthma
- chest injuries following trauma, *when the mechanism of respiration may be impaired*
- heart disease, *when the cardiac output is reduced,* e.g. by:
  — myocardial infarction
  — congestive cardiac failure
- haemorrhage, *when the oxygen-carrying capacity of the blood is reduced*
- preoperatively and postoperatively *when analgesic drugs may have an effect on respiratory function,* e.g. narcotics
- in emergency situations, e.g. cardiac or respiratory arrest, cardiogenic, bacteraemic or haemorrhagic shock, *as cardiac output will fall, reducing available oxygenated blood for the vital organs.*

Except in emergency situations oxygen therapy will be prescribed by a medical practitioner, who will specify both the percentage of oxygen and the method of administration. The administration of oxygen is one of the specific medical treatments: each patient will have individually assessed requirements related to his particular medical problem (BNF 1995).

Oxygen therapy can be administered in the patient's own home under the care of the community nurse or in an institutional setting. The principles for this nursing practice remain the same wherever it takes place. At home, the oxygen cylinder and its associated equipment will be delivered regularly to the patient's home from a central supply, depending on individual health board policy, as prescribed and ordered by the general practitioner.

Equipment

Oxygen supply, e.g. piped oxygen or oxygen cylinder

Reduction gauge as required

Flow meter

Oxygen mask or nasal cannulae as appropriate

Oxygen tubing

Humidifier as appropriate

'No Smoking' signs

Receptacle for soiled disposables.

Oxygen masks

Oxygen masks are designed to give an accurate percentage of oxygen by entraining an appropriate amount of air for a specific flow rate of oxygen. Instructions are available for each type of mask and they should be used accordingly (Bambridge 1993).

Edinburgh mask   The percentage of oxygen is adjusted by the flow rate of the flow meter only.

Hudson mask/Venturi mask   With these masks there are various attachments which can be used to give a more specific percentage if prescribed. The required flow of oxygen for the prescribed percentage is given for each attachment, which may be colour coded (Fig. 34.1).

Figure 34.1   *Oxygen therapy: mask in position*

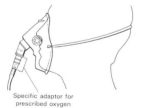

Specific adaptor for prescribed oxygen percentage

Figure 34.2   *Oxygen therapy: nasal cannulae in position*

Nasal cannulae

These are light plastic tubes inserted into each nostril and shaped to fit over the ears to maintain their position. Patients find them less claustrophobic than a conventional mask. They are not suitable for all patients as lower percentages of oxygen are not accurately obtained, and, at higher percentages, humidification is inadequate (Fig. 34.2).

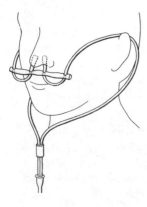

T-piece

Oxygen may be delivered directly into an endotracheal tube or tracheostomy tube via wide corrugated tubing and a T-piece. Adequate humidification is essential.

Oxygen tents

These are used mainly in paediatrics, *when babies and young children would not tolerate masks.* Danger of fire is increased further using this method, *because of the larger area of concentration of oxygen within the oxygen tent, and the difficulty of confining the gas to a small area when nursing the patient.*

Emergency situations

For emergency resuscitation procedures, oxygen may be administered via an Ambubag and resuscitation mask *for a higher percentage of oxygen to be given with assisted ventilation* (see Cardiopulmonary resuscitation, p. 75).

Humidifiers

If is important that the oxygen administered is adequately humidified *to prevent drying of the mucosa of the respiratory tract.* Various humidifiers are available.

When percentages of oxygen above 35% are prescribed, humidifiers which nebulise and warm the water vapour should be used, e.g. Inspiron humidifier, *to help to maintain a healthy bronchial mucosa.*

Guidelines and rationale for this nursing practice

- identify and check the prescription for oxygen therapy *to ensure the correct percentage is administered* (Baxter et al 1993)
- explain the nursing practice to the patient *to gain consent and cooperation and encourage participation in care*
- explain the dangers of smoking to the patient, his family and friends and display appropriate 'No Smoking' signs, *making sure they understand the increasing risk of fire when oxygen is administered*
- at home, hang the notice on the oxygen cylinder, *as a reminder for all the family and visitors*
- collect and assemble the equipment as required *so that everything is at hand*
- help the patient into a comfortable position *so that he will tolerate the oxygen therapy without distress*
- observe the patient throughout this activity *to monitor any adverse effects as well as any improvement in respiratory function*
- fill the humidifier with sterile water to the correct level *so that there is efficient humidification of the inspired oxygen*
- adjust the flow rate of oxygen as prescribed *so that the correct percentage is administered* (Bell 1995)
- observe the flow of oxygen and water vapour through the mask or cannulae before administration *to check that the equipment is working efficiently*
- place the mask in the correct position, and adjust it to fit firmly and comfortably over the patient's nose and mouth (Fig. 34.1) *so that all the oxygen prescribed is administered and as little as possible escapes from the mask*
- remain with the patient as necessary *and help him to maintain the equipment in position*
- top up the level of water in the humidifier as required *to maintain humidification*

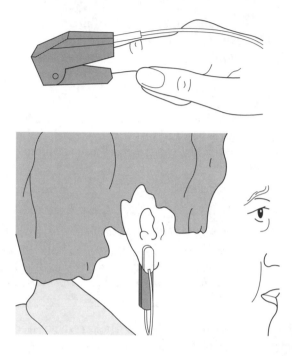

Figure 34.3 *Oxygen therapy: pulse oximeter A Hand sensor B Ear lobe sensor*

- assist the medical practitioner with the estimation of arterial blood gases as required *to evaluate the efficiency of the treatment*
- monitor the saturation levels using pulse oximetry if required *to evaluate the effect of the oxygen administered* (Jones 1995)
- observe all fire precautions *to minimise the risk of fire throughout the practice while oxygen is used*
- ensure that the patient is left feeling as comfortable as possible *so that he will continue to tolerate the oxygen therapy* (Ashurst 1995)
- dispose of the equipment safely *to prevent any transmission of infection*
- document the nursing practice appropriately, monitor after-effects and report abnormal findings immediately, *ensuring safe practice and enabling prompt appropriate medical and nursing intervention to be initiated as soon as possible.*

Pulse oximetry

It is now possible to measure oxygen saturation levels (Sa O_2) by a non-invasive technique. An electronic device called a pulse oximeter measures the absorption of red and infra-red light passing through living tissue. This is normally a specialised sensitive electronic clip which fits comfortably on a finger, a toe or an ear lobe and records the result on the patient's electronic monitor (Fig. 34.3). The oximeter reading closely responds to the arterial blood gas levels, so fewer blood samples are needed for monitoring arterial blood oxygen levels. The fact that a continuous read-out of levels can be observed helps to evaluate the effect of oxygen therapy and, being non-invasive, helps to maintain a safe environment for both the patient and caring staff (Coull 1992).

Arterial blood gas estimation

In intensive care areas, accident and emergency units and during perioperative care the effectiveness of oxygen therapy may be monitored by the medical practitioner assessing the arterial blood gases. The results are recorded in relation to the percentage of oxygen administered. Changes in the percentage of oxygen or methods of administration may be ordered accordingly. Samples of arterial blood are usually obtained from the radial artery, either from an indwelling arterial cannula, or by individual sampling, performed by the medical practitioner. The nurse should maintain observations of the arterial puncture site. There is less need for this monitoring assessment now that pulse oximetry is available (Stoneham et al 1994).

Relevance to the activities of living

Observations and further rationale for this nursing practice will be included within each activity of living as appropriate.

Maintaining a safe environment

The patient's general condition should be observed to identify any deterioration or improvement in his hypoxic state, e.g. degree of drowsiness, level of orientation, level of consciousness. The colour and condition of the patient's skin should be observed for the presence of cyanosis, clamminess or sweating.

Oxygen is a gas which readily supports combustion, so in areas where it is used the risk of fire is greatly increased. Every precaution to prevent fire should be maintained. If possible the patient should be aware of the problem and help in maintaining a safe environment. The dangers of smoking should be explained to him and all his family and visitors. 'No Smoking' signs can help to reinforce this precaution.

Alcohol-based solutions, oils and grease should not be used in areas where oxygen is administered. These volatile substances are readily flammable and the presence of oxygen will increase the risk of fire. All these precautions should be part of the patient's education when therapy is administered in a community setting. All the family and the associated carers should also be involved.

Health authority policy on fire precautions should be familiar to all staff and carers.

The administration of oxygen does not require aseptic technique. However, adequate levels of cleanliness should be maintained to prevent cross-infection, and equipment replaced as necessary. The nurse should wash her hands before commencing and on completion of this nursing practice.

Communicating

Oxygen masks can be a barrier to communication by making it more difficult for the patient to speak and be heard, so there is a risk of misunderstandings. This may cause the patient to remove the mask. The nurse needs good communication skills to help the patient tolerate the procedure during the period of time when it is necessary. The use of closed (direct) questions, for which only a 'yes' or 'no' answer is needed, may help with this.

Breathing

In most instances the need for oxygen therapy indicates that the patient has some difficulty with breathing. Dyspnoea may be relieved by helping the patient into an appropriate comfortable position as his condition allows, e.g. sitting upright, leaning over a bed table supported on a pillow, or sitting in a chair.

The respiration rate should be recorded as frequently as necessary, noting the type and depth of the respirations (Kendrick & Smith 1992).

Patients who have bronchospasm can be helped by medications which induce bronchodilation, either systemically or via a nebuliser as prescribed (*see* Nebuliser therapy, p. 227).

Patients who have chronic obstructive airways disease (COAD) have permanently altered respiratory physiology. The respiratory drive or stimulus for respiration responds only to low arterial blood levels of oxygen, therefore only low percentages of oxygen should be prescribed and administered, e.g. 24–28% oxygen; raising the arterial blood oxygen level too high in these patients could cause respiratory arrest. It is important that the patient and his family understand the importance of not altering the prescribed flow rate. They should be aware of the danger of increasing the amount of oxygen administered.

Eating and drinking

The removal of the mask for drinking should be supervised by the nurse, and will depend on the patient's condition.

It may be possible to change to nasal cannulae at meal times only, using a mask at other times to maintain the accuracy of the oxygen percentage as necessary.

Oxygen, even when adequately humidified, causes the mouth and nasal passages to become dry. Frequent oral and nasal hygiene will be required for the patient's comfort, and to maintain a healthy oropharyngeal mucosa.

Personal cleansing and dressing

The patient may need help with both washing and dressing, depending on his condition.

The inside of the oxygen mask may become wet with condensation. The patient's face can be washed and the inside of the mask dried as appropriate. This will greatly increase the patient's comfort and tolerance of this nursing practice.

Expressing sexuality

The use of a face mask has an adverse effect on the patient's self image. The nurse should use good communication skills to counteract this.

Male patients should be helped to shave daily, as this enables the mask to fit comfortably, as well as preserving self esteem, however 'after shave' should not be used as it is often alcohol based.

An explanation about the dangers of using perfume or make-up during this procedure should be given to female patients. Extra opportunities for washing and drying the face may help to alleviate the feeling of neglect of body image.

Patient education: key points

The reason for the administration of oxygen therapy should be explained to the patient and all the family and carers involved. They should understand that it is a specific part of his treatment.

At home the patient and carers should be shown how to adjust the flow rate to the prescribed rate only, and to fill the humidifier, maintaining a safe environment, as well as how to connect the mask and tubing.

The procedure for changing oxygen cylinders and the personnel involved will depend on health authority policy; carers may be instructed in some instances.

The increased risk of fire should be explained and simple instructions about fire precautions given.

The danger of smoking when oxygen is used should be reinforced continually. Patient and family cooperation is needed for this. They can choose where 'No Smoking' signs should be displayed.

For patients with COAD, everyone should understand the importance of never increasing the prescribed flow of oxygen delivered to the patient. This may need reinforcing if there is a change of carer in the community setting. The reason for this should be part of patient education.

The patient should understand the importance of reporting immediately any changes in respiratory function such as increased dyspnoea, cough, sputum or general feeling of distress.

References

Ashurst S 1995 Oxygen therapy. British Journal of Nursing 4(9): 508–515

Bambridge A 1993 An audit of comfort and convenience of oxygen masks and nasal catheters in the provision of post operative oxygen therapy. Professional Nurse 8(8): 513–518

Baxter K, Nolan K, Winyard J, Goldhill D 1993 Are they getting enough? Meeting the oxygen therapy needs of post-operative patients. Professional Nurse 8(5): 310–312

Bell C 1995 Is this what the doctor ordered. Accuracy of oxygen therapy prescribed and delivered in hospital. Professional Nurse 10(5): 295–300

British National Formulary (BNF) 1995 Oxygen. British Medical Association and the Royal Pharmaceutical Society of Great Britain, March 126–127

Coull A 1992 Making sense of pulse oximetry. Nursing Times 88(32): 42–43

Jones S 1995 Getting the balance right. Pulse oximetry and inspired oxygen concentration. Professional Nurse 10(6): 368–372

Kendrick A, Smith E 1992 Respiratory measurements 2. Simple measurements of lung function. Professional Nurse 7(1): 748–754

Stoneham M, Saville G, Wilson I 1994 Knowledge about pulse oximetry among medical and nursing staff. Lancet 344: 1339–1342

Further reading

Allan D 1989 Making sense of . . . oxygen delivery. Nursing Times 85(18): 40–42

Hayes E 1994 Shock. In: Alexander M, Fawcett J, Runcimen P (eds) Nursing practice — hospital and home: the adult. Churchill Livingstone, Edinburgh, pp 607–609

Heslop A, King M 1994 Let's treat the body and mind. Collaborative rehabilitation for chronic breathlessness. Professional Nurse 10(3): 188–192

Heslop A, Shannon C 1995 Assisting patients living with long-term oxygen therapy. British Journal of Nursing 4(19): 1123–1128

Stables L, Tarry J 1992 Setting nursing standards in hyperbaric oxygen therapy. Intensive and Critical Care Nursing 8(1): 17–23

Young T 1995 Hyperbaric oxygen therapy in wound management. British Journal of Nursing 4(14): 796–803

35 Paracentesis: Abdominal

Learning outcomes

By the end of this section you should know how to:
- prepare the patient for this procedure
- collect and prepare the equipment
- assist the medical practitioner with abdominal paracentesis as required.

Background knowledge required

Revision of the anatomy and physiology of the abdominal organs, with special reference to the peritoneum.

Revision of Aseptic technique (*see* p. 383).

Indications and rationale for abdominal paracentesis

Abdominal paracentesis is the removal of fluid from the peritoneal cavity through a sterile cannula or needle. Sometimes medication may be introduced into the peritoneal cavity by the same route.

This procedure may be performed for the following reasons:
- *to obtain a specimen of abdominal fluid for diagnostic purposes*
- *to relieve intra-abdominal pressure caused by increased fluid within the abdominal cavity.* This symptom is called ascites and may occur in association with several conditions, e.g.:
  - congestive cardiac failure involving dysfunction of the right side of the heart
  - chronic hepatic disease
  - malignant disease with metastases in the liver
- *to introduce medication into the peritoneal cavity,* e.g. cytotoxic therapy for malignant disease.

Outline of the procedure

Abdominal paracentesis is carried out by the medical practitioner using aseptic technique. A mask and sterile gown as well as sterile gloves should be worn.

The site of insertion is midway between the umbilicus and the symphysis pubis along the midline.

The skin is cleansed with antiseptic lotion and a local anaesthetic is administered. The area round the site is covered with sterile towels. A small skin incision is made with a sterile blade, and a trocar and cannula are inserted into the peritoneal cavity. The trocar is removed, allowing fluid to flow through the cannula. Required specimens of abdominal fluid for investigation are collected at this stage by holding the appropriately labelled sterile containers under the flow of fluid, maintaining asepsis. The cannula may be removed and a sterile dressing applied, or it may be stitched in position and attached to sterile tubing and a closed drainage bag, if drainage is to be maintained. A suitable sterile dressing should be applied round the cannula. The flow of drainage fluid is regulated with a gate clamp or roller clamp to prevent too rapid a reduction of intra-abdominal pressure. Initially only 1l of fluid should be allowed to drain before regulating the flow to 100 ml per hour, or as prescribed by the medical practitioner (Lancaster & Stockbridge 1992).

Equipment

Trolley

Theatre mask

Sterile gown

Sterile gloves

Sterile dressings pack

Sterile towels

Sterile bowl

Sterile specimen containers appropriately labelled, completed laboratory forms and a plastic specimen bag for transportation

Antiseptic lotion

Sterile abdominal paracentesis set containing:
- specialised trocar and cannula
- forceps
- blade and holder
- tubing

Local anaesthetic and equipment for its administration

Sterile sutures and needle for stitching the cannula in position

Sterile drainage bag

Gate clip or roller clamp

Disposable tape measure

Measuring jug

Receptacle for soiled disposables.

Guidelines and rationale for this nursing practice

- help to explain the procedure to the patient *to gain consent and co-operation and encourage participation in care*
- ask the patient to empty his bladder immediately prior to the procedure. *This will ensure that the bladder remains within the pelvis, so preventing any risk of perforation when the trocar is inserted*
- ensure the patient's privacy *respecting his individuality and to maintain his self esteem*
- measure and record the patient's abdominal girth before commencing the procedure *to compare with the measurements after abdominal paracentesis*

- help to collect and prepare the equipment *making good use of time and resources*
- help the patient into a suitable, comfortable position. He may sit upright with his back well supported. If possible the legs may be lowered *to allow easier access to the insertion site and to increase the patient's comfort.* A bed which can be adjusted *to allow only the lower limbs to be lowered* is the most suitable. In some instances the medical practitioner may prefer that the patient lies flat. *The chosen position depends on the reason for the abdominal paracentesis*
- help to adjust the patient's clothing *to expose the site of insertion*
- observe the patient throughout this activity *to monitor any adverse effects*
- help to prepare the sterile field as required *to maintain asepsis*
- assist the medical practitioner as required during the procedure
- measure the amount of drainage and adjust the flow of drainage fluid as required *to ensure that the volume drawn does not cause a sudden reduction in intra-abdominal pressure.* Initially only 1 litre of fluid should be removed before regulating the flow to 50–150 ml/hour (Young et al 1988)
- ensure that the patient is left feeling as comfortable as possible in a sitting position, *so that drainage is encouraged*
- dispose of equipment safely *to prevent transmission of infection*
- dispatch labelled specimens of abdominal fluid to the appropriate laboratory with their completed forms immediately *so that investigations can be commenced as soon as possible*
- document the procedure appropriately, monitor after-effects and report abnormal findings immediately *to ensure safe practice and enable prompt appropriate medical and nursing intervention to be initiated.*

Relevance to the activities of living

Observations and further rationale for this nursing practice will be included within each activity of living as appropriate.

Maintaining a safe environment

This is an invasive procedure giving direct access to the peritoneal cavity so all precautions to minimise the risk of infection should be maintained. Asepsis should be maintained and adequate hand washing technique should be practised.

Following the procedure, the site should be observed for any redness or swelling which may indicate infection; this should be reported immediately.

Dressings should be changed as required, using aseptic technique (*see* Wound care, p. 383).

Any leakage of fluid round the cannula should be noted and reported as this may indicate that the cannula is blocked or dislodged.

Safety of staff transporting specimens should be maintained by enclosing containers in plastic specimen bags (*see* Specimen collection, p. 297).

Communicating

Patients do not normally find this procedure too uncomfortable, even during a period of continuous drainage. When the abdominal paracentesis is performed to relieve pressure caused by excess fluid in the peritoneal cavity, the patient is much more comfortable after the procedure is performed. A prescribed analgesic medication should be administered if required.

Breathing

The patient's blood pressure, pulse and respirations should be recorded 4-hourly following this procedure, for 24–48 hours. The frequency of the recordings will depend on the patient's condition and the reason for the abdominal paracentesis.

When a patient has had severe ascites, with a raised intra-abdominal pressure, the blood pressure and pulse should be recorded every half hour for 2 hours immediately following this procedure as a sudden drop in intra-abdominal pressure could cause cardiogenic shock due to rapid vasodilatation. A low blood pressure recording should be reported immediately and the rate of flow of the drainage fluid should be reduced to a minimum. Initially only 1 litre of fluid should be removed before regulating the flow as prescribed by the medical practitioner. This may be 50–150 ml hour, depending on the patient's condition.

Eating and drinking

Fluid intake should be recorded and accurate fluid balance charts maintained. This will enable any reduction or increase in peritoneal fluid to be monitored in relation to the fluid intake and urinary output.

The appetite may have been poor due to the feeling of fullness and discomfort caused by the ascites; patients often experience indigestion due to pressure on the stomach. Depending on the situation, they may have to be encouraged to eat following this procedure, as protein is lost with the peritoneal fluid. Advice from the dietitian may help with the choice of nourishing foods, and the family may be encouraged to help provide favourite treats if appropriate.

Eliminating

The colour and viscosity of the peritoneal fluid should be noted. The presence of blood should be noted and reported, as it may indicate trauma to the abdominal organs during the insertion of the trocar.

The amount of fluid drained should be accurately measured and recorded, and fluid balance charts should be maintained throughout this procedure. Appropriate arrangements for measuring the urine should be made, with the patient's cooperation. The patient may be helped to the toilet, or to use a commode, depending on his condition.

Fluids and electrolytes pass across the peritoneal membrane, so electrolytes may also be lost in the drained ascitic fluid. This could cause hypokalaemia (low potassium levels) or hyponatraemia (low sodium levels). The medical practitioner will monitor the patient's blood chemistry and prescribe replacement potassium and sodium as required. The loss of protein may also be a concern, as this is often present in ascitic fluid (Ryan & Neale 1981).

Drainage of large amounts of excess peritoneal fluid is not performed routinely, as the fluid will reform from the circulation unless the cause itself can be treated. Amounts sufficient to relieve distressing pressure and associated symptoms can be removed without causing problems.

When ascites is caused by abdominal metastases the patient may gain some relief from continuous drainage of the excess peritoneal fluid; this will be prescribed as appropriate.

Measurement of the abdominal girth may help to monitor developing or improving ascites. The bladder should be emptied before the daily measurement, which should be taken at the same position each time. To facilitate accurate measurement, and with the patient's permission, lines may be drawn on each side of the abdomen outlining the path of the tape measure for 1 or 2 cm.

Peritoneal dialysis   A form of abdominal paracentesis is used as one of the treatments for renal failure. Continuous ambulatory peritoneal dialysis (CAPD) uses the properties of the peritoneal membrane as a substitute kidney. A permanent catheter is inserted into the peritoneal cavity. A quantity of sterile dialysis fluid is introduced through the catheter where it remains in the peritoneal cavity for 4–6 hours. The fluid is then allowed to drain out over half an hour. This procedure is repeated continuously over 24 hours, so that nitrogenous waste and excess electrolytes can be eliminated from the body.

The patient may be taught how to introduce his own dialysis fluid and drain the peritoneal fluid using aseptic technique. This method of home dialysis allows the patient to continue a relatively normal lifestyle (Martin 1993).

Personal cleansing and dressing

Depending on the patient's condition he may be able to have a shower while this procedure is in progress; a waterproof dressing can be used to protect the cannula site.

The patient's clothes may have to be adapted to accommodate the cannula and drainage bag.

Controlling body temperature

The temperature should be recorded 4-hourly during and following this procedure to monitor any change in body temperature which might indicate a developing infection. Any abnormality should be reported immediately.

Mobilising

Immediately following this procedure the patient should remain in bed to enable observations of his condition to be maintained. Mobilising may then be encouraged as his condition allows. Patients with a continuous drainage system may need help to maintain a safe environment when mobilising, to prevent infection or disconnection of the tubing. Patients treated with continuous ambulatory peritoneal dialysis (CAPD) for chronic renal failure may roll up their empty bag and tuck it under their waist band once the dialysis fluid is in situ, and then recommence normal activities (Beer 1995).

Expressing sexuality

The presence of an abdominal catheter will present the patient with a feeling of an altered body image. The nurse's attitude and communication skills, both verbal and non-verbal, can help the patient to accept this. The relief of abdominal pressure from excess ascites should help the patient's acceptance. Patients on CAPD should be counselled with their sexual partners. They should be encouraged to seek guidance from local support groups (Cronan 1993).

Patient education: key points	Explain the reason for the procedure and the importance of the patient's position during the insertion of the catheter.

Reassure the patient that she should feel more comfortable once some of the abdominal fluid has drained away.

If the catheter is to remain in situ for a while, explain how the patient can cope with toileting, personal cleansing and dressing, and the help she will be given with this.

The patient should understand the importance of reporting redness, swelling, pain or discomfort at the access site, even after the catheter has been removed.

Patients with renal failure who commence CAPD will undergo a period of specific education from a team of clinical nurse specialists in the CAPD unit. The patient may be admitted for one or two days; increasingly, however, this is carried out on a 'day care' basis. Partners, family and carers will be included in the education programme, which continues until the patient is confident with self-care of CAPD. There will be continued links with the CAPD clinic as well as liaison with the community team.

References

Beer J 1995 Body image of patients with ESRD (experiencing both CAPD and haemodialysis) and following renal transplant. British Journal of Nursing 4(10): 591–598
Cronan N 1993 Management of the patient with altered body image. British Journal of Nursing 2(5): 257–261
Lancaster S, Stockbridge J 1992 PV shunts relieve ascites. Registered Nurse 55(8): 58–60
Martin J 1993 Peritoneal dialysis, prescription for the 90's. British Journal of Nursing 2(3):162–166
Ryan E, Neale G 1981 Procedure in practice. Devonshire Press, Torquay, pp 7–9
Young M E et al 1988 Third spacing. When a body conceals fluid loss. Registered Nurse 51(8): 46–48

Further reading

Miller R, Howie E, Murchie M 1994 The gastro-intestinal system, liver and biliary tract. In: Alexander M, Fawcett P, Runciman P (eds) Nursing practice — hospital and home: the adult. Churchill Livingstone, Edinburgh, pp 116–118
Morrison M, Shandran M, Smithers F 1994 The urinary system In: Alexander M, Fawcett J, Runciman P (eds) Nursing practice — hospital and home: the adult. Churchill Livingstone, Edinburgh, pp 321–323
Roper N, Logan W, Tierney A 1996 The elements of nursing, 4th edn. Churchill Livingstone, Edinburgh, pp 221–222

36 Preoperative Nursing Care

The guidelines in this nursing practice apply to patients experiencing day surgery and those undergoing surgery requiring a longer stay in hospital.

Learning outcomes

By the end of this section you should know how to:
- explain the standard preoperative preparations of a patient who is scheduled for surgery
- describe the nurse's role in looking after a patient prior to surgery.

Background knowledge required

Revision of the cardiopulmonary system.

Review of health authority policy on preoperative preparation of patients.

Indications and rationale for preoperative care

Preoperative nursing care is required *to promote the optimum physical and psychological condition of patients undergoing surgical procedures.*

Guidelines and rationale for this nursing practice

- explain the pre- and postoperative routines to the patient and answer any questions appropriately; the discussion of any fears or anxieties that the patient may have should be encouraged. *Studies by Boore (1978) and Sofaer (1983) have demonstrated that patients' anxiety levels are reduced by receiving information and explanations*
- record the temperature, pulse, respiration, blood pressure and urinalysis, *to give baseline findings with which to compare postoperative observations*
- carry out evacuation of the patient's bowel using suppositories or a specific bowel preparation requested by the surgeon. This is usually requested if the surgical procedure involves the bowel, *as evacuation helps to reduce the risk of contamination of the wound by intestinal organisms*
- offer the sedative which will have been ordered by medical staff the night before surgery, *to help the patient sleep well*
- fast the patient for 4–6 hours prior to surgery so that the stomach is empty, *in order to avoid the risk of regurgitation and the inhalation of gastric contents while under anaesthesia*
- prepare the skin according to health authority policy. This may involve removal of an area of body hair by shaving or depilatory cream; showering or bathing using an antiseptic soap; and putting on a theatre gown, and perhaps

socks and paper pants. *These preparations are used to reduce the risk of a postoperative infection developing.* Research into removal of body hair and use of antiseptic preparations in baths and showers has produced contradictory findings. See Leigh et al (1983), Wells et al (1983), Willford (1983), Winfield (1986), Hayek et al (1987).

- ensure that all underwear has been removed, although paper pants may be worn on some occasions. Nail varnish should be removed from finger- and toenails *so that they can be examined by the anaesthetist for signs of hypoxia,* and make-up should be removed for the same reason. Dentures must be removed *because of the danger of inhaling them and causing asphyxiation.* Health authority policies vary about the removal of spectacles, hairgrips, contact lenses, hearing aids and other prostheses, e.g. wigs, artificial eyes or limbs

- tape the wedding ring to the patient's finger, but all other jewellery and valuables which the patient has brought into hospital should be recorded, put into an envelope, appropriately labelled, and placed in a valuables box or safe. *Metal jewellery may be accidentally lost or may be a cause of harm to the patient, e.g. diathermy burns*

- check the patient's identification verbally and from the identiband and confirm that the consent for operation form has been signed. *This is carried out to comply with legal requirements and hospital policy*

- after the patient has had the opportunity to micturate, administer the premedication ordered by the anaesthetist. *Premedication can help to relax the patient and may dry up secretions*

- leave the patient to rest quietly when the premedication has been given but observe for reaction to premedication drugs. *Rest may encourage relaxation and maximise the effect of the premedication.* In day surgery units premedication is often only offered to patients who appear to have high anxiety levels

- when the porter from the theatre reception area arrives to collect the patient, accompany them to the theatre reception area, and hand the patient over to the care of a theatre nurse. There is usually a form with a checklist which the ward nurse and theatre nurse will confirm. The patient may travel to theatre on a hospital bed or on a theatre trolley, according to health authority policy. *Research studies have demonstrated that a known person accompanying the patient helps reduce anxiety* (Boore 1978).

Relevance to the activities of living

Maintaining a safe environment

Preoperative skin care may vary, as each surgeon has his own theories about any necessary skin preparation to help avoid infection of the wound. Putting clean linen on the bed for the patient's return from theatre is another measure which helps to prevent infection.

It is essential that there is careful identification of the patient to ensure that the patient has the correct operation. Patient safety while under the influence of premedication is the nurse's responsibility.

It is also the nurse's responsibility to ensure that the patient's valuables are listed and safely stored.

Communicating

Information and explanations are an important part of the nurse's responsibility for patients in surgical wards. Research has shown that explanations prior to surgery can help reduce the incidence of postoperative pain and complications (Boore 1978).

For patients experiencing day surgery, preadmission booklets are essential as much of the information given at the outpatient clinic may be forgotten or misunderstood by the patient.

A brief description of what to expect in the immediate postoperative period can often be reassuring to the patient, especially if equipment such as urethral catheters, wound drains or intravenous infusion will be in use.

When the patient is being anaesthetised, hearing is the last sense to disappear, so staff should ensure that the content of conversation in the vicinity of the patient will not increase anxiety.

Breathing

The patient should be encouraged to stop smoking before surgery, to enable the lung fields to be as clear as possible and lessen the susceptibility to pulmonary infection. Breathing exercises should be explained to the patient. These consist of encouraging the patient to sit as upright as possible and to breathe in deeply through his nose, expanding the chest and abdominal wall as much as possible. This allows good inflation of the lungs. On exhaling, the chest and abdominal walls should be allowed to relax and then extra air pushed out of the lungs. The wound can be supported if necessary.

Eating and drinking

As mentioned in the Guidelines, the patient should be fasted for 4–6 hours prior to surgery to avoid the danger of inhaling gastric contents while the cough reflex is reduced during general anaesthesia. If this has not been possible, e.g. in an emergency admission, it may be necessary to pass a nasogastric tube and aspirate the stomach contents (*see* Gastric aspiration, p. 143).

It is especially important that day surgery patients know the length of time they have to fast and the reasons for this.

Research has shown that prolonged periods of fasting reduce blood glucose levels to below normal range and also cause the patient to become dehydrated. This can impair the healing process and reduce the body's ability to cope with the trauma of surgery (Hamilton-Smith, 1972).

Eliminating

It is necessary for the patient to have an empty bladder and rectum, especially if muscle relaxant drugs are going to be used during surgery, because of the risk of contaminating the theatre table with excrement and the attendant risk of infecting the surgical wound. In addition, in abdominal surgery a full bladder is more liable to be damaged; in emergency surgery, the bladder may be catheterised to obviate this potential complication.

Patients for day surgery may have to carry out the required bowel preparation at home if this is prescribed by the surgeon. Nurses need to ensure that the patient knows how to use any suppositories or enema supplied for this purpose.

Personal cleansing and dressing

As mentioned in the Guidelines, special skin preparation may be required, although some research has shown that the bacterial skin count is lower when skin cleansing is done in theatre rather than some hours prior to surgery.

The discussion about removal and method of removal of body hair from around the site of surgery is ongoing and unresolved.

Mobilising

The patient should receive some teaching preoperatively about postoperative exercises to prevent such complications as pressure sores, deep venous thrombosis and chest infections. Nursing staff should ensure that the physiotherapist has visited the patient to give this teaching or, in the case of day surgery patients, that they have knowledge of these exercises.

Patients considered to be at risk of developing a deep vein thrombosis may be fitted with antiembolitic stockings as a prophylactic measure.

Expressing sexuality

Having to remove all personal clothing, jewellery, make-up, nail varnish and dentures can make the patient feel that personality and personal dignity are threatened. An explanation for these procedures should be given, together with the assurance that as soon as possible after surgery the patient's wishes regarding cleansing and dressing will be met.

Sleeping

The patient's normal sleeping pattern may be disturbed by the unaccustomed noise of the ward, change of environment, or by anxiety, and every possible means should be used to reduce or remove the cause of anxiety and promote comfort. Medication may be ordered to promote sleep on the night prior to surgery.

Dying

It is not uncommon for a patient to fear dying while anaesthetised. The patient should be helped to verbalise and discuss this fear and to realise that, with modern technology, such an occurrence is rare.

Many patients facing surgery benefit from attention to their spiritual needs by the hospital chaplain, who is a member of the caring team.

Patient education: key points

It is important that patients undergoing day surgery should have obtained beforehand all the information and knowledge necessary for them to successfully undergo their surgery. This will probably involve nurses at the outpatient clinic, in the community and in the day surgery unit. Written material should be provided to reinforce the verbal information given. Patients will need to carry out at home many of the preoperative preparations required such as bowel preparation, skin preparation and fasting.

References

Boore J 1978 Prescription for recovery. Royal College of Nursing, London
Hamilton-Smith S 1972 Nil by mouth? Royal College of Nursing, London
Hayek L J, Emerson J M, Gardner A M N 1987 A placebo controlled trial of the effect of preoperative baths or showers with chlorhexidine detergent on postoperative wound infection rates. Journal of Hospital Infection 10(2): 165–172
Leigh D A, Stronge J L, Marriner J, Sedgwick J 1983 Total body bathing with 'Hibiscrub' in surgical patients. A controlled trial. Journal of Hospital Infection 4(3): 229–235
Sofaer B 1983 Pain relief — the importance of communication. Nursing Times 79(48): 32–35
Wells F C, Newsom S W, Rowlands S C 1983 Wound infection in cardiothoracic surgery. Lancet 1: 1209–1210
Willford P S 1983 Hair removal — shave, preps, depilation and other preoperative considerations. Are they really necessary? Journal of Operating Room Research Institute 3(3): 26–28
Winfield V 1986 Too close a shave? Nursing Times Journal of Infection Control Nursing 82(10): 64–68

Further reading

Carrie L, Simpson P 1988 Understanding anaesthesia. Heinemann, London
Hallstrom R 1994 Is preoperative skin shaving outdated? Short report. Nursing Times 90(11): 11–12
Jones I 1995 Skills update. Pre-surgery preparation. Community Outlook 4(8): 18–19
Kalideen N 1990 Preparing skin for surgery. Nursing 4(15): 28–29
Llewellyn T 1990 Preoperative skin preparation. Surgical Nurse 3(2): 24–26
Lovett P, Stanton S, Hennessy D, Cashman J 1994 Pain levels and analgesia after surgery. British Journal of Nursing 3(4): 159–162
Markanday L 1994 Day surgery. Brief encounters. Nursing Times 90(7): 38–44
Roper N, Logan W, Tierney A 1996 The elements of nursing, 4th edn. Churchill Livingstone, Edinburgh
Schwartz-Barcott D, Fortin J, Kim H 1994 Preparation of patients for pain after surgery. Short report. Nursing Times 90(41): 12
Thomas E 1989 Preoperative fasting — a question of routine? Nursing Times 83(49): 46–47
Torrance C 1991 Preoperative nutrition, fasting and the surgical patient. Surgical Nurse 4(4): 4–9
Wachstein J 1987 Care of the elderly surgical patient. Geriatric Nursing and Home Care 7(4): 12–14
Winfield U 1986 Too close a shave? Nursing Times 82(10): 64, 67–68

37 Postoperative Care

In the case of day surgery, many of the Guidelines described here will be carried out by the community nurse, the patient or carers at home.

Learning outcomes

By the end of this section you should know how to:
- explain the general postoperative care of a patient
- describe the nurse's role in carrying out general postoperative care.

Background knowledge required

Revision of the clinical features of shock.

Revision of the physiology of wound healing.

Review of health authority policy on postoperative care.

Indications and rationale for postoperative care

Postoperative nursing care is required to monitor the patient's condition in order *to prevent and identify any problems that may occur after a surgical procedure.*

Guidelines and rationale for this nursing practice

When receiving the patient back into the ward:

- check that the airway is patent and that the patient is breathing adequately. Usually the patient is conscious before leaving the recovery room *but if he is heavily sedated the tongue may slip back and obstruct the airway*
- record the temperature, pulse and blood pressure and compare the results with the patient's preoperative recordings. *This will give some indication of the stability of the patient's condition*
- observe the wound and any drains which may be present, e.g. Redivac, corrugated drain, *to ensure there are no problems such as haemorrhage*
- check, if an intravenous infusion is present, that it is functioning according to medical staff instructions
- read the patient's theatre notes to confirm the surgical procedure which has been carried out and ascertain any instructions from the surgeon or anaesthetist, e.g. positioning of the patient, oxygen therapy
- ensure that the patient is lying in as comfortable a position as possible, and that the limbs are positioned in a manner which will not endanger muscle and nerve tissue. *These measures can help to control pain levels*
- administer analgesics as required by the patient and as prescribed by the

medical staff. *Several research studies have demonstrated that patients rate being in pain as the most anxiety-provoking issue when undergoing surgery* (Seers 1987, Biley 1989).

Continuing postoperative nursing:

- record blood pressure, pulse and respiration rates until they are within normal range and stable. *This usually indicates the reduction of physiological stress induced by surgery*
- assist the patient to wash and change into his own nightwear and offer a mouthwash *to aid comfort and recovery of sense of individuality*
- encourage the patient to sit up in bed well supported by pillows (unless contraindicated) and move around as much as he is able, helping him out of bed when blood pressure recordings are satisfactory. *These measures help minimise the risk of complications such as skin breakdown and deep venous thrombosis*
- allow graduated amounts of fluid unless contraindicated (e.g. by the presence of a nasogastric tube), then gradually introduce solid food if there is no vomiting and if bowel sounds are present, *to rehydrate the patient and to help restore blood glucose levels to within the normal range*
- record the amount and time when the patient passes urine and has a first bowel movement *as constipation is a common postoperative problem because of immobility, dehydration and the use of narcotic analgesics*
- ensure that the patient has adequate periods of rest *as this will aid recovery*
- give encouragement and support to the patient and any explanation or information that may be requested
- the breathing exercises described in the appropriate section on page 271 should be encouraged *to help avoid the problems mentioned.*

Relevance to the activities of living

Maintaining a safe environment

All precautions must be taken for prevention of infection, e.g. a strict aseptic technique should be used when carrying out wound care. An appropriate wound dressing which will promote an ideal healing environment should be prescribed.

While the patient is under the influence of anaesthesia and analgesics safety is of prime importance and is a nursing responsibility.

Communicating

Hearing is one of the first senses to return after anaesthesia.

Adequate explanations, support and encouragement must be available to the patient at all times. Patient education about surgery and its after-effects must be well planned and carried out by an appropriately qualified member of staff, preferably prior to surgery, and reinforced in the postoperative period.

Pain control should be well planned and frequently evaluated.

Breathing

Chest infections and pulmonary embolism are potential problems for patients undergoing surgery; patient education prior to surgery about suitable exercises and deep breathing can help to prevent these complications.

The complication of haemorrhage should be detected by monitoring the wound, pulse, blood pressure and the patient's colour.

Eating and drinking

Fluids should be limited to 3 litres for the first 24 hours after surgery because of the excess production of antidiuretic hormone as a result of surgery; thereafter, unless contraindicated, fluid intake should be encouraged.

A gradual return to a normal diet, high in protein and vitamins, should be encouraged to promote wound healing.

Antiemetics may be prescribed if the patient is suffering from nausea and vomiting.

Eliminating

Anaesthesia can alter bladder muscle tone and may cause difficulty in micturition. It has been demonstrated that anaesthesia can lead to excess secretion of antidiuretic hormone, and it may take 24–48 hours for renal function to return to normal. If the patient's bladder becomes very distended, catheterisation may be necessary, although all other activities to encourage micturition are attempted first.

If the surgery has involved handling the intestines, abdominal distension caused by large amounts of flatus can result, causing extreme discomfort. Sometimes a paralytic ileus develops; the clinical features are abdominal distension, vomiting and absence of bowel sounds, and must be reported immediately.

As with the bladder muscle, some forms of anaesthesia can have an effect on the muscle layer of the bowel; bowel function may take 24–48 hours to return to normal. If the patient has not had a bowel movement by the third postoperative day, a bulk-forming laxative or evacuant suppositories may be administered.

Personal cleansing and dressing

Adequate assistance should be given in the immediate postoperative period but the patient should be encouraged to be independent as soon as possible.

The appearance of the skin over the pressure areas and the appearance of the skin around the wound site should be observed.

Mobilising

The patient should have been taught preoperatively about the importance of movement in bed to prevent pressure sores and the development of deep vein thrombosis. Antiembolitic stockings may be appropriate. The rate of mobilisation will vary depending on the type of surgery carried out, the general condition of the patient, and personal response to the stress of surgery. A nursing assessment should enable the nurse and patient to plan the most suitable programme of mobilisation for that individual.

Working and playing

Surgery may affect the patient's ability to return to former employment or hobbies or sport. Encouragement and support should be maintained while alternatives are found.

Expressing sexuality

If surgery results in an altered body image the patient may require ongoing support and encouragement to adjust to and accept the change.

Sleeping

The patient's normal sleeping patterns may be altered after surgery due to observations being carried out or because of pain, anxiety, discomfort, noise or connection to unusual equipment. Medication to induce sleep may be prescribed but only after other measures have been tried, e.g. helping the patient to find a more comfortable position, relieving pain, giving a hot soothing drink, listening to concerns.

Patient education: key points

Depending on the surgical procedure performed, the hospital patient may require a planned education programme delivered by an appropriately experienced nurse.

All patients should be informed about ways of reducing the risk of occurrence of the common postoperative complications.

Day surgery patients and their carers assume a large degree of responsibility for postoperative care, and staff must ensure that they are able to cope with this before allowing the patient to be discharged. Close liaison should be maintained with the community nursing service (*see* Transfer of patients between care settings, p. 339).

References

Biley FC 1989 Perceptions of stress in preoperative patients, Journal of Advanced Nursing 14(7): 575–581
Seers K 1987 Perceptions of pain. Nursing Times 83(48): 37–39

Further reading

Adams J, Sicard G, Allan B 1994 Perioperative MI diagnostic test devised. Short report. Nursing Times 90(12): 10

Carr F 1989 Waking up to postoperative pain. Nursing Times 85(3): 38–39

Closs SJ 1990 An explanatory analysis of nurses' provision of postoperative analgesic drugs. Journal of Advanced Nursing 15(1): 42–49

Firth F 1991 Pain after day surgery. Nursing Times 87(40): 72–76

Gilchrist B 1990 Washing and dressing after surgery. Nursing Times 86(50): 71

Gleeson C 1995 How was it for you? Nursing Standard 9(22): 51

McHenry C 1991 Silent suffering. National Association of Theatre Nurses 1983 Code of Practice. Nursing Times 87(46): 21

McIntosh C 1994 Do nurses provide adequate postoperative pain relief? British Journal of Nursing 3(7): 342–347

Stevenson C 1994 Massage brings benefit after surgery. Clinical update. Nursing Times 90(4): 10

Vaughan B 1988 Discharge procedures: discharge following surgery. Nursing Times 84(15): 28–33

Williams P 1985 Hospital at home. Journal of District Nursing 4(2): 4–6

38 Pulse

Learning outcomes

By the end of this section you should know how to:

- prepare the patient for this nursing practice
- locate, assess, measure and record the radial pulse
- locate the major pulse points of the body.

Background knowledge required

To help you palpate the pulse and interpret the results, it is necessary to have some knowledge of the structure and function of the cardiovascular system, particularly the heart, conduction system and the arteries.

Some indications and rationale for assessing the radial pulse

A pulse is the rhythmic expansion and recoil of the elastic arteries caused by the ejection of blood from the left ventricle. It can be palpated where an artery near the body surface can be pressed against a firm structure, e.g. bone. It may be assessed for the following reasons:

- on admission *to ascertain the patient's pulse and assess whether or not it is within the normal range for the person's age*
- preoperatively *to ascertain the patient's baseline pulse rate, rhythm and quality so that comparisons can be made with postoperative assessments*
- postoperatively *to monitor the rate, rhythm and quality as indicators of the patient's cardiovascular stability and to compare the findings with the preoperative baseline data*
- *to help estimate, in general terms, the degree of fluid loss when the level of body fluids is lowered*, e.g. after excessive vomiting, excessive diarrhoea, or haemorrhage. In the event of large fluid loss from the body the pulse is thready and rapid. Severe electrolyte imbalance causes impaired cell function and cardiac arrhythmias
- *to compare with baseline admission assessments to help evaluate the effect of treatment on patients who have cardiovascular or pulmonary disease.* The majority of patients with these problems will have pulse irregularities which should stabilise with treatment
- *to monitor the patient who is receiving a blood/blood product intravenous infusion.* Elevated pulse and temperature are among the first signs of reaction to infusion.

Equipment

Watch with a seconds hand

Guidelines and rationale for this nursing practice

- explain the nursing practice to the patient *to obtain consent and cooperation. Patients should be encouraged to be active partners in care*
- ensure that the patient is in a position which is as comfortable and relaxed as possible. *This will help the nurse obtain a true baseline measurement*
- observe the patient throughout this activity for any signs of discomfort or distress. *This should allow the nurse to intervene immediately in the event of an adverse reaction*
- locate the radial artery, place the first and second fingers along it and press gently. *Sufficient pressure should be applied to allow the artery to be against an underlying bone so that the pulse of blood passing through the artery can be felt but care must be taken not to press too hard or the artery may be occluded. See* Relevance to activities of living
- count the pulse for 60 seconds *to allow sufficient time to detect any irregularities or other defects. See* Relevance to activities of living
- document the findings appropriately, comparing past recordings, and report abnormal findings immediately *to enable early intervention to improve the problem.*

Sites of major pulse points of the body

Although the pulse assessment is usually made using the radial artery, there are other sites where an artery near the body surface can be pressed against an underlying bone or other firm body structure. The other major sites are (Fig. 38.1):

— temporal
— carotid
— brachial
— radial
— femoral
— popliteal
— posterior tibial
— dorsalis pedis.

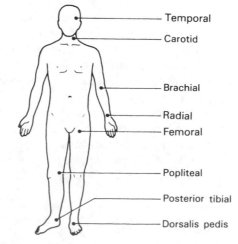

Figure 38.1 *Major pulse points*

Relevance to some of the activities of living

Breathing

Rate   The resting adult normally has a pulse rate of 60–100 beats per minute. Tachycardia (rapid pulse rate) can be a result of pain, anger, fear or anxiety, all of which stimulate the sympathetic nervous system. It can also occur in some heart diseases, anaemia, fever and during exercise, all of which require greater amounts of oxygen and so increase the cardiac output. Bradycardia (slow pulse rate) occurs in any condition which stimulates the parasympathetic nervous system e.g. in patients who have raised intracranial pressure; it also occurs in fit athletes who develop a very efficient heart muscle action.

Rhythm   The rhythm should be regular; any irregularities should be noted. It should be observed whether the irregularities occur at regular or irregular intervals.

Quality   The pulse pressure is the difference between systolic and diastolic pressure. The force is a reflection of the pulse strength. The pulse is usually recorded as being normal, bounding, weak and thready, or absent.

Elasticity   The elastic recoil of the artery wall should be noted. The artery of a healthy young adult feels flexible and non-tortuous; quite different from that of an elderly patient suffering from a condition such as arteriosclerosis, whose artery will feel hard and cord-like.

The pulse rate is much higher in babies and young children than in adults, because they have a higher metabolic rate. In children and young adults it is fairly common to find an irregular increase in rate on inspiration and decrease on expiration.

Occasionally a pacemaker 'fires' before the sinoatrial node; the resulting decrease in filling time of the heart chambers causes a pause in the rhythm which can be detected when assessing the pulse.

Eating and drinking

The level of the body fluids can affect the pulse rate, as can electrolyte imbalance.

A drop in the level of body fluids, e.g. as a result of haemorrhage, will lead to a rapid, thready and weak pulse.

Controlling body temperature

Fever causes the rate of the pulse to be raised because of the need for greater supplies of oxygen. Hypothermia can cause a slowing down of the rate because of the need to keep the body's core temperature as high as possible.

Mobilising

Exercise increases the rate of the pulse, because of the increased demand from muscles for oxygen and nutrients and the increased production of waste products.

Working and playing

Occupations which demand physical exertion result in an increased pulse rate, as do hobbies such as active participation in sport.

Dying

The peripheral pulses are often difficult to palpate in the dying patient because of the gradual non-function of the various cardiopulmonary mechanisms, and may be absent in the period immediately prior to death.

Patient education: key points

It is helpful to explain to patients that their pulse rate will increase with exercise. If they wish to palpate their own pulse they should be shown the correct way to do this and the results monitored by staff until it is demonstrated that the patient is competent.

Further reading

Alexander M, Fawcett J, Runciman P 1994 Nursing care — hospital and home: the adult. Churchill Livingstone, Edinburgh

Cluroe S 1989 Blood transfusions. Nursing 3(40): 8–11

Nursing Standard 1988 Finger on the pulse. Nursing Standard (Wall Chart) 2(47): 22–23

Marieb E 1989 Human anatomy and physiology. Benjamin Cummings, California

Roper N, Logan W, Tierney A 1996 The elements of nursing, 4th edn. Churchill Livingstone, Edinburgh

39 Rectal Examination

Learning outcomes	By the end of this section you should know how to: • prepare the patient for this procedure • collect and prepare the equipment • assist the medical practitioner as requested.
Background information required	Revision of the anatomy and physiology of the sigmoid colon, rectum and anus.
Indications and rationale for rectal examination	Rectal examination is used as a diagnostic aid when there is: • *rectal bleeding* • *severe constipation* • *severe diarrhoea* • *pain in the anal or rectal area* • *suspected enlarged prostate gland* • *suspected rectocele.*
Outline of the procedure	The medical practitioner will put a disposable glove on his dominant hand and apply some lubricant to his fingertips. He will then insert one or two fingers into the patient's rectum and perform the examination. On completing the examination he will remove the glove by turning it inside out as he takes it off. He may insert a lubricated rectal speculum and, using the light source, carry out a visual examination. He may also take an anal or rectal swab for laboratory examination.
Equipment	Tray Disposable gloves Sterile rectal speculum (Fig. 39.1) Water-soluble lubricant Protective covering for the bed Receptacle for soiled disposables Swabs Sterile laboratory swab in container Light source.

Figure 39.1 *Rectal speculum*

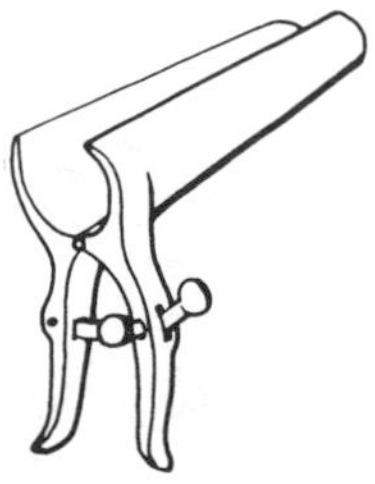

Guidelines and rationale for this nursing practice

- help explain the procedure to the patient *to gain consent and cooperation*
- collect and prepare the equipment *for efficiency of practice*
- assist the patient into the position requested by the medical practitioner, ensuring privacy. *This is usually the left lateral position*
- observe the patient throughout this activity *to detect any signs of discomfort or distress*
- assist the medical practitioner as requested
- ensure the patient is left feeling as comfortable as possible. If any bleeding is likely as a result of the examination ensure that the patient's underwear is protected
- dispose of the equipment safely *for the protection of others*
- document the examination in the patient's records, monitor after-effects and report abnormal findings immediately *to provide a written record and assist in the implementation of any action should an abnormality or adverse reaction to the practice be noted.*

Relevance to the activities of living

Maintaining a safe environment

The nurse and medical practitioner should wash their hands before commencing and on completion of the procedure.

Communicating

This can be a painful and embarrassing procedure for the patient so a careful explanation of the necessity for this examination should be given.

Breathing

It should be explained to the patient that he can help himself relax while the examination is taking place by breathing in and out slowly and deeply.

Eliminating

An empty rectum facilitates the examination but when there is rectal bleeding it is not advisable to administer suppositories or an enema.

Personal cleansing and dressing

Always ensure that the patient's anal area is clean and dry after this examination.

Expressing sexuality

This procedure can be embarrassing for the patient, so the nurse must ensure that there is maximum privacy while the examination is being conducted.

Patient education: key points

A careful explanation should help gain the patient's cooperation and help him to relax which, in turn, will reduce the discomfort of the examination.

The patient should be informed about who to contact if severe pain, discharge or bleeding is experienced after the examination.

Futher reading

Alexander M, Fawcett J, Runciman P 1994 Nursing practice—hospital and home: the adult. Churchill Livingstone, Edinburgh

Bradley C 1994 Which machine? Infection Control Supplement, Nursing Times 90(13): 67–70

Lawler J 1991 Behind the screens. Churchill Livingstone, Edinburgh

Roper N, Logan W, Tierney A 1996 The elements of nursing, 4th edn. Churchill Livingstone, Edinburgh

Singh H, Bowditch M, Dennison A, Shorthouse A 1994 Sigmoidoscopy with a view. British Journal of Surgery 81: 1795

Wicks J 1994 Handle with care. Infection Control Supplement, Nursing Times 90(13): 67–70

40 Skin Care

Learning outcomes	By the end of this section you should know how to:
	▪ prepare the patient for this nursing practice
	▪ collect the quipment
	▪ carry out skin care.

Background knowledge required	Revision of the anatomy and physiology of the skin.
	Revision of the predisposing factors for development of a pressure sore.
	The health authority policy regarding risk assessment, care implementation and criteria for the use of aids to prevent pressure sores should be reviewed.
	Revision of moving and handling a patient (p. 219) and active and passive exercises (p. 129).

Indications and rationale for skin care	This care involves the maintenance of a patient's skin viability by ensuring skin cleanliness, relieving skin capillary pressure, ensuring adequate nutritional status and monitoring of potential problems. Skin care is indicated for every patient, but specific circumstances increase the need for care when:
	▪ a patient is incontinent
	▪ a patient's mobility is impaired temporarily or permanently, e.g. a bedfast, paralysed or unconscious patient
	▪ a patient has a poor nutritional status
	▪ a patient has impaired peripheral circulation

Equipment	Appropriate risk assessment scale, e.g. Norton, Waterlow or Braden (Bergstrom et al 1987)
	Aid for pressure relief.

Guidelines and rationale for this nursing practice	▪ explain the nursing practice to the patient *to gain consent and cooperation*
	▪ ensure the patient's privacy *to reduce anxiety*
	▪ observe the patient throughout this activity *to note any signs of distress or discomfort*
	▪ assess the risk factor of the patient developing a pressure sore, utilising one of the assessment scales such as the Norton Scale (Fig. 40.1) or Waterlow Scale (Fig. 40.2) (p. 290) *to permit preventative care to be implemented*. This should be performed as part of the initial assessment process and at regular

		A		B		C		D		E		Total Score
		Physical Condition		Mental condition		Activity		Mobility		Incontinent		
		Good	4	Alert	4	Ambulant	4	Full	4	Not	4	
		Fair	3	Apathetic	3	Walk/help	3	Sl. limited	3	Occasionally	3	
		Poor	2	Confused	2	Chairbound	2	V. limited	2	Usually/ur.	2	
Name	Date	V. bad	1	Stuporous	1	Bedfast	1	Immobile	1	Doubly	1	

Figure 40.1 *Norton Scale (Reproduced with permission from Roper N, Logan W, Tierney A 1985 The elements of nursing, 2nd edn. Churchill Livingstone, Edinburgh)*

Instructions for use

1. Identify the most appropriate description of the patient (4, 3, 2, 1) under each of the five headings (A to E) and total the result.

2. Record the 'score' with its date in the patient's notes or on a chart.

3. Assess weekly and whenever any change in the patient's condition and/or circumstances.

With a 'score' of 14 and below the patient is 'At Risk' denoting need for intensive care, i.e. 1–2 hourly changes of posture and the use of pressure-relieving aids.

Note: When oedema of the sacral area has been present a rise of score above 14 does not indicate less risk of a lesion.

Figure 40.2 *Waterlow Scale*

Build/weight for height		Visual skin type		Continence		Mobility		Sex Age		Appetite	
Average	0	Healthy	0	Complete	0	Fully mobile	0	Male	1	Average	0
Above average	2	Tissue paper	1	Occasionally	1	Restricted/	1	Female	2	Poor	1
Below average	3	Dry	1	incontinent		difficult		14–49	1	Anorectic	2
		Oedematous	1	Catheter/	2	Restless/	2	50–64	2		
		Clammy	1	incontinent		fidgety		65–75	3		
		Discolour	2	of faeces		Apathetic	3	75–80	4		
		Broken/spot	3	Doubly incontinent	3	Inert/traction	4	81+	5		

Special risk factors:
(1) Poor nutrition eg terminal cachexia	8	
(2) Sensory deprivation eg diabetes, paraplegia, cerebrovascular accident	5	**Assessment value**
(3) High dose anti-inflammatory or steroids in use	3	At-risk = 10
(4) Smoking 10+ per day	1	High risk = 15
(5) Orthopaedic surgery/fracture below waist	3	Very high risk = 20

Directions for use:

1 Assess the patient, circling the number in each category in which the patient fits
2 Add up all the numbers, including 'special risk factors'
3 If the total places the patient within the 'at risk', 'high risk' or 'very high risk' areas, turn the card over and read the suggested preventive aids listed on the back
4 Record the circled numbers in the patient's documentation, giving the total and the date
5 Assess each patient every third day, unless the need to reassess the patient earlier becomes evident

intervals throughout his care when the patient's condition alters (Waterlow 1992, Bale 1994)

- identify individual patient problem areas, such as a patient with peripheral vascular disease whose affected limb may be at greater risk than the rest of his body *as there is increased risk of the development of a pressure sore* (Torrance 1983)
- when a risk factor is noted, institute preventive skin care (Torrance 1983) *which will reduce the risk of development of a pressure sore*
- relieve the pressure exerted on the skin surface by regularly changing the patient's body position (Lowthian 1987) *to prevent devitalisation of healthy tissue*
- support the patient's body and limbs in natural positions *to promote comfort and prevent damage, and maintain joint and muscle movement* with passive and active exercises (p. 129)
- a patient who is assessed as having a high risk factor will require frequent position changes, such as 2-hourly, *to relieve pressure of the soft tissues against bone* (Bale 1994). A turning chart may be used to record the time, position of the patient and the signature of the nurse or carer
- reduce the pressure, friction and shearing forces on the skin by the use of any of the recommended aids available such as static load distribution, posture changing or dynamic load distribution beds or mattresses (Lowthian 1995) *which reduce the contributory factors of pressure sore development*
- cleanse the skin of an incontinent patient or a patient who is perspiring profusely *as the numbers of microorganisms will be greatly increased.* Use soap with caution *as the alkaline content tends to dry the skin and deplete it of its natural oils*
- thoroughly dry the skin by patting gently. *These measures will decrease the numbers of skin microorganisms and reduce the development of infected skin tissue* (Roper et al 1996)
- examine and classify (Box 40.1) the patient's skin during the nursing practice for signs of hyperaemia or loss of integrity *which signifies the development of a pressure sore* (Reid & Morison 1994)
- *reduce shearing and friction forces exerted on a patient's skin* by using a skilled moving and handling technique when repositioning him, and proper positioning of the patient to prevent him from sliding down in the bed or chair
- maintain or improve, when appropriate, the patient's nutritional status, using the services of a dietitian if necessary, *as poor nutritional and hydration status greatly increases the risk of pressure sore development* (Bale 1994)
- educate the patient about preventive care for pressure sore development when his condition permits (Thomas et al 1990); for example, a patient nursed in traction can assist in pressure relief measures. *Cooperation and care by the patient are vital in the overall prevention of pressure sores* (Morison 1992)
- after giving any of the forms of care above, ensure the patient is left feeling as comfortable as possible *to ensure quality of patient care*
- dispose of used equipment safely *to reduce any health hazard*
- document the nursing practice appropriately, monitor after-effects and report

Box 40.1   **The UK consensus classification of pressure sore severity**

Stage 0

No clinical evidence of a pressure sore
0.0 Normal appearance intact skin
0.1 Healed with scarring
0.2 Tissue damage, but not assessed as a pressure sore

Stage 1

Discoloration of intact skin (light finger pressure applied to the site does not alter the discoloration)
1.1 Non-blanchable erythema with increased local heat
1.2 Blue/purple/black discoloration. The sore is at least stage 1

Stage 2

Partial-thickness skin loss or damage involving epidermis and/or dermis
2.1 Blister
2.2 Abrasion
2.3 Shallow ulcer, without undermining of adjacent tissue
2.4 Any of these with underlying blue/purple/black discoloration or induration. The sore is at least stage 2

Stage 3

Full-thickness skin loss involving damage or necrosis of subcutaneous tissue but not extending to underlying bone, tendon or joint capsule
3.1 Crater, without undermining of adjacent tissue
3.2 Crater, with undermining of adjacent tissue
3.3 Sinus, the full extent of which is not certain
3.4 Full-thickenss skin loss but wound bed covered with necrotic tissue (hard or leathery black/brown tissue or softer yellow/cream/grey slough) which masks the true extent of tissue damage. The sore is at least stage 3. Until debrided it is not possible to observe whether damage extends into muscle or involves damage to bone or supporting structures

Stage 4

Full-thickness skin loss with extensive destruction and tissue necrosis extending to underlying bone, tendon or joint capsule
4.1 Visible exposure of bone, tendon or capsule
4.2 Sinus assessed as extending to bone, tendon or capsule

Third digit classification
for the nature of the wound bed

x.x0 Not applicable: intact skin
x.x1 Clean, with partial epithelialisation
x.x2 Clean, with or without granulation, but no obvious epithelialisation
x.x3 Soft slough, cream/yellow/green in colour
x.x4 Hard or leathery black/brown necrotic (dead/avascular) tissue

---

Box 40.1   **Cont'd**

Fourth digit classification
for infective complications

x.xx0   No inflammation surrounding the wound bed
x.xx1   Inflammation surrounding the wound bed
x.xx2   Cellulitis bacteriologically confirmed

---

abnormal findings immediately *providing a written record and assisting in the implementation of any action should an abnormality or adverse reaction to the practice be noted.*

Relevance to the activities of living

Maintaining a safe environment

All equipment should be clean or disposable and all precautions taken to prevent cross-infection. The nurse should wash her hands before commencing, and on completion of, the nursing practice.

Equipment which is used to relieve pressure must be checked at regular intervals to maintain its working condition. The equipment should be kept clean and dry, both when in use and when in storage, to reduce microbial growth which could act as a source of infection to the patient.

If a pressure sore develops, cleansing and dressing of this wound must involve aseptic technique (see p. 383). A sore is a break in skin continuity and is therefore at risk of infection. Numerous dressing materials and agents are available. The dressing of choice should be one which will provide maximum patient comfort and promote wound healing.

Sensory impairment to the skin, such as occurs in an unconscious or paralysed patient, may predispose to the development of a pressure sore.

In some local authorities the responsibility for regular pressure area care of a chronically ill individual at home has been deemed social care and is delivered by home carers (Nazarko 1995).

Communicating

It is important that the patient and, when appropriate, the relatives, are educated about pressure sores and their prevention. The preventive and educational process should be a team approach utilising the nurse, physiotherapist, occupational therapist, social worker and doctor. An educational leaflet such as that suggested by Morison (1992) or the Department of Health (1994) will assist in the information and education process of both the patient and carers.

Breathing

A patient who has impairment of his cardiovascular system, even for a short period of time, is at increased risk of developing a pressure sore due to the reduced perfusion of the skin tissue (Torrance 1983).

Eating and drinking

The patient's nutritional status should be assessed by the dietitian and appropriate intervention implemented as poor nutritional status will increase the risk of pressure sore development (Bale 1994). The nurse may offer the patient high-calorie, high-protein drinks, unless otherwise instructed, to supplement the diet he is already eating. At home the nurse will require the assistance of the carer in monitoring and encouraging the patient to maintain/improve his nutritional status. If the patient is unable to maintain a satisfactory nutritional status by the oral route, nasogastric or parenteral nutrition may be required.

Eliminating

A patient who is incontinent must have his skin kept as free of contamination as possible. Problems of eliminating may be overcome by bladder or bowel training programmes or by treating the underlying cause, e.g. urinary retention with overflow can manifest as urinary incontinence. Following incontinence, the skin should be washed and dried thoroughly without vigorous rubbing, as this can cause maceration of the skin tissue (Roper et al 1996). Soap should be used with caution because it has drying and oil-reducing effects; skin which is dry and lacking in natural oils will break down more readily. A barrier cream may be used, but with caution, as it may interfere with the oxygen and moisture exchange of the skin. The patient who is identified as incontinent must be assessed by a knowledgeable professional in continence care who can plan and implement individualised care (Swaffield 1994).

Personal cleansing and dressing

The nurse should use the form of assessment she is familiar with to calculate the patient's risk factor for the development of a pressure sore.

When a patient is confined to bed, the use of a bedcage can greatly reduce the pressure created by the bed linen on the body. Sheets and blankets should be left loose at the edges of the bed, while the use of a duvet can greatly reduce the weight of bed linen on the patient's body. Bed linen should be maintained in a clean, dry and wrinkle-free condition.

Capillary pressure, shearing and friction forces are known to be some of the predisposing factors in the development of a pressure sore, and care must be instituted to reduce these factors. The capillary pressure can be relieved by altering the patient's body position at regular intervals, such as 2-hourly, or more frequently depending on the individual patient's 'at risk' assessment (Lowthian 1987). Shearing and friction forces exerted on the patient's skin tissue can be reduced by utilising a skilled moving and handling technique and positioning of the patient to prevent sliding in any direction while in bed or in a chair (Waterlow 1992). Adjusting the mattress to maintain the patient's knees in a slightly flexed position while the thighs remain supported, or the use of a padded footboard, can be of help to reduce sliding.

Attention must be paid to the patient's clothing: buttons, zips, belts and even hard objects like loose change in pockets have been known to produce a pressure sore.

Controlling body temperature

A patient suffering from hypothermia has an increased risk of developing a pressure sore due to the effect of the temperature change on the cardiovascular system and perfusion of the skin tissue.

Mobilising

Early ambulation is of great benefit in the prevention of a pressure sore.

A patient who is using an aid to mobility is susceptible to the development of a pressure sore at the point of contact of the aid with the body; for example, a patient who uses a pair of crutches may develop redness of his hands due to the alteration in distribution of body weight. Involuntary muscle movements and joint contracture interfere with body positioning and can create and increase in shearing and friction forces of the patient's skin tissue, resulting in increased risk of the development of a pressure sore.

Working and playing

A pressure sore may increase the patient's rehabilitation period and may have resultant effects on his social status. The nurse must implement care to prevent patient boredom, depression and anxiety about his family's social needs. The social worker may need to be involved in this intervention.

Expressing sexuality

The nurse must provide adequate privacy during the nursing practice. The patient's individual wishes should be observed when possible, to help maintain his self esteem.

Sleeping

Skin care for the prevention and treatment of a pressure sore must be maintained throughout the 24-hour period. At home this may require the assistance of the carer when the community nurse is not present.

Patient education: key points

The patient and carers should be given information regarding the implemented care to reduce the risk of pressure sore development.

A patient who will permanently be at risk of pressure sore development must take an active role in the preventative care. This may involve the nurse in teaching the patient how to regularly inspect his skin tissue, such as in the use of a mirror to assess skin areas which are difficult to access.

Where prolonged/permanent use of pressure relieving aids by a patient is implemented, the patient and carers should be given information on the safe continued care of the equipment and on appropriate action should a fault occur.

References

Bale S 1994 Wound healing. In: Alexander M, Fawcett J, Runciman P (eds) Nursing practice — hospital and home: the adult. Churchill Livingstone, Edinburgh

Bergstrom N, Braden B, Laguzza A 1987 The Braden scale for predicting pressure sore risk. Nursing Research 36(4): 205–210

Department of Health 1994 Relieving the pressure: your guide to pressure sores. HMSO, London (patient/carers information leaflet available from the Department of Health)

Lowthian P 1987 The practical assessment of pressure sore risk. Care, Science and Practice 5(4): 3–7

Lowthian P 1995 Pegasus Airwave and Bi-Wave Plus. British Journal of Nursing 4(17): 1020–1024

Morison M 1992 A colour guide to the nursing management of wounds. Wolfe, London

Nazarko L 1995 Community care deskilling. Nursing Management 2(4): 9–10

Reid J, Morison M 1994 Towards a consensus: classification of pressure sores. Journal of Wound Care 3(3): 157–160

Roper N, Logan W, Tierney A 1996 The elements of nursing, 4th edn. Churchill Livingstone, Edinburgh, pp 245–251

Swaffield J 1994 Continence. In: Alexander M, Fawcett J, Runciman P (eds) 1994 Nursing practice — hospital and home: the adult. Churchill Livingstone, Edinburgh

Thomas A, Krowskop S, Noble G, Noble P 1990 Pressure sore management and the recumbent person. In: Bader D (ed) Pressure sores: clinical practice and scientific approach. Macmillan, London

Torrance C 1983 Pressure sores: aetiology, treatment and prevention. Croom Helm, Beckenham

Waterlow J 1992 A policy that protects: the Waterlow pressure sore prevention/treatment policy. In: Horne E, Cowan T (eds) Staff Nurse's survival guide, 2nd edn. Wolfe, London

Further reading

Banks S, Bridel J 1995 A descriptive evaluation of pressure-reducing cushions. British Journal of Nursing 4(13): 736–746

Crow R 1988 The challenge of pressure sores. Nursing Times 84(38): 68–73

Davies K 1994 Pressure sores: aetiology, risk factors and assessment scales. British Journal of Nursing 3(6): 256–262

Dawes H, Small D, Glen E 1990 Adding computers to the armoury (describes computerised history-taking and assessment of incontinent patients). Nursing Times 86(46): 68–69

Department of Health 1993 Pressure sores: a key quality indicator — a guide for NHS purchasers and providers. HMSO, London

Docherty J (ed) 1995 Clinical guideline — pressure area care: a report from a working party set up by the Clinical Resource and Audit Group (CRAG). CRAG, Edinburgh

Douglas D, Watret L 1995 Auditing pressure sore risk assessment. Journal of Wound Care 4(4): 189–191

Flanagan M 1993 Pressure sore risk assessment scales. Journal of Wound Care 2(3): 162–167

Irvine L 1988 Incontinence in the young woman. Senior Nurse 8(3): 16–18

Macaulay M, Henry G 1990 Drop in and do well (discusses establishment of a continence clinic). Nursing Times 86(46): 65–66

McSweeney P 1989 Continence: prevent, retrain, treat, contain. Nursing Times 85(46): 68–69

Mowlam V, North K, Myers C 1986 Managing faecal incontinence. Nursing Times 82(48): 55–59

Roper N, Logan W, Tierney A 1990 The elements of nursing, 3rd edn. Churchill Livingstone, Edinburgh, pp 218–225

Rough M, Brooks H 1995 The prevention of pressure sores after hospital discharge. Community Nurse 1(4): 27–28

Santy J 1995 Hospital mattresses and pressure sore prevention. Journal of Wound Care 4(7): 329–332

Walsh M, Ford P 1989 Nursing rituals — research and rational actions. Heinemann Nursing, Oxford, ch 7

41 Specimen Collection

General information is given on the collecting of specimens, followed by specific additional information. The section 'Relevance to the activities of living' refers to all specimens.

Learning outcomes

By the end of this section you should know how to:
- identify the need for laboratory investigations
- facilitate the obtaining of the necessary specimens
- know the appropriate containers for each type of specimen
- arrange the correct storage and delivery of the specimens to the laboratory.

Background knowledge required

Revision of appropriate microbiology.

Review of local policies referring to the collection and transportation of specimens.

Indications and rationale for collecting specimens

A specimen may be required:
- *as an aid to the diagnosis of disease*
- *to monitor the effect of treatment*
- to permit laboratory culture *to identify pathogenic microorganisms and determine drug sensitivity.*

Equipment

Appropriate container clearly labelled with patient's details

Equipment to enable collection of the specimen

Laboratory form

Plastic specimen bag for transportation.

General guidelines and rationale for this nursing practice

- explain the nursing practice to the patient *to gain consent and cooperation. Patients should be encouraged to be active partners in care*
- ensure the patient's privacy *to help maintain dignity and sense of 'self'*
- ensure the appropriate precautions are observed to reduce the risk of contact with body fluids during the collection and transportation of the specimen (Hart, 1991)
- collect the specimen at the most appropriate time *to facilitate obtaining accurate results.* This time will vary depending on the specimen, e.g. the

optimum time for collection of a specimen of urine for culture is from the first voiding of the bladder in the morning
- ensure that no substance which might cause inaccurate results has been used prior to collection, *to avoid interference with accurate results*; for example a specimen of sputum could be adversely affected by the patient using an antiseptic mouthwash before giving the specimen
- ensure sufficient quantities of the specimen have been collected *to allow accurate results*
- avoid contamination of the specimen by the hands of the nurse or patient *as this could invalidate the results of the culture*
- avoid contamination of the outside of the container with the specimen substance *as this could pose a health risk to anyone handling the specimen*
- ensure the patient is left feeling as comfortable as possible after the collection of the specimen
- dispatch the labelled specimen container immediately to the laboratory with the completed form. *Delay may alter the reliability of any results obtained*
- document this nursing practice appropriately, monitor after-effects and report abnormal findings immediately *so that appropriate measures can be instigated to relieve the problem.*

Swab collection

Specific equipment

Sterile swab

Disposable gloves

Sterile water for nose swab

Sterile vaginal speculum for vaginal swab

Sterile lubricating jelly for vaginal swab

Spatula for throat swab.

Specific guidelines and rationale for these nursing practices

Wound swabs
- obtain a specimen before the wound is washed *so that the specimen material is not contaminated by washing agent*
- rotate the swab in the wound *to obtain a sufficient quantity for examination.*

Throat swabs
- help the patient to sit in an appropriate position *to facilitate a good view of the faucial tonsils*
- depress the patient's tongue with a spatula *to facilitate access to the site*
- speedily and gently rub the swab over the faucial area
- avoid touching any other area of the mouth as the swab is being removed *so that the specimen will not be contaminated.*

Ear swabs
- help the patient to sit in a comfortable position with the head slightly tilted to the unaffected side

- gently pull the adult pinna upwards and backwards to straighten the external canal. *This facilitates the insertion of the swab to obtain a specimen of discharge*
- insert the swab into the external canal and rotate gently *to ensure the swab is well coated with the discharge.*

Nasal swabs

- help the patient sit in a comfortable position *to allow access to the nasal cavity*
- moisten the swab in sterile water before insertion into the nose *to make the procedure more comfortable for the patient as the nasal cavity can be dry*
- insert the swab into the nose rotating it as it moves upwards towards the tip of the nose.

Vaginal swabs

- help the patient into an appropriate position *to allow access to the vagina*
- gently insert a lubricated speculum into the vagina to separate the vaginal walls. *This allows the area to be swabbed to be visualised*
- introduce the swab into the high vaginal area and rotate it gently. Charcoal-impregnated swabs should be used if a trichomonas infection is suspected *as the organism survives for longer in this medium.*

Penile swabs

- help the patient into a comfortable position *to allow access to the penis*
- retract the prepuce *to allow the area to be swabbed to be visualised*
- rotate the swab gently in the urethral meatus *to collect a sample of secretions.*

Faeces

Specific equipment

Disposable gloves

Bedpan

Sterile spatula

Sterile container

Receptacle for soiled disposables.

Specific guidelines and rationale for this nursing practice

- request the patient to defaecate into a clean bedpan, ensuring that the faecal matter does not become contaminated with urine *as this could affect the analysis results*
- use a spatula or implement provided to fill about one third of the specimen container with faecal material
- if the faeces are being tested for occult blood, follow the instructions on the packaging in which the occult blood testing equipment is supplied.

Urine

Specific equipment

Sterile container

Disposable gloves

Bedpan or urinal may be necessary

Sterile receiver may be necessary to receive the specimen

Washing equipment to wash the surrounding tissue

Midstream specimens of urine — sterile tinfoil bowl

Catheter specimens of urine — sterile needle, syringe, alcohol-impregnated swab (Fig. 41.1)

24-hour urine collection — large glass sterile container with lid.

Specific guidelines and rationale for this nursing practice

- to facilitate the collection of a midstream specimen of urine, ask the patient to start passing urine to flush out the urethra *so that urethral organisms will not interfere with analysis*
- collect the middle section of the stream directly into the container or, for a female, into a sterile bowl and then pour into the container

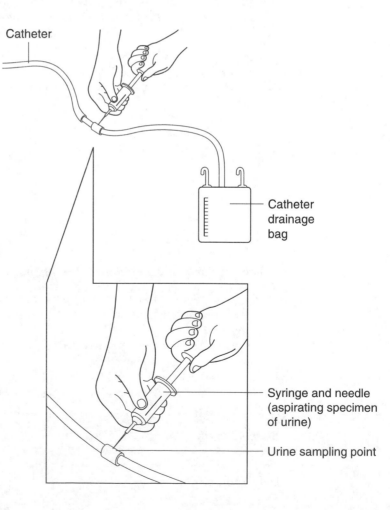

Catheter

Catheter drainage bag

Syringe and needle (aspirating specimen of urine)

Urine sampling point

Figure 41.1 *Collecting a specimen of urine when a catheter is in position*

- to facilitate the collection of a catheter specimen of urine, wipe the catheter with an alcohol-impregnated swab
- connect the needle to the syringe and insert it into the special marked section of the collecting bag tube. *This section is made of special self-sealing material so the needle will not damage it.* Some collecting tubes now have a special port to which the syringe connects directly.
- withdraw the required amount of urine into the syringe and then transfer it to the sterile container
- to commence a 24-hour collection, ask the patient to void his bladder and discard the urine *so that the patient and staff know the exact time the collection commences*
- collect all urine passed in the next 24-hours.

Cervical smear

Specific equipment

Disposable gloves

Lubricating gel

Vaginal speculum

Container with appropriate fixative

Glass slide

Cervical spatula or brush

Medical wipes/tissues.

Specific guidelines and rationale for this nursing practice

- help the patient into the most appropriate position *to facilitate the collection of the specimen*
- put on the disposable gloves
- lubricate the spatula
- gently insert it into the vagina and open it slowly until the cervix can be visualised
- insert the brush or spatula and rotate it twice round the cervix, ensuring it is at the entrance (Fig. 41.2)
- transfer the cells to the glass slide immediately and insert in the container with the fixative
- close the speculum and withdraw it gently
- offer tissues to the patient for her to clean the outside of the vagina and then provide privacy for dressing.

Relevance to the activities of living

Maintaining a safe environment

Thorough cleansing of the patient's genitalia must be carried out prior to the collection of the specimen to reduce the number of contaminants from outside the urinary and intestinal systems. Antiseptics should not be used for cleansing as this would alter the number of pathogenic microorganisms, leading to inaccurate laboratory results.

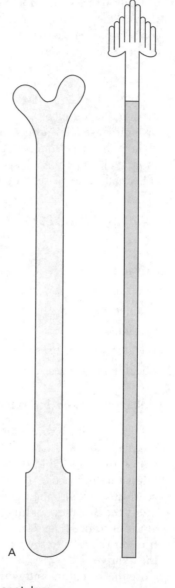

A

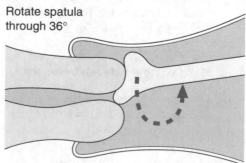

Rotate spatula
through 36°

Figure 41.2 *Cervical
smear
A Cervical spatula and
brush
B Correct use of cervical
spatula*

B

Human tissue and body fluids such as urine and faeces can act as a health hazard to the staff handling the specimen, therefore gloves can be worn during collection to prevent staff contamination. The specimen container should only be half to a third full and checked for lid security to reduce the problem of leakage. The use of a plastic specimen container bag for transportation will help to prevent any health hazard to the staff, should accidental breakage of the specimen container occur. When a patient requires source isolation all precautions prior to, during and following specimen collection must be maintained.

Once collected, the specimen should be dispatched immediately to the laboratory. Should there be a delay the specimen must be stored at 4°C in a special refrigerator to reduce further growth of the pathogenic microorganisms. Urine specimen containers which contain boric acid crystals can be used when a delay in the dispatch of the specimen is anticipated, as boric acid acts as a urine preservative.

A catheter specimen of urine should not be collected by disconnecting the drainage bag from the catheter or by taking the specimen from the outlet tap of the urine drainage bag. The former method has the potential of allowing pathogenic microorganisms to have access to the urinary system; the latter will not give a specimen of urine which will contain the 'true' pathogenic microorganisms present in the urinary system. Care has to be taken during the collection of a catheter specimen of urine to prevent the accidental stabbing of the nurse's finger by advancing the needle too far and going through the drainage tubing.

Communicating

The patient should be given an easily understood explanation as to how and why the specimen collection is required. The laboratory results should be conveyed to the patient as soon as possible. Both of these actions will reduce patient anxiety.

A patient who has a urinary tract infection, or has just had surgery to the urinary system, may suffer urinary muscle spasm and/or pain. The medical practitioner may prescribe appropriate analgesics and antispasmodics which can be of great benefit to the patient.

Eating and drinking

A patient who is suspected of having a bacterial or viral infection of the urinary or intestinal systems may suffer from thirst, nausea, vomiting and/or loss of appetite. The nurse will require to initiate the appropriate nursing intervention to help the patient.

Eliminating

Frequent micturition should be encouraged when a urinary infection is suspected. This will reduce the time the pathogenic microorganisms have for multiplication within the patient's urinary system.

When collecting a specimen, the urine and/or faeces should be observed for colour, amount, consistency and any obvious abnormality.

A faecal specimen may be requested for bacterial or viral studies, but can be requested for biochemical analysis such as testing for the presence of faecal occult blood. This test is now carried out at ward level by a nurse using a commercial biochemical testing kit such as Haemocult. The nurse should acquaint herself with the manufacturer's recommendations for use.

A stool chart may be initiated when a patient has a suspected intestinal infection. This records the frequency, colour, consistency and amount of faecal matter passed by the patient. The stool chart can be used as an aid to diagnosis and assists in the assessment of the effect of treatment.

Sleeping

A patient with a suspected infection of the urinary or intestinal systems may suffer from an increase/urgency of micturition and defaecation, which may interrupt sleeping. The nurse should assist the patient with this problem by initiating the appropriate nursing intervention.

Expressing sexuality

A clear explanation of the reason for the specimen should be given to the patient and he should be allowed as much privacy as possible.

Many patients will not have had any sexual experience; sufficient time must be given to explanations and counselling of these patients.

Permitting other people to be involved in body functions such as eliminating is alien to many people's culture and this needs to be handled with great sensitivity.

Patient education: key points

An explanation of the method and reasons for collecting the specimen will help the patient understand how and why it is necessary. This is particularly important if the patient is in the community and collecting the specimen at home.

If the specimen is collected at home the patient will need clear instructions about the storing of the specimen and where and when to deliver it so that it arrives at the laboratory in the optimum condition.

Reference

Hart S 1991 Blood and body fluid precautions. Nursing Standard 5: 25–27

Further reading

Anderson L, May D 1995 Has the use of cervical, breast and colorectal cancer screening increased in the United States. American Journal of Public Health 85(6): 840–842

Byles J, Redman S, Sanson-Fisher R 1995 Effectiveness of two direct-mail strategies to encourage women to have cervical smears. Health Promotion International 10(1): 5–16

Lawler J 1991 Behind the screens. Churchill Livingstone, Edinburgh

Miller B 1995 Failures of cervical cancer screening. Editorial. American Journal of Public Health 85(6): 761

Roper N, Logan W, Tierney A 1996 The elements of nursing, 4th edn. Churchill Livingstone, Edinburgh

Sasieni P 1995 Cervical screening: what is the point? Letter. Lancet 244

42 Stoma Care

Learning outcomes

By the end of this section you should know how to:

- prepare the patient for this nursing practice
- collect and prepare the equipment
- carry out stoma care for the patient
- help the patient accept and care for the stoma himself, both at home and in an institutional setting.

Background knowledge required

Revision of the anatomy and physiology of the digestive system, with special reference to the small and large intestine.

Review of health board policy regarding the role of the stoma care nurse and the available literature for patient education in an institutional and community setting.

Knowledge of the information and level of counselling given to the patient before the operation to create a stoma.

Indications and rationale for stoma care

A stoma is an opening from the small or large intestine onto the surface of the abdomen through which the bowel contents are diverted for excretion. (Fig. 42.1) A stoma is formed following surgical intervention *for treatment of intestinal disease*. Different names are used according to the site of the stoma (Crooks 1994).

Stoma care involves cleansing of the stoma and surrounding skin, and the provision of a suitable appliance for the safe collection and disposal of excreta, *in order to enable the person to resume normal activities of living as soon as possible.*

A colostomy is an opening from the colon, usually the transverse or descending colon, and may be required:

- *for patients who have malignant disease of the rectum or colon*
- *for patients who have diverticular disease of the colon*
- *for patients who have inflammatory disease of the intestine*, e.g. Crohn's disease or ulcerative colitis (Kelly 1994).

An ileostomy is an opening from the ileum and may be formed for the same reasons as a colostomy, but is more often formed *for patients who have inflammatory disease of the intestine*, e.g. Crohn's disease or ulcerative colitis. In some cases a temporary stoma may be formed *so that once the disease has resolved, the stoma may be closed and the intestine anastomosed to function as before.*

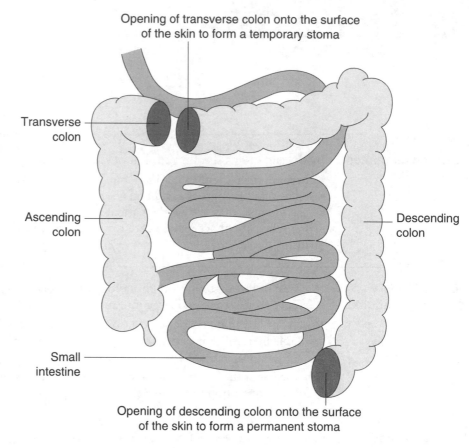

Opening of transverse colon onto the surface
of the skin to form a temporary stoma

Transverse
colon

Ascending
colon

Descending
colon

Small
intestine

Figure 42.1 *Sites which may be chosen for colostomy*

Opening of descending colon onto the surface
of the skin to form a permanent stoma

A jejunostomy is an opening from the jejunum.

An urostomy is an opening from the bladder or ureters into a segment of the ileum, which is used as a channel for the urine to be diverted through an abdominal stoma. This is also known as an ileal conduit and may be required *for treatment of malignant disease of the bladder* (Leaver 1994).

Equipment	Trolley or tray
	A bowl of warm water
	Tissues or paper towels
	Material for protecting the skin area round the stoma, e.g. Stomahesive, karaya gum
	Suitable appliance (stoma pouch)
	Scissors
	Measuring jug
	Gloves (non-sterile)

Figure 42.2 *Examples of disposable stoma bags*
A Closed pouch
B Open lower end to permit emptying of contents

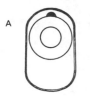

A

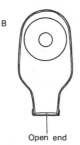

B

Open end

Barrier cream for protecting the skin around the stoma

Deodorant as required

Receptacle for soiled disposables.

Stoma appliances

There is a wide range of appliances available and, with the guidance of a stoma care nurse, the patient chooses the one most suitable for his needs. Bags may have pre-cut apertures or they may have to be cut to fit individually. They may be closed pouches or open-ended to allow emptying (Fig. 42.2). Some are two-piece appliances with a semi-rigid circular aperture on which a bag can be clipped, allowing for changing or emptying (Black 1994a).

Immediately postoperatively the surgeon will have placed a clear plastic appliance over the stoma, probably incorporating a suitable backing to protect the skin. This allows observation of the stoma and its function. Protective backing also allows removal of the appliance without too much discomfort to the patient during the postoperative period. It may be 2–5 days before the appliance needs to be changed for the first time.

Karaya gum-backed appliance   This appliance may have a circle of karaya gum pre-cut, when the appropriate size to fit the stoma should be chosen; otherwise a hole should be prepared by cutting the karaya backing to a suitable size. The gum must be moistened before applying to the skin (see manufacturer's instructions).

Skin protective wafer, e.g. Stomahesive   This is a square wafer in which a hole is cut to fit snugly round the stoma. A pouch with an adhesive backing is prepared to fit over the stoma and adhere to the wafer (see manufacturer's instructions).

Protective cream   Occasionally protective barrier creams or gels may be prescribed for patients who have particularly sensitive skin. These should be massaged into the skin until dry and non-greasy, and any surplus cream wiped off before the new appliance is fitted.

Deodorants   These can range from sprays to concentrated deodorants where only one drop is needed. The stoma care nurse should be consulted about preparations most suitable for the patient's needs.

Guidelines and retionale for this nursing practice

- explain the nursing practice to the patient *to gain consent and cooperation and encourage participation in care* (Kelly 1994)
- ensure the patient's privacy *to maintain self esteem and prevent embarrassment*
- collect and prepare the equipment *so that everything is ready*
- help the patient into a comfortable position *to reduce any distress and to help him see the area of the stoma*
- help to adjust clothing to expose the patient's abdomen in the area of the

stoma *for easy access and so the patient can observe the practice* (Allison 1995)
- don gloves *to prevent any contamination from body fluids*
- place a paper towel appropriately *to protect the surrounding area from spills or leakage*
- observe the patient throughout this activity *to monitor any adverse effects*
- empty the appliance and measure its contents if required *for evaluation of elimination fluid balance*
- gently remove the appliance and protective backing *to expose the stoma area*
- wash the skin around the stoma with warm water only. *Soap may cause skin irritation*
- encourage the patient to look at his stoma and explain what you are doing *so that he gradually accepts his change of body image and to encourage early independence* (MacGinley 1994)
- observe the colour and condition of the stoma and the surrounding skin *to evaluate the wound healing process*
- dry the skin around the stoma thoroughly *to maintain healthy intact skin and prevent excoriation*
- prepare the appliance as required by cutting the aperture of the bag and the skin protective wafer if necessary *so that it is tailored to fit the individual stoma*
- apply any prescribed protective creams if required and remove surplus cream *to prevent any excoriation of the surrounding skin area*
- place the new appliance in position *so that it fits comfortably, and allows no leakage round the stoma* (Fig. 42.3)
- seal an open-ended bag with an appropriate closure *to prevent leakage*
- ensure that the patient is left feeling as comfortable as possible *to limit distress and promote the healing process*
- dispose of waste products and soiled appliances according to health authority policy *to prevent transmission of infection*
- document the nursing practice appropriately, monitor after-effects, and report abnormal findings immediately. *This will ensure safe practice and enable prompt appropriate medical and nursing intervention to be initiated.*

Figure 42.3 *Positioning an appliance over a stoma*
A Removing protective covering from adhesive ring before placing appliance over stoma
B Applying a stoma pouch. The open-ended pouch is sealed with a clip ready for use; when the clip is removed, the stoma pouch can be emptied without removing the appliance from the skin

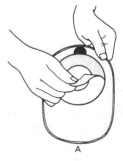
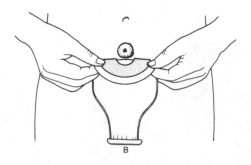

Relevance to the activities of living

Observations and further rationale for this nursing practice will be included within each activity of living as appropriate.

Maintaining a safe environment

In the postoperative period, the abdominal wound should be dressed separately using aseptic technique, and covered with plastic sealant spray or a sterile dressing, before stoma care is performed (*see* Aseptic technique, p. 383).

Care of the stoma itself is not a sterile practice, but high standards of cleanliness should be maintained. Stoma care should be regarded as a form of toileting and appropriate hand washing performed. Patient education should reflect this as he is helped to look after his own stoma under the guidance of the stoma care nurse and others involved with his care.

The contents of the stoma bag should be emptied into the toilet or Clinamatic. The soiled bags should be treated as clinical waste. Once home, the patient will be instructed to wrap the bags in newspaper when they have been emptied and rinsed. They should be placed in the dustbin for disposal, although in some health authority areas a special service is available for removal and disposal of soiled bags.

Communicating

An important part of the patient's postoperative care should be to help him care for the stoma himself. It is helpful for all nursing staff to know the level of counselling given to each patient before the operation, and the involvement of the stoma care nurse in this instruction. The nurse should encourage the patient to talk about the stoma, and create an environment for him to ask questions about any worries he has, while performing stoma care for him initially and then while helping him learn to care for the stoma himself. There should be good liaison between the ward staff and the stoma care nurse, so that the patient feels he can discuss his concerns freely. Literature about his particular type of stoma should be readily available from the stoma care nurse, and discussions can be a useful aid for communication and patient education (Black 1994b).

Details of local support groups and a visit from someone successfully coping with a stoma can help the patient with his own adjustment to the stoma.

Initially, the patient may find the smell of flatus and excreta from the stoma difficult to accept. It should be explained that once a normal diet is established he will soon find out which foods appear to make the flatus worse, and exclude them. Once the stoma is established and functioning normally, unpleasant odour will be less of a problem. Local deodorant can be used, and some appliances are fitted with deodorant filters to cope with the problem. Advice from the stoma care nurse should be sought. The most important way of helping the patient is for the nurse to indicate by her non-verbal communication that she is not upset by a normal bodily function taking place in a different area of the body.

If the patient normally uses spectacles, he should be encouraged to wear them initially to watch while stoma care is performed, and later so that he can see properly to do it himself.

Eating and drinking

Once the patient is allowed a normal diet the stoma will discharge faecal material more frequently. By a process of observation the patient should be encouraged to notice the effect which different foods have on faecal elimination. In this way he may be able to adjust his diet so that a more solid stool is formed. This process may take several weeks and the stoma care nurse will continue to give help and advice about appropriate diet when the patient is at home.

Eliminating

The presence of a stoma completely changes the way in which faecal material is eliminated from the body and the patient has to be helped to adjust to this.

Preoperatively the patient should be involved with the discussion and decision of the site for his stoma. The stoma care nurse, the surgeon and the ward nursing staff should all be involved with this important preoperative preparation, in their appropriate roles.

In the immediate postoperative period, the patient has no control over faecal material eliminated through a stoma; this is an added problem about which he has to learn. Initially faecal material is fluid when expelled through the stoma, as the water absorption function of the colon may have been bypassed. After 2–3 weeks, when the patient is able to eat a normal diet, a semisolid stool may be formed, especially when the stoma is a colostomy in the transverse or descending colon. Eventually the frequency of bowel function can be reduced and controlled and almost resemble normal bowel movement, to the extent that a stoma bag need not be worn continuously.

Drainage from an ileostomy, on the other hand, is liquid and rich in digestive enzymes which can cause excoriation and erosion of the skin. The discharge flows almost continuously, requiring constant wear of an appliance unless an ileal pouch (a reservoir below the skin surface) has been constructed. Odour problems, fear of soiling and skin complications are more common with an ileostomy, and an open-ended bag which can be emptied regularly is the most suitable appliance. Eventually, however, there is usually some control over the frequency of bowel function.

Appliances should be emptied or changed as often as necessary to prevent over-filling and leakage onto the surrounding skin area (usually one-third – one-half full, or they become heavy and unwieldy). Any redness, swelling or abnormalities of the stoma or the surrounding skin area should be reported.

Initially, the faecal fluid should be measured and observed for any abnormalities. Abnormal excreta should be kept for observation and reported.

An urostomy is formed to allow urine to be excreted through an abdominal stoma. This may be collected directly into a suitable stoma bag, or a catheter may be incorporated so that a closed drainage system may be used. Whichever system is used, the bag chosen should have facilities for frequent emptying (*see* Catheter care, p. 94). The principles of stoma care remain the same.

Personal cleansing and dressing

The patient may feel that the stoma is a threat to his cleanliness. Shower or bathing facilities should be available as soon as his condition allows, and prior to that a bed bath given as often as required. Stoma care should be coordinated with showering or bathing whenever possible; the appliance can be emptied and removed and the skin area washed first, and the new appliance fitted afterwards. This may not be possible with an ileostomy or urostomy, and in these instances the appliance should be emptied, or changed and replaced, before showering or bathing.

While the patient is learning how to care for the stoma, comfortable clothes which give easy access to the stoma should be worn. Modern appliances are comfortable and unobtrusive so no permanent change in clothing style should be needed. Advice from the stoma care nurse and the appropriate support group can be helpful.

Working and playing

Once the patient has recovered from the operation and is able to cope with the stoma it is hoped that he will return to his normal lifestyle. Even swimming is possible, using a small temporary appliance. Helpful advice can be obtained from the stoma care nurse and support groups.

Expressing sexuality

A stoma, especially if it is permanent, is a major insult to the patient's body image and he may become withdrawn and depressed. His acceptance by the hospital staff will be the first step in giving the patient confidence in himself. He should choose which of his friends and relatives he tells about the stoma, and their acceptance will help his rehabilitation. Counselling before the operation and constant support from all concerned will boost his morale, and help him overcome the almost inevitable initial revulsion.

Patients who have a stoma following resection of the lower bowel may have problems with sexual function. Men may become impotent, and women may have dyspareunia, and sexual partners should be included in counselling before and after surgery. Inevitably the presence of an abdominal stoma appliance calls for additional thoughtfulness and ingenuity during sexual intercourse. Counselling from the stoma care nurse, the surgeon and the appropriate support group will help in this situation, which may only be temporary (Black 1994c).

Sleeping

Stoma care should be performed prior to the patient settling for the night, as this will prevent the need to empty or change an appliance and thus disturb sleep.

Once the patient is eating a normal diet, and has adjusted to his own requirements, it is unlikely that the stoma will need any attention during the night. A larger bag can be used overnight, which may be helpful for patients who have an ileostomy.

Patient education: key points

Before, during and after admission, patient education will be shared with the stoma care nurse, who should have very close links with the nursing staff in both the institution and community.

Patient education begins prior to stoma surgery with counselling and decision making about the site of the stoma, related to the patient's individual problems and the activities of living.

There should be shared decision making between the stoma nurse and the patient about the most appropriate stoma appliance. The method of application, retention, and changing of the appliance should be explained and supervised until the patient is confidently self caring.

The importance of adjusting the diet to suit the changed elimination process should be explained, and advice given to help the stoma to operate efficiently as soon as possible.

The patient should understand the importance of reporting immediately any redness, swelling or pain at the site, or general feeling of illness or distress, which may need medical help. A telephone 'help line' can reduce anxiety in the first few weeks.

The address of a local support group should be given to the patient; a visit from a member who has a functioning stoma can help increase confidence in his own self care.

References

Allison M 1995 Comparing methods of stoma function. Nursing Standard 9(24): 25–28
Black P 1994a Choosing the correct stoma appliance. British Journal of Nursing 3(11): 545–550
Black P 1994b Management of patients undergoing stoma surgery. British Journal of Nursing 3(5): 211–216
Black P 1994c Problems in stoma care. British Journal of Nursing 3(14): 707–711
Crooks S 1994 Foresight leads to improved outcome. Stoma care nurses role in siting stomas. Professional Nurse 10(20): 89–92
Kelly M 1994 Patients' decision making in major surgery. The case of total colectomy. Journal of Advanced Nursing. Nursing Times 90(42): 48–51
Leaver R 1994 The Mitrofanoff pouch. A continent urinary diversion. Professional Nurse 9(11): 748–753
MacGinley K 1994 Nursing care of the patient with altered body image. British Journal of Nursing 3(22): 1098–1102

Further reading

Corless R 1992 Caring for a homosexual man undergoing a colostomy formation. British Journal of Nursing 1(10): 501, 503–506
Haywood Jones I 1994 Stoma care (skills update). Community Outlook 4(12): 22–23
Kelly M 1992 Colitis. Routledge, London
Kelly M, Henry T 1992 A thirst for practical knowledge. Stoma care patients' opinions of the services they receive. Professional Nurse 7(6): 350–356

Kinsman S 1992 The perils of stoma sponsorship (for stoma care posts). British Medical Journal 385: 671

Mayberry J, Mayberry M 1993 Practice nurses and chronic diseases of the gastrointestinal tract. Practice Nurse 2(4): 176–178

Sadler C 1992 Working together. Better relations are needed between stoma care nurses and volunteer support groups. Nursing Times 88(22): 61–62, 64–66

43 Suppositories

Learning outcomes	By the end of this section you should know how to: ▪ prepare the patient for this nursing practice ▪ collect and prepare the equipment ▪ administer rectal suppositories ▪ describe some of the types of suppositories and their function.
Background knowledge required	Revision of the anatomy and physiology of the colon, rectum and anus. Revision of medicine administration, particularly checking the medication against the prescription (*see* p. 1).
Indications and rationale for administering suppositories	A suppository is a cone or cylinder of a medicinal substance which can be introduced into the rectum and will eventually dissolve and may be absorbed through the rectal mucosa. It is used: ▪ *to relieve constipation* ▪ *to evacuate the bowel prior to surgery or certain investigations* ▪ *to treat haemorrhoids or anal pruritis* ▪ *to administer medication, e.g. antibiotics, bronchodilators, analgesics.*
Equipment	Tray Disposable gloves Medical wipes/tissues Water-soluble lubricant Protective covering Receptacle for soiled disposables Prescribed suppository. Suppositories are of value in evacuating the rectum. Glycerine suppositories lubricate dry, hard stools and have a mild stimulant effect on the rectum. Other suppositories with a stimulant effect are Beogex and Bisacodyl. Medication is well absorbed through the rectal mucosa. For many years, it has been a common way to administer medication in Europe, but it is only recently that it has become an acceptable route of administration to patients in the UK.

Guidelines and rationale for this nursing practice

- explain the nursing practice to the patient *to gain consent and cooperation*
- ensure the patient's privacy and assist him into the left lateral position with his buttocks near the edge of the bed *to allow ease of access to the rectal sphincter*
- observe the patient throughout this activity *for any signs of distress or discomfort*
- place the protective covering under the patient's buttocks *in case of soiling by faecal matter*
- check with the prescription sheet and with a qualified member of staff that the suppository is the correct one and is being administered to the correct patient *to avoid mistakes occurring*
- squeeze some lubricating gel onto a medical wipe/tissue and lubricate the end of the suppository *for ease of insertion*
- put on the disposable gloves *for your protection*
- part the patient's buttocks with the non-dominant hand *to allow easier access to the anal sphincter*
- with the dominant hand insert the suppository into the rectum in an upward and slightly backward direction *to follow the natural line of the rectum* (Fig. 43.1)
- push the suppository in gently as far as possible with the middle finger *to optimise the effect*

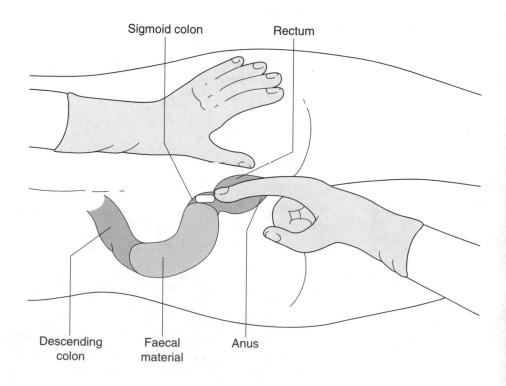

Sigmoid colon   Rectum

Descending colon   Faecal material   Anus

Figure 43.1 *Insertion of rectal suppository*

- withdraw the gloved finger
- wipe the patient's anal area with a medical wipe/tissue *to clean any soiling*
- remove the protective covering
- remove the gloves
- provide a bedpan or commode or assist the patient to the toilet when this is required. To reduce embarrassment for the patient try to provide as much privacy as possible, remembering that curtains do not act as sound or smell filters
- ensure the patient is left feeling as comfortable as possible *maintaining the quality of this practice*
- dispose of the equipment safely *to prevent transmission of infection*
- document this nursing practice appropriately, monitor after-effects and report any abnormal findings, *ensuring safe practice and enabling prompt appropriate medical and nursing intervention to be initiated.*

Relevance to the activities of living

Communicating

It is important to explain clearly to the patient the reason for and method of action of the suppository.

Eliminating

If the suppository is being given to evacuate the rectum, the patient must have ready access to a bedpan, commode or toilet, and any necessary assistance should be given. Bedpans should be used as a last resort as patients can find it difficult to use a bedpan and this can aggravate an existing problem of constipation.

Expressing sexuality

Many patients find the administration of suppositories embarrassing so an adequate explanation should be given and maximum privacy must be provided.

Patient education: key points

An explanation should be given about the reasons for administering medication via the rectal route as this route of administration may be unknown to the patient.

The patient may require education in the self administration of suppositories.

If suppositories are being prescribed to relieve constipation it may be appropriate to discuss ways in which increased exercise, fluid and diet may relieve this problem. A self-completed bowel chart may be useful for helping to resolve the problem of constipation.

Further reading

Brown M, Everett I 1990 Gentler bowel fitness with fibre. Geriatric Nursing 1: 26–27

Campbell J 1994 Suppositories. Skills update. Macmillan Magazines, London

Laming E 1994 A preventable problem. Journal of Community Nursing 8(7): 28–35

Lawler J 1991 Behind the screens. Churchill Livingstone, Edinburgh

Roper N, Logan W, Tierney A 1996 The elements of nursing, 4th edn. Churchill Livingstone, Edinburgh

White T 1995 Dealing with constipation. Nursing Times 91(14): 57

44 Tepid Sponging

Learning outcomes

By the end of this section you should know how to:

- prepare the patient for this nursing practice
- collect and prepare the equipment
- carry out tepid sponging.

Background knowledge required

Revision of the anatomy and physiology of the skin with special reference to the role of the skin in the maintenance of body temperature.

Revision of Body temperature (*see* p. 57), Bed bath (*see* p. 29) and Mouth care (*see* p. 209).

Indications and rationale for tepid sponging

This practice is commonly used *to promote the comfort of a pyrexial patient.* Tepid sponging is the application of warm water to a patient's skin surface to promote the dispersal of body heat when the body temperature is raised, by utilising the principles of evaporation and conduction (Walsh 1992).

A patient may show the manifestation of pyrexia when there is:

- invasion by pathogenic microorganisms
- disease of the nervous system
- a metabolic disorder
- malignant/neoplastic disease.

Equipment

Equipment for temperature recording (*see* p. 57)

Equipment for mouth care (*see* p. 209)

Basin of warm water (30–33°C)

Lotion thermometer

Disposable face cloths or similar items

Three bath towels

Pyjamas or gown

Bed linen

Trolley or adequate surface for equipment

Receptacle for soiled disposables

Receptacle for soiled pyjamas or gown if it belongs to the patient

Receptacle for soiled bed linen.

Guidelines and rationale for this nursing practice

This practice could be undertaken at home by a carer following a demonstration and instruction by the nurse responsible for the patient's care.

- explain the nursing practice to the patient *to gain consent and cooperation*
- wash the hands *to reduce the risk of cross-infection*
- collect and prepare the equipment required *to ensure all equipment is available and ready for use*
- ensure the patient's privacy *to reduce anxiety*
- observe the patient throughout this activity *to note any signs of distress*
- help the patient into a comfortable position *permitting the patient to assist during the practice*
- assess and record the patient's body temperature *providing a baseline measurement before the practice*
- remove excess bed linen and bed appliances if in use, but leave the patient covered with a bed sheet *allowing easy access to the patient during the practice and maintaining privacy for the patient*
- help the patient to remove the pyjamas or gown *as a pyrexia can cause physical debility*
- check the temperature of the basin of water using the lotion thermometer *as the use of cold water can create localised vasoconstriction* (Childs 1994)
- without using friction *to prevent further increase of the skin temperature*, slowly sponge the patient's body with a wet face cloth as suggested in bathing in bed (*see* p. 29)
- gently pat the patient's skin dry, if required. It is preferable to leave the water to evaporate, *assisting in the temperature reduction* (Walsh 1992)
- change all bed linen *to remove damp cold material and enhance patient comfort*
- help the patient to dress in pyjamas or gown *generating a feeling of security and well-being*
- remake the patient's bed with a reduced level of bed linen *promoting contact with the environmental temperature, thus enhancing the reduction in the patient's temperature*
- assess and record the patient's body temperature *to note the effectiveness of the practice*
- help the patient with mouth care if desired *enhancing the overall benefit of the practice*
- ensure that the patient is left feeling as comfortable as possible *confirming the quality of care delivered*
- dispose of the equipment safely *to reduce any health hazard*
- document the nursing practice appropriately, monitor after-effects and report abnormal findings immediately *providing a written record and assisting in the implementation of any action should an abnormality or adverse reaction to the practice be noted.*

Relevance to the activities of living

Maintaining a safe environment

Although tepid sponging does not require aseptic technique, all equipment should be clean or disposable and all precautions be taken to prevent cross-infection. The nurse should wash her hands before commencing and on completion of the nursing practice.

The patient should be observed throughout the nursing practice for any sign of an adverse reaction such as shivering and/or an increase in respiration rate. If these arise the nurse must stop the tepid sponge, cover the patient with a blanket and report the adverse reaction immediately.

Disorientation with regard to time can be caused by pyrexia; the nurse may therefore need to assist the patient with actual or potential problems as they are identified.

Communicating

The patient may suffer from irritability and anxiety due to the effect of the pyrexia, and the nurse should assist the patient to reduce these problems by attending promptly to his needs. The patient's relatives may require an explanation from the nurse for the reason for the patient's anxiety and irritability. Should the patient be at home the carer could be given the responsibility of implementing this practice to enhance the comfort of the patient.

Eating and drinking

Following a tepid sponge the patient may be offered a cool drink. It may help him to feel cooler but it also assists in the prevention of dehydration and reduces the discomfort caused by a dry mouth. As the patient's metabolic rate is increased during pyrexia, drinks containing protein and carbohydrate are of benefit.

Personal cleansing and dressing

A patient who requires a tepid sponge is, in most circumstances, perspiring freely. It enhances patient comfort if the clothing to be worn and the bed linen are made from a non-synthetic fabric such as cotton, as this has a high moisture absorption rate.

The patient's clothing and bed linen should be changed as they become damp with perspiration.

Controlling body temperature

A patient whose body temperature is 39.5°C and above has the problem of impairment to the temperature-regulating mechanisms within the body. Tepid sponging is one of the nursing practices which may help to reduce this problem.

The patient's body temperature is assessed and recorded prior to and following this nursing practice to evaluate the effect of the tepid sponge.

Mobilising

Patient movements prior to, during and following the tepid sponge should be kept to a minimum as body temperature is lowest during periods of relative inactivity.

Sleeping

An environment conducive to resting and sleeping should be provided throughout the day to decrease the patient's activity.

Patient education key points

The patient should be informed of the effect of the tepid sponge on body temperature.

The carer may be taught how to carry out this nursing practice.

References

Childs C 1994 Temperature control. In: Alexander M, Fawcett J, Runciman P (eds) Nursing practice — hospital and home: the adult. Churchill Livingstone, Edinburgh

Walsh M 1992 Temperature regulation. In: Royle J, Walsh M (eds) Watson's Medical-surgical nursing and related physiology, 4th edn. Bailliere Tindall, London

---

Further reading

Brunner L, Suddarth D 1992 The textbook of adult nursing. Chapman & Hall, London, pp 81–82

Roper N, Logan W, Tierney A 1996 The elements of nursing, 4th edn. Churchill Livingstone, Edinburgh, pp 274–277

45 Toileting

Learning outcomes

By the end of this section you should know how to:
- prepare the patient for this nursing practice
- collect and prepare the equipment
- provide facilities for the patient to empty his bladder or bowel, at home or in an institutional setting.

Background knowledge

Revision of the anatomy and physiology of the urinary system, with special reference to micturition.

Revision of the anatomy and physiology of the rectum and anus with special reference to defaecation.

Review of health authority policy regarding disposal of excreta and the control of infection for both community and institutional care.

Indications and rationale for toileting

Toileting is the provision of appropriate facilities *for the patient to micturate or defaecate*. This may be a toilet, a commode, a bedpan or urinal.

A bedpan, urinal or commode should be provided *for patients who are confined to bed or only allowed up for short periods*.

Assistance to the toilet should be provided *for patients who are too frail or immobile to be self-caring in relation to toileting*.

Equipment

Bedpan, urinal, commode or toilet, as appropriate

Toilet paper

Disposable cover for bedpan or urinal

Gloves

Measuring jug

Bedpan disposer, e.g. Clinamatic

Bedpan washer for non-disposable equipment

Facilities for hand washing

Facilities for communicating the patient's need for toileting to the nurse, e.g. bell

Appropriate aids for lifting and handling, e.g. Ambulift

Receptacle for soiled disposables.

Bedpan

For female patients a bedpan may be used for micturition and defaecation. For male patients it may be used for defaecation; a urinal should be offered at the same time for micturition. Toilet ware may be disposable or non-disposable; non-disposable equipment is usually made of stainless steel. Disposable equipment is increasingly being used.

Disposable bedpan   This should be placed in a rigid bedpan holder and taken to the bedside under a disposable cover. The used bedpan should be flushed in the bedpan disposer according to the manufacturer's instructions. The holder should be washed and dried before storing

Stainless steel bedpan   This should be warmed under hot water, dried and covered with a disposable cover. The used bedpan should be placed in the bedpan washer and flushed according to the manufacturer's instructions. It should be washed and dried before storing, and regular sterilisation should be performed according to health authority policies. Within the community, waste should be disposed of in the toilet and equipment cleansed according to local infection control policy.

Urinal

This is used for male patients for micturition, and should be covered with a disposable cover when taken to and from the patient. Like a bedpan, it may be disposable or non-disposable and, after use, is processed in the same way.

Commode

This is a mobile chair constructed to hold a bedpan which can be taken to the bedside for the patient's use. It may be constructed to transport the patient to the toilet so that the commode seat fits over the toilet seat. Many mechanical lifting aids incorporate a commode seat so that the patient may be taken safely to the ward toilet or use it as a conventional commode (see manufacturer's instructions) (Professional Development Unit 1995). A commode can be made available for patients at home to maintain independence, or as a temporary help for toileting if access to the bathroom is difficult.

Guidelines and rationale for this nursing practice

Guidelines are given for the provision of a bedpan to a female patient and a urinal to a male patient.

The provision of a bedpan for a female patient

- explain this nursing practice to the patient *to gain consent and cooperation and encourage participation in care*
- ensure that the patient knows how to request a bedpan when needed *to reduce anxiety about this activity of living*
- respond immediately to the patient's request for a bedpan *to prevent incontinence and patient distress*

- don a plastic apron after washing hands *to prevent any contamination*
- don plastic gloves *to prevent contamination from body fluids*
- collect and prepare the bedpan, carrying it to the bedside under a disposable cover *to maintain her self esteem and reduce embarrassment*
- ensure the patient's privacy *to respect her individuality* (Glen & Jownally 1995)
- observe the patient's condition throughout this activity *to monitor any adverse effects*
- help the patient into a comfortable sitting position, supporting her back with pillows *so that she will be in the best position for micturation*
- help the patient to adjust her clothing *to expose the buttocks and perineum*
- help to lift the patient's buttocks by placing a hand under the lower lumbar region, using a safe lifting technique or mechanical aid. Two nurses may be needed, depending on the patient's condition, *for safe lifting and handling* (RCN 1993)
- slide the bedpan into position with the shaped rim under the patient's buttocks *so that it is safely in place*
- adjust the patient's pillows *to ensure she is sitting comfortably*
- leave the patient to use the bedpan, ensuring privacy *to maintain her self esteem*
- remain in the vicinity *to be available when the patient is ready*
- assist with wiping the perineum and/or anus if necessary *to maintain healthy skin in the area*
- remove the bedpan *once toileting is complete*
- give the patient a bowl to wash her hands *for her own personal hygiene and to prevent cross-infection* or help her to the wash hand basin if more appropriate
- ensure that the patient is left feeling as comfortable as possible *to minimise any distress*
- observe the contents of the bedpan *for any abnormalities; these should be reported and the bedpan saved for inspection*
- measure the urine and retain a labelled specimen *for ward testing if required* (*see* Urine testing, p. 357) (Daffurn et al 1994)
- dispose of the equipment safely *to prevent transmission of infection*
- wash hands using good hand washing technique *to maintain a safe environment*
- document the nursing practice appropriately and report abnormal findings immediately. *This will ensure safe practice and enable prompt appropriate medical and nursing intervention to be initiated.*

Guidelines for providing a commode

These are in principle the same as those for using a bedpan. Once the prepared and covered commode is taken to the bedside the patient should be helped out of bed *to sit on the commode in privacy*, and guidelines followed as for a bedpan. Help from one or two nurses may be needed *to assist the patient in and out of bed, depending on the patient's condition and mechanical aids used for safe lifting and handling* (Corlett et al 1992).

The provision of a urinal for a male patient

- explain this nursing practice and *gain the patient's consent and cooperation*
- ensure that the patient knows how to request a urinal when needed *to reduce anxiety about this activity of living*
- collect and prepare the urinal and take it to the bedside under a disposable cover *to maintain his self esteem and reduce embarrassment*
- ensure the patient's privacy *to respect his individuality*
- help the patient to place the urinal in position if required *so that no urine is spilled*
- remain in the vicinity *to be available when the patient is ready*
- remove the urinal and proceed as for guidelines for providing a bedpan.

Relevance to the activities of living

Observations and further rationale for this nursing practice will be included within each activity of living as appropriate.

Maintaining a safe environment

To prevent cross-infection and to maintain adequate standards of hygiene a separate area should be designated for storage and disposal of equipment used for toileting.

Adequate hand washing facilities should be available for both patients and staff in this area and beside the patient's toilets. Good hand washing technique should be maintained to prevent cross-infection. Gloves should be worn to prevent contamination from body fluids. Nurses should be knowledgeable about related health authority practices.

All equipment should be washed and dried immediately after use, to prevent cross-infection.

Plastic aprons should be worn by nursing staff when providing toilet facilities; these should be removed or changed after this nursing practice to prevent cross-infection.

Maintaining the patient's privacy for eliminating sometimes conflicts with the need to maintain the safety of his environment. The nurse must make sure that there is no danger of the patient falling when using a bedpan or commode and that he can be safely left on the ward toilet. The decision about which facilities are used for toileting depends not only on the patient's condition, but also on his orientation and mobility.

Communicating

Good communication skills by the nursing staff can prevent the patient worrying about toilet arrangements. He should be shown the patients' toilets or told how to ask for a bedpan, urinal or commode by the nurse who admits him, and the reason for these arrangements should be explained. A bell or other means of requesting assistance should be available as required and requests for toilet facilities should be acted on immediately.

Eliminating is a private activity of living: the nurse's attitude and non-verbal communication when performing this nursing practice can affect the way the patient accepts the need for particular toilet arrangements.

Eating and drinking

For the patient's own comfort and for the maintenance of personal hygiene, toilet facilities followed by hand washing should be offered before meals for all patients who are not self-caring.

Eliminating

Urine should be measured and the results recorded for patients whose fluid balance is being monitored. Patients who are self-caring, but whose urine is to be measured, should be shown how to place a bedpan over the toilet seat and use that for micturition, so that the nurse can measure the urine. Urine should be observed for any abnormalities and tested as required (*see* Urine Testing, p. 357).

Patients' bowel movements should be recorded, so that problems of constipation or diarrhoea can be monitored. Any abnormalities should be reported immediately (*see* Specimen collection, p. 297).

The patient's condition will dictate whether a bedpan or commode is used when he is confined to bed. However, the stress of using a bedpan may be considerable for some patients, and a commode should be available if possible.

Male patients should be given a urinal for micturition when they require a bedpan or commode for defaecation.

Patients with problems of continence should be helped to use appropriate toilet facilities at frequent intervals; any request for toileting should be answered immediately, so that the patient may regain adequate bladder control (Pomfret & Haslam 1994). If the patient is mobile, his bed and chair should be within easy reach of an available toilet to encourage continence. The assistance of one or two nurses may be needed. Patients with a continuing continence problem should have a full continence assessment carried out (refer to health authority policy).

At home, the toilet area can be adapted to promote independence — by the use of rails or by raising the seat, or by using a toilet frame (Fig. 45.1). The arrangements will be discussed and implemented by the primary health care team (White 1994).

Personal cleansing and dressing

The nurse may have to help the patient to wipe or wash and dry the anus, vulval area and perineum following defaecation.

This should always be done so that the wiping or washing is from front to back, away from the urethra, and the paper towel renewed after each wipe. For women in particular it is important that no bacteria from the rectal area reach the urethra, as this may cause a urinary tract infection. Careful perineal toilet should prevent this (*see* Bed bath, p. 31).

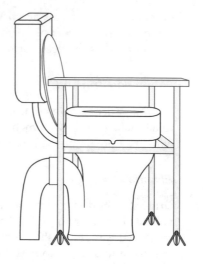

Figure 45.1 *Use of hand rails and raised seat to promote independence at home*

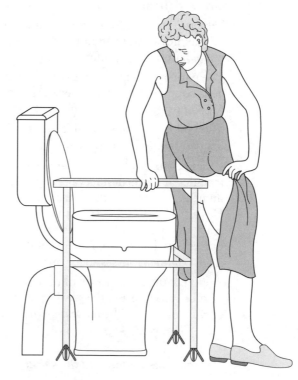

Figure 45.2 *Adaptation of clothing for ease of access for toileting*

To maintain independence, clothes can be adapted for ease of access for toileting, using folding skirts and extra velcro fastenings (Fig. 45.2). The community team can help with appropriate advice.

Controlling body temperature

During toileting the patient should be kept warm with adequate clothing and covers, as well as footwear. This is particularly important in the ward toilet, or on the bedside commode. Elderly people, particularly, become cold very quickly, and the nurse should ensure that patients are not left exposed for more than the minimum time required for toileting.

The temperature of ward areas and toilet areas should remain at an environmentally comfortable level.

Mobilising

The choice of toilet arrangements for a particular patient, and the decision to use mechanical aids, may depend on the patient's individually assessed activity of mobilising. The choice of arrangements should be discussed and accepted by the patient. At home, special adjustments, e.g. rails, raised seat, may be made to the toilet area, (Barker et al 1994).

Expressing sexuality

When a patient needs help with toilet requirements it is an invasion of his privacy. The nurse may have to touch areas of the body which would normally be socially unacceptable, and may cause embarrassment to the patient. The nurse's attitude and good communication skills will help to alleviate some of the embarrassment felt by the patient although he may never be completely happy about this nursing practice. Urinary incontinence can also have an adverse effect on body image and be associated with sexual dysfunction (Winder 1994).

Sleeping

Toilet facilities should be offered just before the patient is settled for the night, so that maximum comfort is achieved. The nurse should also assure the patient that if he needs help for toileting during the night it will be readily available, ensuring that his bell or other means of communication is at hand.

Patient education: key points

The importance of regular toileting should be explained and if necessary reinforced with simple aids such as adapted clothing and the help of carers.

The reason for the use of mechanical aids for help with toileting should be explained.

Maintaining a healthy perineal area, and efficient safe cleaning of the area, should be emphasised. This may be achieved using something as simple as wet wipes or as specialised as a bidet.

The availability of special equipment to aid continence should be discussed with the patient according to his individual needs, as part of continuing care in an institutional setting or included in goals for discharge to community care. This may include adaptation to the toilet area in his home.

When a patient has had a full continence assessment, a plan of care should be discussed with the patient and mutually agreed with the community team.

References

Barker A, Cassar S, Gabbett J et al 1994 Handling people: equipment, advice and information. Disabled Living Foundation, London

Corlett E, Lloyd P, Tarling C et al 1992 The guide to handling patients, 3rd edn. National Back Pain Association / RCN, London

Daffurn K, Hillman K, Bauman A et al 1994 Fluid balance charts; do they measure up? British Journal of Nursing 3(16): 816–820

Glen S, Jownally S 1995 Privacy: a key nursing concept. British Journal of Nursing 4(2): 69–72

Pomfret I, Haslam J 1994 Continence management (a beneficial partnership). Community Outlook, March 23–26

Professional Development Unit 1995 12:1 Lifting and handling, knowledge and practice. Nursing Times (suppl) 91(1): 1–4

RCN 1993 Code of practice for the handling of patients. RCN advisory panel for back pain in nurses. Royal College of Nursing, London

White H 1994 Choosing continence aids. British Journal of Nursing 3(22): 1158–1163

Winder A 1994 Incontinence and sexuality. Community Outlook, August: 21–22

Further reading

Barron A 1990 The right to personal space. Nursing Times 86(27): 28–33

Health and Safety Executive 1992 Manual handling: guidance and regulations. HMSO London

Mantle J 1994 Essential education: re-educating the pelvic floor muscles. Journal of Community Nursing, December: 14–20

Professional Development Unit 1995 12:2 Lifting and handling, the role of the nurse. Nursing Times (suppl) 91(2): 1–4

Roper N, Logan W, Tierney A 1996 The elements of nursing, 4th edn. Churchill Livingstone, Edinburgh, pp 199–230

Walsh M, Ford P 1989 Nursing rituals, research and rational actions. Heinemann Nursing, Oxford, pp 68–69

46 Tracheostomy Care

There are two parts to this section:

1 **Removal of respiratory tract secretions via a tracheostomy tube**
2 **Changing a tracheostomy tube**

The concluding subsection, 'Relevance to the activities of living' refers to both practices.

Learning outcomes

By the end of this section you should know how to:

- prepare the patient for this nursing practice
- collect and prepare the equipment
- care for a patient who has a tracheostomy tube in situ.

Background knowledge required

Revision of the anatomy and physiology of the larynx, trachea and bronchus.

Revision of Aseptic technique (*see* p. 383).

Review of health authority policy on care of a patient with a tracheostomy.

Indications and rationale for tracheostomy care

Tracheostomy is the surgical procedure of creating an artificial opening into the trachea to relieve an obstruction of the airway (e.g. tumour, acute infection). This procedure is almost always performed in an operating theatre. The artificial airway is maintained with a suitable tube; this requires to be aspirated, cleaned and changed:

- *to ensure that the tube remains patent*
- *to reduce the risk of respiratory infection.*

1 Removal of respiratory tract secretions via a tracheostomy tube

Equipment

Tray

Sterile disposable gloves

Sterile suction catheters with a thumb control

Sterile container and water for flushing the catheter and tubing

Receptacle for soiled disposables

Suction apparatus, e.g. portable machine or centralised suction.

Guidelines and rationale for this nursing practice

- explain the nursing practice to the patient, if possible, *to gain consent and cooperation. Patients should be encouraged to participate actively in care*
- ensure the patient's privacy *to maintain dignity and sense of 'self'*
- collect the equipment *for efficiency of practice*
- assist the patient to a suitable position *for ease of access to the tracheostomy tube*
- observe the patient throughout this activity *for any signs of discomfort or distress*
- fill the sterile container with sterile water *to flush the suction catheter*
- open the end of the pack containing the connecting end of the suction catheter and connect it to the tubing of the suction machine
- put a disposable glove on the dominant hand
- slide the cover off the catheter and rinse it through with sterile water *to lubricate it*
- insert the catheter into the tracheostomy for 20–25 cm with the gloved hand and without any suction (Fig. 46.1)
- withdraw the catheter, applying suction by covering the thumb control hole, and rotate the catheter as this is being done. If the mucus is tenacious and difficult to remove, medical staff may order 5–15 ml of sterile normal saline to be dripped into the tracheostomy before suction is applied. *This loosens the mucus for easier removal*
- allow the patient to rest and re-oxygenate before repeating insertion of the catheter
- dispose of the catheter at the end of the practice after rinsing it and the tubing with sterile water

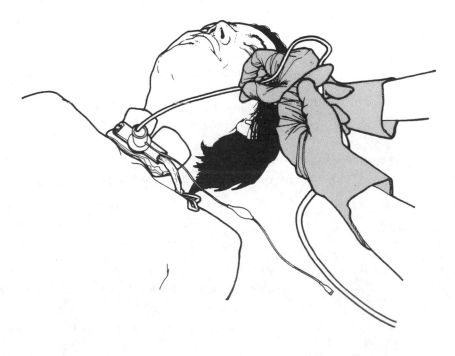

Figure 46.1 *Aspirating respiratory tract secretions via a tracheostomy tube (Reproduced with permission from Chilman A, Thomas M (eds) 1987 Understanding nursing care, 3rd edn. Churchill Livingstone, Edinburgh)*

- ensure that the patient is left feeling as comfortable as possible
- dispose of the equipment safely *for the protection of others*
- document the nursing practice appropriately, monitor after-effects, and report abnormal findings immediately *to provide a written record and enable prompt intervention should an adverse reaction to the procedure be noted.*

2 Changing a tracheostomy tube

Equipment

Tray or trolley

Sterile dressings pack

2 sterile tracheostomy tubes, taped and with an obturator

Sterile KY jelly

Sterile tracheal dilators

Sterile scissors

Protective pad

Container of sodium bicarbonate solution in which to put the soiled silver tracheostomy tube

Disposable gloves

Instrument brush

Receptacle for soiled disposables.

Plastic disposable tracheostomy tubes are normally used nowadays for temporary tracheostomies. Silver tubes are still preferred by most surgeons and patients for use in permanent tracheostomies because the wide range of sizes and types makes it possible to choose the one most suitable for each patient (Fig. 46.2).

Guidelines and rationale for this nursing practice

- explain the nursing practice to the patient *to gain consent and cooperation. Patients should be encouraged to be active participants in care*
- ensure the patient's privacy *to maintain dignity and sense of 'self'*

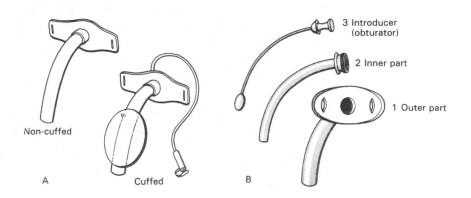

Figure 46.2
Tracheostomy tubes in common use
A Disposable
B Non-disposable

Non-cuffed

A   Cuffed   B

3 Introducer (obturator)

2 Inner part

1 Outer part

- collect and prepare the equipment *for efficiency of practice*
- assist the patient to a suitable position *to allow this practice to be carried out*
- observe the patient throughout this activity *for any signs of discomfort of distress*
- open the dressings pack and the tracheostomy tube pack
- check that the obturator fits. Check particularly that it can be easily removed *as it blocks the airway once the tube is in situ*
- lubricate the end of the tube and obturator *for ease of insertion*
- make a slit in the end of the protective pad *so that it will easily wrap round the tube*
- put on the disposable gloves *for your and the patient's protection*
- remove the soiled tube with a smooth outward and downward motion, discarding it into the receptacle for disposables if it is plastic, or putting it into a container of sodium bicarbonate solution if it is silver. *The sodium bicarbonate loosens any dried areas of secretion.* Ensure that the tube is well rinsed after sodium bicarbonate has been used
- remove the gloves *to allow more dextrous hand movements*
- hold the new tube by the tapes and insert it smoothly from below in an upwards, in and down movement into the trachea. *This follows the line of the stoma*
- immediately remove the obturator while holding the tube in place *to free the airway*
- tie the tapes at the side of the patient's neck. *This is a more comfortable position than the back*
- slide the protective pad into position round the stoma
- ensure that the patient is left feeling as comfortable as possible
- dispose of the equipment safely *for the protection of others*
- if a silver tube is used clean the soiled tube using the brush and gloved hands
- record this nursing practice appropriately, monitor after-effects, and report abnormal findings immediately *providing a written record and enabling prompt intervention should an adverse reaction to the practice be noted.*

Relevance to the activities of living

Maintaining a safe environment

All precautions must be taken for the prevention of infection, as the air inhaled via the tracheostomy tube bypasses the protective ciliated epithelium of the nose, and so the risk of pulmonary infection is increased.

The wound must also be protected from sources of infection.

Thorough hand washing should be carried out, preferably using an antiseptic detergent.

The suction catheter must be inserted gently, and the prescribed suction pressure must not be exceeded or the tracheal mucosa may be traumatised.

Tracheal dilators should be available when changing the tube of a patient with a newly-formed tracheostomy, in case there is difficulty inserting the new tube. This is a rare occurrence.

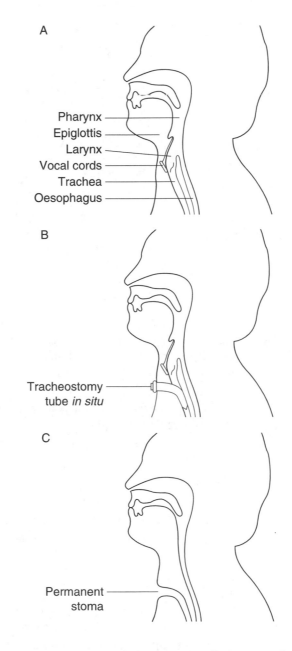

Figure 46.3
Tracheostomy
A Anatomy of the head
and neck
B Temporary
tracheostomy
C Permanent
tracheostomy after
laryngectomy

Care must be taken to maintain a clear airway at all times, as the tube interferes with the normal cough reflex. The need for suctioning may be detected visually (the appearance of laboured breathing, increase in rate, change in pattern), aurally (moist, gurgling sounds) or by auscultation (low-pitched, loose rattling).

Communicating

A tracheostomy reduces the function of the vocal cords, so the patient may have

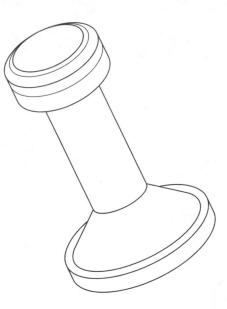

Figure 46.4 *Stoma button for permanent tracheostomy*

a problem with verbal communication; the use of a pad of paper and pencil may partially overcome this. A bell must always be available for the patient to summon assistance.

If it is envisaged that the tracheostomy will be permanent, a teaching programme to educate the patient to change his own tube may be planned and implemented by suitably qualified staff.

Breathing

The purpose of a tracheostomy is to aid the patient's breathing, but the nurse must be vigilant to ensure the patency of the tube at all times.

If a silver tracheostomy tube is used, it will have an inner lining. It may be sufficient to remove this on alternate days and clean it thoroughly with sodium bicarbonate solution, sterilise and re-insert it after applying suction to clear the outer tube.

Eating and drinking

As the trachea is in close proximity, anatomically, to the upper alimentary organs, the presence of a tracheostomy tube may cause apprehension about swallowing, and education and encouragement should be given to the patient to maintain dietary intake.

Personal cleansing and dressing

Advice may be required about the most suitable type of clothing to wear around the stoma and about skin care of the stoma area, especially if the tracheostomy is permanent. The tapes should be tied at the side of the neck, not over the cervical spine where the knot causes discomfort.

Expressing sexuality

A permanent tracheostomy may cause the patient to have psychological problems due to altered body image. A talk with someone who has successfully adjusted to life with a tracheostomy can help.

Sleeping

Initially the patient may be unwilling to sleep, fearing that the tube may become blocked; reassurance that staff are available and observing may have to be given to relieve such anxiety.

Patient education: key points

Patients require planned education to help them cope with the anxiety which most people experience when they first have a tracheostomy. If the tracheostomy tube does not have a speaking flap they will need help and advice about alternative ways of communicating.

Patients who have permanent tracheostomies will require a structured teaching programme of self-care.

Further reading

Allan D 1987 Making sense of tracheostomy. Nursing Times 83(45): 36–38
Clarke L 1995 Care study: A critical event in tracheostomy care. British Journal of Nursing 4(12): 676–682
Roper N, Logan W, Tierney A 1996 The elements of nursing, 4th edn. Churchill Livingstone, Edinburgh
Thurston-Hookway F, Sneddon S 1989 Care after laryngectomy. Ear, Nose and Throat 3: 35

47 Transfer of Patients Between Care Settings

Learning outcomes	By the end of this section you should know how to: • prepare the patient and carer for transfer to another care setting • complete patient transfer documentation.
Background knowledge required	Carers (Recognition and Services) Act 1996 Revision of health authority policy on transfer of patients. UKCC 1995 Discharge of patients from hospital. Department of Health 1989 Discharge of patients from hospital. Department of Health 1991 The patients' charter.
Indications and rationale for patient transfer	The NHS and Community Care reforms have resulted in a much greater focus on the appropriate use of available services for patient care. Thus the patient may be transferred between institutional and community settings within the statutory health and social care agencies or in the voluntary or private/independent sectors, *as is judged appropriate for his individual needs and benefit.*
Outline of the procedure	Patient transfer (rather than discharge) is the term used in this section as it demonstrates a continuum rather than a cessation of care. The procedure may be simple or complex, depending on the needs of the patient and carer. However the systematic approach to care — namely assessment, planning, implementation and evaluation — may be used as a framework for the patient transfer process. • The assessment phase involves the collection of data pertinent to the patient/carer. A variety of sources may be used to build up an holistic picture of the patient and his caring environment. Some of this information will already have been collected at the patient admission assessment • The planning stage utilises the assessment data to provide a plan of transfer. Liaison with other agencies to request/discuss their input will also be carried out at this stage of the process • The implementation phase involves putting the plan into action and completing patient transfer documentation • The evaluation stage of the transfer procedure is essential in order to assess the effectiveness of the process and to identify any difficulties or problems.

Guidelines and rationale for this nursing procedure

General principles will be given, followed by guidelines for planning and implementing the transfer process. Some of the guidelines may not be applicable for patients transferring from community to institutional settings.

Principles

- the patient and carer should be involved in all stages of the transfer process *enabling consideration and discussion of their needs prior to the transfer plan being completed and implemented* (Department of Health 1991, Worth & Tierney 1994)
- patient transfer is normally a multi-disciplinary procedure which may involve social, voluntary and private care agencies as well as different health care professionals, *ensuring an holistic approach to patient transfer*
- good communication is an essential part of the patient transfer process *as poor communication patterns affect continuity of care on transfer from community to institutional settings as well as from institutional to community care* (Evers 1991, Sollitt 1992)
- it is essential that there be early involvement and liaison with staff from the receiving care setting (this may be a hospital ward, a nursing home or the patient's own home). Some areas have a designated liaison nurse who provides a link between institutional and community care *to promote continuity of care* (Worth & Tierney 1994)
- at least 48 hours' notice of transfer from institutional to community care should be provided. In addition patients should not be transferred immediately prior to a weekend or public holiday *in order that adequate community care support services can be organised* (Saville & Bartholomew 1994, Worth & Tierney 1994)
- an evaluation system should be in place *to judge the effectiveness of the patient transfer process* (McHale 1995).

Planning patient transfer

- discuss care needs with the patient and carer *to ascertain their views and requirements, and involve them in the decision process*
- plan and initiate any teaching programmes for the patient/carer. Examples may include a self-medication programme for patients being transferred from institutional to community care (Fuller 1995) or a lifting and handling teaching session for carers *to prepare the patient/carer for tasks which they will be required to undertake in the community*
- consult, liaise, and refer to appropriate care agencies (health, social, voluntary or private). If the patient has complex care needs it may be necessary to invite all relevant personnel to a case conference *to ensure that support services are in position prior to transfer*
- order any equipment or patient aids *to ensure that the receiving care setting meets the patient's needs*
- if the patient has complex needs and is being tranferred from institutional care it is of value to organise a home assessment visit prior to transfer. This would

involve the patient, carer and district nurse as well as other relevant personnel such the occupational therapist, physiotherapist and social care staff *to enable the patient's needs to be assessed within his own environment, and to enable assessment of the carer's ability to provide care.*

- arrange for transport between care settings *to ensure that transport is appropriate for the patient's needs*
- order any medicines and assess the patient's ability to administer medications. If deficits are identified then a teaching programme may have to be initiated for the patient/carer and/or patient compliance devices introduced. This should be done in conjunction with the pharmacist *to ensure that a small supply of medicines is available for the immediate transfer period and that the patient/carer is able to administer the medicines correctly*
- consult with carers about access arrangements to the patient's home on the day of transfer *to enable access arrangements to be made in advance of transfer*
- give an approximate expected time of arrival to the patient/carer and any other personnel who require this information (for example district nurse and home-help) *to enable the caring network to be organised.*

Implementing the transfer process

- complete patient transfer documentation and retain a copy (see Table 47.1) *to provide a permanent record of the transfer process*
- ensure that medical staff have completed a transfer form for the patient's general practitioner. This usually comprises a summary of diagnoses, treatments and medication *and provides a permanent summary of admission details*
- send documentation to personnel in the receiving care setting. This should be carried out according to local health authority policy but may involve internal mailing system, postal service, delivery by patient/carer, fax or computer network. In the future patient-held records (which stay with the patient as he moves between care areas) may be the way in which information is communicated *thus enabling the sharing of information between care settings*
- discuss any medication with the patient. This includes reinforcing information provided by medical staff such as the reason for the drug, dosage, timing/frequency and route of administration as well as any special instructions. The use of a personal medical record card may be of value to some patients (Whyte 1994) *to reinforce the information given on the container label and facilitate understanding*
- check that the patient has all his personal belongings *to ensure that no property is lost during transfer*
- arrange any follow-up outpatient appointment *so that the patient is aware of follow-up care*
- provide details of the receiving care setting (named nurse and contact number).

Relevance to the activities of living

The material provided under each of the activities gives an indication of the type of information which could be shared between care settings.

Table 47.1   **Checklist of contents for transfer documentation**

Social data
Patient details — name, date of birth, address, telephone number, occupation, housing and any dependants
Carer details — name, address, telephone number, occupation, any relevant health problems or disabilities, other dependants and ability/willingness to care

Health data
Diagnosis (including patient/carer's knowledge and understanding of the diagnosis)
Disability/impairment
Prognosis (if applicable)
Medication (including any specialised instructions or medicine aids)
Treatments (this might include details of procedures such as wound care or catheter management)

Patient/carer's needs
These will be specific to the service user and should be decided in conjunction with the patient/carer (for more information *see* Relevance to the activities of living)

Support services
Details of care/therapy provided by other services in the current care setting (such as dietitian, physiotherapist or occupational therapist)
Information — name, contact number and type of input — on any support services arranged for post-transfer period (including commencement date)
Most care settings will have a directory of services in the local area. For information on national services contact NHS Helpline (national information service set up by government)

Financial data
Details of welfare benefits (either in place or applied for)

Equipment data
Details of equipment either in place or requested (indicate source of equipment)

Health promotion/patient education
Provide a summary of:
- health promotion activities
- information on any education programmes.

Enclose a copy of patient education or health promotion literature given to the patient
All documentation should be signed and dated by the named nurse responsible for the patient's care.

Maintaining a safe environment

Information related to any risk factors should be recorded. This might include:

- difficulties related to self-administration of medications
- the patient being at risk from falls
- infection which may put the patient or his carers at risk. If appropriate the MRSA status of the patient should be given (*see* Isolation nursing, p. 185)
- any sensory deficit which may put the patient at risk.

Whilst a patient may function effectively within his existing environment, in a new care setting he may be at risk (for example by becoming disorientated).

Communicating

The patient's ability to communicate and understand information, as well as any deficit such as hearing, sight or speech difficulties, should be noted. Provide information on equipment such as hearing aids or spectacles which the patient may require to communicate effectively.

It is essential that staff communicate with the patient/carer to ensure that they are fully informed and understand all aspects of the transfer. All anxieties or concerns should be discussed and documented.

Breathing

Record any difficulties which the patient has with breathing, as well as treatments such as inhalers or oxygen therapy. For the patient being transferred to the community, arrangements should be made for the delivery of oxygen cylinders and teaching provided for the patient/carer on its use and precautions.

Eating and drinking

The nutritional status of the patient can affect the healing process, so any problems should be documented. Information should be provided on any special dietary requirements and whether there has been input from a dietitian.

Provide information on the patient's ability to feed herself and about equipment required to aid this activity.

Eliminating

Bladder and bowel function is an essential activity: like nutrition it may be affected by a change in environment or illness.

A record of the patient's present bladder and bowel pattern should be given, together with any difficulties related to function, including abnormal patterns such as diarrhoea, constipation or urinary incontinence.

Any investigations should be documented.

A record of necessary continence aids or toilet equipment should be given.

The patient may have begun a teaching programme (such as bladder training) which requires to be continued in the receiving care setting.

Personal cleansing and dressing

The patient's ability to carry out this activity should be described, and a record given of the assistance the patient requires as well as equipment such as bathing aids (Seymour 1995).

The patient may be at risk from pressure sores: the risk factors and score (*see* Skin care, p. 290) should be documented along with the plan of care and any special equipment required. If pressure sores are present, a full description (including tracings) should be documented as baseline data for staff in the receiving care setting.

The condition of the patient's mouth may affect his health; any problems such as ulceration, oral infection or problems with dentition plus details of treatment should be described.

Mobilising

The following should be documented.

- any deficit in the patient's ability to mobilise
- information on any rehabilitation programmes
- equipment required to aid mobility
- the level and type of assistance required from another person
- active/passive exercises which require to be followed up in the receiving care setting.

Working and playing

Information on relevant social activities may be of importance.

The patient's employment status may also be of importance if, because of his illness, time off is required or unemployment a possibility.

Day care attendance and/or activities should be recorded.

Expressing sexuality

Concerns regarding change in body image caused by the illness should be discussed and documented.

Sexual issues require tact and diplomacy. The patient may discuss issues of a highly confidential nature and it may not always be appropriate to document this information. Advice on how to approach the issue of sexuality is given by Van Ooijen (1995).

Sleeping

A change in environment or anxiety about her health is likely to have an impact on the patient's normal sleep pattern. Any difficulties and treatments should be recorded.

Dying

Patients may think about death during an episode of illness. Such thoughts may be transitory, or may be longer-lasting when the patient has a life-threatening or terminal illness. It is important that staff in the receiving care environment are aware of the information and understanding which the patient has about his condition and prognosis. Outline any counselling initiated with the patient.

Patient education: key points

Education for the patient and carer will be dependent on the needs identified in the planning phase of transfer. Patient education may take the form of:

- health promotion initiatives
- teaching, demonstration and supervision of a practical procedure, such as administration of insulin
- literature on a specific illness or disease such as myocardial infarction. This would be used in conjunction with discussion
- verbal discussion to evaluate understanding (for example of an illness or medicines).

Details of patient education programmes should be recorded in the transfer documentation.

References

Department of Health 1989 Discharge of patients from hospital. Health circular 89/5.HMSO, London
Department of Health 1991 The patients' charter. HMSO, London
Evers HK 1991 Issues in community care services. Nursing Standard 5(21): 29–31
Fuller D 1995 Simplifying the system: assessing drug administration methods. Professional Nurse 10(5): 315–317
McHale SA 1995 Implementation of a patient discharge policy. Professional Nurse 10(9): 590–592
Saville R, Bartholomew J 1994 Planning better discharges. Journal of Community Nursing 8(3): 10–14
Seymour J 1995 Bathing aids: handling and lifting in the home. Nursing Times 91(8): 53–54
Sollitt L 1992 Working together. Journal of Community Nursing 6(3): 9–11
UKCC 1995 Discharge of patients from hospital: Registrar's letter 18/1995. UKCC, London
Van Ooijen E 1995 How illness may affect patients' sexuality. Nursing Times 91(23): 36–37
Whyte LA 1994 Medication cards for elderly people: a study. Nursing Standard 8(48): 25–28
Worth A Tierney A 1994 Community nurses and discharge planning. Nursing Standard 8(21): 25–30

48 Unconscious Patient

Learning outcomes

By the end of this section you should know how to:

- maintain an adequate airway for the unconscious patient
- care for the unconscious patient in such a way that his activities of living are appropriately maintained despite almost total dependency.

Background knowledge required

Revision of the anatomy and physiology of the nervous system with special reference to the brain.

Review of health authority policy relating to the care of the unconscious patient.

Indications and rationale for care during a state of unconsciousness

Nursing intervention is required when a patient's level of consciousness is such that, *unaided, he can no longer maintain a clear airway; his normal protective reflexes are so reduced that he can no longer maintain the safety of his environment; and he is unable to perform everyday activities of living.*

The unconscious state is most commonly associated with:

- patients who have a cerebral vascular accident, *when areas of brain tissue will be damaged and have a diminished blood supply,* e.g.:
  — cerebral haemorrhage
  — cerebral embolus or ischaemia
  — subarachnoid haemorrhage
- patients who have taken an overdose of analgesic drugs *which will affect the function of the brain cells*
- patients who have a traumatic head injury *as brain cells may be damaged by the injury*
- patients who have a brain tumour *causing pressure and damage to the brain*
- patients who are in a comatose state caused by:
  — severe infection *as hyperpyrexia may affect brain cell function*
  — hypothermia *because severe temperature change reduces brain cell activity* (Toulson 1994)
  — uncontrolled diabetes mellitus (hyperglycaemia or hypoglycaemia) *which may result in reduced brain cell function*
- patients who have received prescribed anaesthetic medication during and following surgery *which affects the patient's neurological state*
- patients in the terminal stage of illness *when cerebral function is diminished.*

Equipment

Bed with a detachable head

Padded cot sides

Guedel disposable airway

Ambubag with valve and mask

Equipment for assessing level of consciousness

Equipment for oral, pharyngeal or tracheal suction

Equipment for oxygen therapy

Equipment for nasogastric feeding

Mouth care tray

Eye care tray

Catheter care tray

Equipment for endotracheal intubation if required.

(Details of the equipment for specific nursing practices can be found in the relevant sections of this book.)

Equipment for assessing the level of consciousness

- Pencil torch to assess eye pupil size and reaction
- Consciousness level chart, e.g. Glasgow coma scale.

The Glasgow coma scale   enables the assessment of level of consciousness to be made, using a numbered scale. The assessment is of motor activity, e.g. limb movements, verbal responses, reaction to pain, and pupil reactions to light (Fig. 48.1). This scale is now used in many health authorities; each area may have documentation of the scale of recordings presented in a different way, and may incorporate other recordings on the same chart. This has been permitted without infringement of copyright (Allan 1984).

Guidelines and rationale for this nursing practice

The most important aspect of nursing is the maintenance of a clear airway while the reason for the patient's unconsciousness is diagnosed and treated *so that the patient's respiratory function is as efficient as possible under the circumstances.*

- remove any dentures which may be present *to avoid obstruction of the airway*
- turn the patient into a semi-prone position or onto his side, with his neck extended *to prevent the tongue from slipping back and occluding the airway, and also to prevent any secretions from flowing into the trachea when the swallowing reflex is absent*
- observe the patient throughout this activity *to monitor any adverse effects*
- perform oral and pharyngeal suction, or endotracheal suction if appropriate *to prevent aspiration of bronchial or oral secretions* (*see* Tracheostomy care, p. 331)
- insert a plastic airway if required, *to help maintain an adequate airway*
- administer oxygen therapy as prescribed *to prevent hypoxia* (*see* Oxygen therapy, p. 255)
- position the patient's limbs *to maintain his position comfortably and to allow an adequate flow of blood circulation to all his extremities*

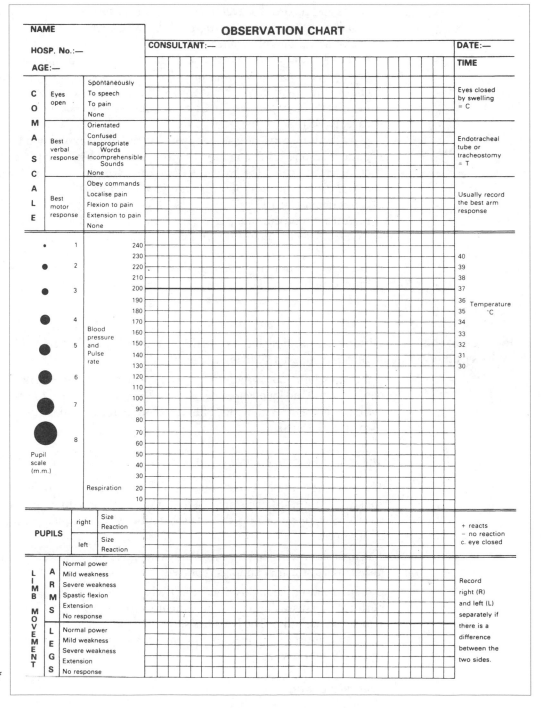

Figure 48.1
Glasgow coma scale: chart for documenting assessment of patient's level of consciousness

- assess and record the level of consciousness every 2 hours if appropriate *to monitor and evaluate his progress* (Ellis & Cavanagh 1992)
- perform oral and pharyngeal suction every 2 hours or as frequently as required, either directly or through the airway as appropriate *to reduce the level of secretions to a minimum, thus preventing any danger of aspiration*
- change the position of the patient to alternate sides every 2 hours *to maintain healthy tissue at pressure areas and to aid the expansion of each lung* (*see* Skin care, p.000)
- provide all nursing care as frequently as required, explaining the care to the patient despite his unconscious state and ensuring his privacy before commencing care. *The patient will be completely dependent for all his needs and the nurse must respect his individuality and maintain his dignity at all times* (Hancock 1992)
- record the temperature, pulse, respiration rates and blood pressure as frequently as required *to maintain observations and record any change in his condition*
- document all nursing practices appropriately and report abnormal findings immediately *to ensure safe practice and enable prompt appropriate medical and nursing intervention to be initiated.*

Relevance to the activities of living

Observations and further rationale for this nursing practice will be included within each activity of living as appropriate.

A patient who is unconscious is at or near the totally dependent end of the dependence – independence continuum. Nursing staff have to assist, or perform for him, the various activities of living until he fully regains consciousness (Roper et al 1996).

Maintaining a safe environment

The patient should be nursed on a firm bed in an area where he can be constantly observed. This may be in a single cubicle with a nurse to provide special care, or a bed near the nurses' station where frequent observations can be maintained.

The area should be well lit so that any change in the patient's colour can be noted, and abnormal findings reported.

Cot sides should be in position expect when nursing practices are being performed. This will prevent the patient from falling if he is restless or in a semiconscious state. The cot sides should be padded to prevent the patient damaging himself on any hard equipment, and pillows placed appropriately can be used effectively.

Communicating

The level of consciousness should be assessed 2-hourly or as ordered by the medical practitioner. Before beginning the assessment the nurse should ensure that the patient is as comfortable as possible in the circumstances. The response to verbal commands and the movement of limbs may be impaired if the patient is uncomfortable or in pain, which may also affect pupil reactions (Chudley 1994).

It is essential to make sure that the patient has no major hearing problem. A profoundly deaf patient will not respond to any verbal instructions, and may be less comatose than the nurse realises. He may become restless and frightened when regaining consciousness as explanations of his surroundings and nursing interventions have not been heard.

A nursing assessment of the patient should be obtained from his family, especially if the patient is unconscious on admission; this should also include his social and family background. It is a great help to communication if the nurse knows the patient's forename or nickname as he may not readily respond to a formal approach such as 'Mr Smith'. It is also a help to know something about the patient's family and interests. Individualised care is enhanced when the nurse is able to chat about the grandchildren, or the dog, or the latest pop records even when there is no immediate response from the patient. This also helps the family to feel that the nursing remains individualised and personal.

The nurse should talk to the patient at every opportunity, even if he appears deeply unconscious. She should try to orientate the patient to his surroundings even where there appears to be no response. He should be told where he is and why, and should be told what day it is, and the date and time as appropriate.

Before commencing any nursing intervention the nurse should introduce herself and explain what is to happen, and should continue to reinforce this throughout the time she is with the patient.

The use of touch as a means of communication is helpful to both the patient and the nurse when caring for the unconscious patient. Physical contact with friends or relatives can help to reorientate a patient as he regains consciousness. Relatives should be encouraged to sit beside an unconscious patient and hold his hand as well as talk to him, whenever they visit (Carruthers 1992).

The patient's response to pain should be noted as part of the assessment of the level of consciousness. This can be done by squeezing the lobes of the ears, squeezing the back of the heel on each side of the achilles tendon, or applying pressure to the fingernail bed. None of these actions will cause damage to the patient but he will react if he feels the pressure as pain. The way his limbs move in response to pain should be noted and recorded on the assessment chart.

Eye care should be carried out 2-hourly. The inability to blink prevents the eyes from being bathed in lacrimal fluid, and the unconscious patient is at risk of developing corneal ulcers if the eyes are not treated regularly (*see* Eye care, p. 135).

The nursing plan should indicate how and when nursing care is carried out, and should include the position of the patient for each period of turning (Murdoch 1994).

Breathing

A clear airway should be maintained until the patient has fully recovered consciousness and has an adequate swallowing and cough reflex.

The respiration rate should be recorded as frequently as necessary, but at least every 4 hours. The depth and the pattern of respiration should also be noted, as well as any evidence of a cough or cough reflex.

The blood pressure and pulse rate should be recorded at least every 4 hours or as frequently as necessary, as any abnormalities may indicate a change in intracranial pressure.

Oral and pharyngeal suction should be performed every 2 hours or as required to clear the airway of secretions. Suction should be performed before turning the patient, as this will prevent secretions from draining into the trachea when he is moved. The amount and consistency of the secretions should be noted and any purulent or bloodstained secretions reported. If the airway is not adequately maintained with routine measures, and the patient has excess secretions which are difficult to clear, the medical practitioner may intubate the trachea with an endotracheal tube, and the patient will breathe through this tube.

The patient's position should be changed 2-hourly, so that he lies on alternate sides. This helps to ensure equal expansion of each lung over 24 hours, and helps with the drainage of any bronchial secretions.

Eating and drinking

Nutrients and fluids may have to be given by nasogastric tube or intravenously. The nasogastric route is used when possible, and a nasogastric tube should be passed initially to prevent any inhalation of the stomach contents. When the presence of bowel sounds is established the medical practitioner may prescribe nasogastric feeds (*see* Nutrition, p. 237).

The patient should have frequent mouth care to maintain a healthy oropharyngeal mucosa, and this should be performed every 2 hours (*see* Mouth care, p. 209).

Fluid intake should be recorded and fluid balance charts maintained to monitor the level of hydration and prevent dehydration.

Eliminating

The unconscious patient is incontinent of both faeces and urine.

Male patients may be fitted with an external sheath catheter, and observations should be maintained for any sign of bladder distension. Catheterisation should be performed for female patients to prevent incontinence increasing the risk of tissue damage to pressure areas. Catheterisation may also be prescribed for male patients who have a prolonged period of unconsciousness.

Catheter care should be performed regularly, and bladder washouts may be prescribed (*see* Catheterisation: urinary, p. 94).

Urinary output should be recorded and fluid balance charts maintained, as this helps to monitor the patient's renal function.

Bowel movements should be noted and recorded. Constipation may be more of a problem than diarrhoea for the unconscious patient, and suppositories or enemas may be prescribed regularly (*see* Suppositories, p. 315).

Personal cleansing and dressing

The nursing plan should include a daily bed bath and any additional washing as required to keep the patient clean and comfortable and his skin in good condition. The nails should be cut short to prevent abrasions caused by scratching, and his hair should be kept clean and tidy (*see* Bed bath, p. 30).

Clothing may have to be adapted to suit the patient's requirements, depending on the reason for his condition. It may not be suitable for him to wear his own clothes, but they should be worn if possible to retain his individuality — this is often a source of comfort to relatives.

The patient's position should be changed every 2 hours to maintain his skin in good condition. An appropriate pressure-relieving mattress system may be needed in addition to position changes (Johnson 1994) (*see* Skin care, p. 289).

Controlling body temperature

The temperature should be recorded 4-hourly, or more frequently as required. Any abnormalities should be reported immediately. Damage to the hypothalamus and its temperature-regulating centre can cause abnormal temperatures to occur.

The bed covers should be adapted to keep the patient comfortably warm. Unconscious patients may show signs of hypothermia, and the nurse should feel the temperature of the feet and hands and note the colour of the skin when observing or working with the patient, (*see* Body temperature, p. 57).

Mobilising

The unconscious patient should be turned every 2 hours so that the tissues under the pressure areas are kept healthy and the blood circulation is maintained to all areas of the body (*see* Skin care, p. 289).

Passive exercises may be performed three times a day, under the guidance of the physiotherapist if possible (*see* Exercises: active and passive, p. 129). This helps to prevent muscle contractions occurring. In addition, light splints may be applied to the lower limbs for patients who are unconscious for a period of time. There are made individually for each patient by the physiotherapist. If possible the nurse should consult the physiotherapist for guidance on the most suitable method of helping to maintain the patient's musculoskeletal system in good condition, so that when he regains consciousness his mobility is not impaired by any muscular or skeletal abnormalities.

The feet should be supported to prevent drop-foot occurring. This can be done by using well-placed sandbags, but specialised splints or sheepskin bootees are more efficient — the guidance of the physiotherapist is helpful.

The semi-prone position (Fig. 48.2) is the most suitable position for maintaining a clear airway, but it is not so suitable for carrying out various nursing activities. The lateral position is preferable and it is still possible to maintain an adequate airway.

Figure 48.2
Unconscious patient: the semi-prone position (Reproduced with permission from Roper N, Logan W, Tierney A 1985 The elements of nursing, 2nd edn. Churchill Livingstone, Edinburgh)

Figure 48.3
Unconscious patient: the lateral position

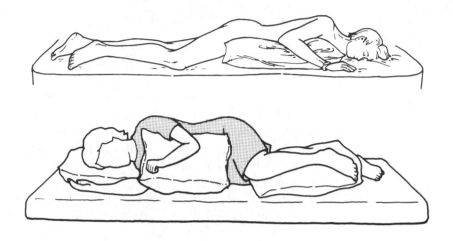

In the lateral position the patient is turned onto his side; his head may be placed on a low pillow with the neck extended. The spine should be extended, and pillows placed at the back to maintain his position. The uppermost leg should be flexed and brought forward to be supported on a pillow clear of the extended lower leg; this prevents internal rotation of the hip and any constriction of blood flow to the lower leg. Pillows should not be placed between the legs. The lower arm should be flexed with the palm facing up and the uppermost arm brought forward and supported on a pillow (Fig. 48.3).

Working and playing

It is important for the people looking after an unconscious patient to learn as much as possible about his interests; it may even be possible to arrange tapes of his favourite music to be played in an attempt to evoke a response.

When suitable, visits from friends and relatives should be encouraged so that they can talk to him about his hobbies or particular interests.

Expressing sexuality

Although superficially the AL of expressing sexuality may not seem relevant to an unconscious patient, ensuring that, for example, the hair is combed and that a male patient is shaved shows respect for the patient's personal identity and can be of inestimable comfort to the family; in fact, they may wish to assist with these activities.

Sleeping

The nursing of a dependent patient can appear to be constant. If possible , any nursing interventions should be arranged to coincide with the time when the patient's position is changed. This is particularly important for patients who show signs of cerebral irritability when handled. It may be beneficial to all unconscious patients to adapt the care so that a period of activity is followed by a long resting period.

Dying

Although an unconscious patient is not necessarily expected to die, the family often associates the apparent unresponsiveness with imminence of death. It is important to listen to the family's concerns, and to explain the cause of unconsciousness and the prognosis, in terms appropriate to the circumstances. When a patient's death is imminent, the family should be encouraged to share their feelings with the nursing staff.

Patient education: key points

Education primarily involves the family. Explanations of the rationale for nursing interventions and expected outcome should be shared with the family.

The family should be encouraged to talk to the patient about his interests and hobbies, reinforced with tapes and music if appropriate. They should understand that hearing is the first communication link which returns as the patient recovers consciousness

The family should also be encouraged to touch the patient and hold his hand, and may wish to help with some of the nursing care. They should be made to feel welcome at the bedside.

References

Allan D 1984 Glasgow coma scale. Nursing Mirror 158(23): 32–34
Carruthers A 1992 A force to promote bonding. Therapeutic touch and massage. Professional Nurse 7(5): 297–300
Chudley S 1994 The effects of nursing care on intracranial pressure. British Journal of Nursing 3(9): 454–459
Ellis A, Cavanagh S 1992 Aspects of neurological assessment using the Glasgow coma scale (research into the pattern of errors made by nurses when assessing neurological patients). Intensive and Critical Care 8(2): 94–100
Hancock K 1992 Caring is a gift of the heart (personal account of sub-arachnoid haemorrhage). Journal of Neuroscience Nursing 24(2): 110–112
Johnson J 1994 Pressure area risk management in a neurological setting. British Journal of Nursing 3(18): 926–935
Murdoch A 1994 The unconscious patient. In: Alexander M, Fawcett J, Runciman P (eds) Nursing practice — hospital and home: the adult. Churchill Livingstone, Edinburgh, ch. 30
Roper N, Logan W, Tierney A 1996 The elements of nursing, 4th edn. Churchill Livingstone, Edinburgh, pp 389–393
Toulson S 1994 Treatment and prevention of hypothermia. British Journal of Nursing 3(13): 662–666

Further reading

Allan D (ed) 1988 Nursing and the neurosciences. Churchill Livingstone, Edinburgh, ch. 4, pp 64–75
Erikson S, Hopkins MA 1987 Grey areas. Informed consent in paediatric and comatose adult patients. Heart Lung 16(3): 323–325
Frawley P 1990 Neurological observations. Nursing Times 86(35): 29–34
Tosch P 1988 Patients' recollections of their post-traumatic coma. Journal of Neuroscience Nursing 20(5): 290–295

49 Urine Testing

Learning outcomes	By the end of this section you should know how to: • prepare the patient for this nursing practice • collect the equipment required • carry out testing of urine.
Background knowledge required	Revision of the anatomy and physiology of the urinary system with special reference to the formation of urine. Revision of the manufacturer's instructions for the chemical reagents to be used.
Indications and rationale for testing urine	Testing urine is the assessment of the constituents of urine by observational, biochemical and mechanical means: • *to aid in the diagnosis of disease* • *to assist in the monitoring of disease and treatment* • *to assist in the assessment of the health of an individual* • *to exclude pathology.*
Equipment	Clean, dry container for urine sample Bottle of reagent strips and/or reagent tablets Test tube if appropriate and test tube rack Pipette Jug for volume measurement Bedpan or urinal Watch with seconds hand Trolley, tray or adequate surface for equipment Receptacle for soiled disposables Disposable gloves.
Guidelines and rationale for this nursing practice	• explain the nursing practice to the patient and obtain his consent and cooperation *to inform the patient about the practice and ensure that he is aware of his rights as a patient* • instruct or assist the patient to collect urine in the clean, dry container the next time he empties his bladder *as this will ensure that the urine specimen is fresh and uncontaminated before testing*

- collect and prepare the equipment *to ensure that the equipment is available and ready for use*
- wash the hands *to reduce cross-infection and contamination by the nurse's hands*
- apply gloves *to protect the nurse's hands from body fluid contamination*
- measure the volume of urine if the patient has a fluid balance chart *which will ensure accurate fluid balance monitoring*
- observe and note any sediment present in the urine *as this may indicate an abnormality of the patient's renal tract*
- observe and note the colour of the urine *as an unusual colour of the urine may indicate an abnormality*
- check the date of expiry on the container of reagent strips and/or reagent tablets *to prevent inaccurate results due to out-of-date reagents.*

Reagent strips

- remove a reagent strip, being careful not to touch the test squares on the strip *as contamination of the reagent strip may give a false reading*
- immerse the reagent strip fully in the urine: note the time *to permit assessment of results at the correct time*
- read the reagent strip after the recommended time has elapsed *to ensure accurate results*
- note the results, *providing an accurate written record.*

Reagent tablet

- remove a reagent tablet from the bottle, placing it on a clean dry surface *as contamination by moisture could give a false reading* (Allwood 1990)
- prepare the urine sample as recommended by the manufacturer *as an incorrectly prepared specimen will alter the final results of the test*
- utilise the reagent tablet as instructed by the manufacturer *to provide accurate results*
- note the result of the test after the recommended time *to ensure an accurate written record.*

Reagent strip and tablet

- dispose of the equipment safely *reducing any hazard to staff amd other equipment*
- document the nursing practice appropriately and report abnormal findings immediately *to provide a written record and assist in the implementation of any action should an abnormal result be noted.*

Relevance to the activities of living	*Maintaining a safe environment*

Although testing urine does not require aseptic technique, all equipment should be clean or disposable and all precautions be taken to prevent cross-infection.

The nurse should wash her hands before commencing and on completion of the nursing practice.

All chemical reagents should be stored in a locked cupboard or drawer to comply with health and safety at work regulations and the control of substances hazardous to health regulations (Department of Health 1989).

When a patient is asked to collect a specimen of urine for routine testing, the container to be used must be clean and dry. It is essential that the container is free from contaminating substances as this may lead to inaccurate results (Royal College of Nursing 1990).

Once the urine sample has been obtained it should be tested immediately. Urine constituents can alter when left exposed to the environment, which may predispose to inaccurate results.

The manufacturer's instructions for care and storage should be followed precisely. These chemical reagents are liable to degradation over a period of time or when storage conditions are not adequate. It is essential that the lid of the container is replaced securely following removal of a reagent strip or tablet, as these are particularly sensitive to changes in temperature and humidity (Allwood 1990). The chemical reagents should be handled carefully. Touching the test square or tablet could introduce contaminants which may alter the results obtained. When using a reagent strip, hold the strip horizontally or place over the urine container. This will prevent any excess urine dripping onto the nurse's hand and proving a health hazard to the member of staff. Holding the strip horizontally will also prevent mixing of the urine between the test squares which could lead to inaccurate results.

It is important that the reagent strip or tablet test is read at the time specified by the manufacturer. Reading the test too late or too soon would give inaccurate results.

Communicating

The patient will require a full and easily understood explanation as to why the urine specimen is required and how to collect the specimen.

The nurse should familiarise herself with any medications the patient may be taking, as certain drugs can affect the test.

Eliminating

Fresh urine from a healthy individual should not have an offensive odour, but decomposing urine will smell like ammonia. A patient whose urine is found to have a 'sweet smell' may be investigated further for diabetes mellitus. Urine smelling of fish can be an indication of infection of the urinary system.

The normal colour of urine ranges from pale straw to dark amber, and the colour of a patient's urine will vary according to the amount of fluid taken into the body (Marieb 1990). The type and amount of urine constituents also affect the colour of urine, e.g. dark coloured urine can be an indication of dehydration or the presence of bile pigments — a manifestation of liver or biliary tract disease.

Certain drugs alter the colour of a patient's urine.

Haematuria is the term used to describe blood in the urine. This can vary from microscopic haematuria, i.e. detected only by testing, through to frank haematuria, i.e. an obvious red coloration. Blood in the urine is suggestive of disease or damage to the renal system (Morrison et al 1994).

Glycosuria is the term used when there is sugar in the urine; it is suggestive of diabetes mellitus.

Proteinuria is the term used when there is protein in the urine, which can be a manifestation of acute or chronic renal disease.

When the body metabolises fat, ketones are one of the products of this metabolism. Ketones are acidotic; if excessive metabolism of fat persists, a state of metabolic acidosis develops which if untreated can lead to coma and death. At a certain stage of acidosis, the ketones are excreted by the urinary system; when they are identified in urine they may be indicative of excessive fasting or uncontrolled or poorly controlled diabetes mellitus.

Specific gravity is a measure of the concentration of the substances dissolved in the urine — the normal range is 1.005–1.025. A single measurement of the specific gravity of urine provides little information as the specific gravity varies depending on the state of hydration of the body. Urine which continually measures a low specific gravity is a manifestation of renal damage or diabetes insipidus. The pH of a urine sample is an indicator of kidney function in maintaining the acid–base balance within the body.

Expressing sexuality

Micturition is an activity associated with privacy and collecting a specimen of urine is usually an unfamiliar experience for the patient, therefore providing privacy and giving an adequate explanation of the practice will be conducive to an uncomplicated collection of the specimen.

When asking a female patient for a urine specimen it is necessary to ask her if she is menstruating, as the menstrual flow may give a falsely positive urine blood result (Bowker 1986).

Patient education: key points

Should the patient be collecting the urine specimen unassisted, ensure that he is aware of the importance of placing the urine in a clean, dry, leakproof container for transport to the doctor's practice or hospital.

Inform the patient of the results and any action required should an abnormality be detected.

A patient or carer may require to be taught this nursing practice; the nurse should therefore devise a suitable educational programme.

References

Allwood M 1990 Quality assurance in urine testing: the role of the hospital pharmacy. In: Newall R, Howell R (eds) Clinical urinalysis: the principles and practice of urine testing in the hospital and community. Ames Division, Miles Limited, Buckinghamshire

Bowker C (ed) 1986 Focus on urinalysis.

    1. Anatomy and physiology of renal tract. Nursing Times (suppl.) 81(17): 1–6

    2. Collection of urine samples. Nursing Times (suppl.) 81(20): 1–6

    3. Urine testing. Nursing Times (suppl.) 81(23): 1–6

    4. Case history — diabetes: urine tests for glucose and ketones. Nursing Times (suppl.) 81(26): 1–6

    5. Proteinuria. Case history — liver function tests: differential diagnosis of jaundice: urine tests for bilirubin and urobilinogen. Nursing Times (suppl.) 81(29): 1–6

    6. Regulation of water balance-specific gravity: urinary pH: urinary tract infection: haematuria. Nursing Times (suppl.) 81(32): 1–6

Department of Health 1989 The control of substances hazardous to health: guidance for the initial assessment in hospitals. HMSO, London

Marieb E 1990 Human anatomy and physiology. Benjamin Cummings, New York

Morrison M, Shandran T, Smithers F 1994 The urinary system. In: Alexander M, Fawcett J, Runciman P (eds) Nursing practice — hospital and home: the adult. Churchill Livingstone, Edinburgh

Royal College of Nursing 1990 Urinalysis — a critical analysis (video). Healthcare Productions, London

Further reading

Ames Division Aids to diagnosis — a short technical manual, 3rd edn. Bayer Diagnostics UK, Slough (available from Bayer Diagnostics UK Limited, Stoke Court, Stoke Poges, Slough SL2 4LY)

Roper N, Logan W, Tierney A 1996 The elements of nursing, 4th edn. Churchill Livingstone, Edinburgh, pp 208–212

50 Vaginal Examination

Learning outcomes

By the end of this section you should know how to:

- prepare the patient for this procedure
- collect and prepare the equipment
- describe the various positions which enable this examination to be carried out most easily
- assist the examiner as necessary.

Background knowledge required

Revision of the anatomy and physiology of the female reproductive system.

Indications and rationale for a vaginal examination

The vagina can be examined visually or digitally for the following reasons:

- *to assess the position, size, texture or appearance of the cervix and vagina*
- *to obtain a swab from the cervix or vagina*
- *to obtain a cervical smear for cytological examination* (*see* Specimen collection, p. 297)
- *to administer treatment to the cervix or vagina*
- *to determine the site of a haemorrhage.*

Outline of the procedure

The examiner puts on a pair of disposable gloves and applies some water-soluble lubricant to the dominant hand. Two or three fingers of the dominant hand are then inserted into the vagina and the uterus palpated through the abdominal wall with the non-dominant hand. This is known as a digital or bimanual examination.

For a visual examination of the vagina and cervix the examiner will insert a lubricated speculum — usually a Sims' or Cusco's — into the vagina (Fig. 50.1). The speculum is gently opened to separate the vaginal walls to enable inspection of the vagina and cervix; a good light is required for this. A pair of vulsellum forceps may be used to hold the cervix while it is examined. A pair of swab-holding forceps and some swabs may be necessary to wipe away any blood or vaginal discharge which might be obstructing inspection of the mucosa. After the examination the speculum is closed and removed gently from the vagina.

Equipment

Tray or trolley

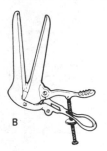

Figure 50.1 *Cusco's vaginal speculum (Reproduced with permission from Chilman A, Thomas M (eds) 1987 Understanding nursing care, 3rd edn. Churchill Livingstone, Edinburgh)*

For digital examination:
— disposable gloves
— water-soluble lubricant
— medical wipes/tissues
— receptacle for soiled disposables

For visual examination, in addition to the above:
— sterile vaginal speculum
— sterile vulsellum forceps
— sterile swab-holding forceps
— swabs
— light source.

The position of the patient

There are several suitable positions for this procedure. The position of choice is usually the one most convenient for the medical practitioner and the patient:

The recumbent position   The patient lies on her back with her knees drawn up and separated and the sides of her feet resting on the bed (Fig. 50.2).

The left lateral position   The patient lies on her left side with her knees flexed and her buttocks near the edge of the bed.

The knee–chest position   The patient kneels on the bed with her thighs vertical. Her head is turned to one side and her chest rests on a pillow.

The lithotomy position   The patient's buttocks are at the end of the table or couch. The thighs are flexed on the trunk and the legs flexed on the thighs. Supports attached to the table or couch keep the patient's legs in the correct position. To avoid injury to the patient, both legs must be lifted gently into position at the same time (Fig. 50.2).

Guidelines and rationale for this nursing practice

- help to explain the procedure to the patient *to gain her consent and cooperation.* Ensure that the woman is aware of her pelvic anatomy and physiology
- ensure as much privacy as possible for the patient *as the majority of patients are very embarrassed about having this examination*
- collect and prepare the equipment *for efficiency of practice*

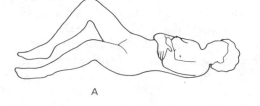
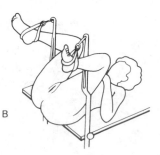

Figure 50.2 *Two common positions used for vaginal examination A Recumbent position B Lithotomy position*

A

B

- assist the patient into the agreed position *for ease of examination*
- observe the patient throughout this activity *to detect any signs of discomfort or distress*
- assist the examiner and the patient as necessary
- ensure that the patient is left feeling as comfortable as possible afterwards *with protection for her underwear if there is any risk of discharge from her vagina*
- dispose of the equipment safely *for the protection of others*
- dispatch any specimens to the laboratory with the completed form and in a plastic specimen bag
- document this procedure, monitor after-effects and report abnormal findings immediately.

Relevance to the activities of living

Maintaining a safe environment

Nowadays, examiners are advised to use a disposable vaginal speculum to prevent any possibility of infecting staff or subsequent patients with HIV, which causes the disease condition AIDS. Because of the current limited knowledge about HIV, the nurse should wear disposable gloves when there is a risk of contact with vaginal discharge or soiled equipment.

Communicating

If the patient can cooperate by relaxing as much as possible, it makes it easier for the examiner to carry out this examination. A clear explanation of why the examination is necessary and how the patient can relax, e.g. by deep breathing, will help to ensure relaxation.

Breathing

Slow, regular, concentrated deep breathing will help the patient to relax the abdominal and perineal muscles.

Eliminating

The patient should be given the opportunity to empty her bladder before the examination. This makes it easier for the examiner to palpate the uterus, and it is more comfortable for the patient, who is usually feeling apprehensive.

Personal cleansing and dressing

If treatment is to be given during the examination which may result in vaginal discharge, the patient should have prior information so that appropriate underwear will be worn.

Expressing sexuality

Many patients find this examination stressful and embarrassing. The best privacy possible should be provided and the patient should be covered as much as possible. The examination should be carried out with the surroundings as calm and relaxed as possible. Some patients may appreciate the opportunity to observe the examination by means of a mirror or a small camera fixed to the examiner's head and a screen to which the pictures are transmitted.

Women who have had no heterosexual experiences and women who have suffered from abuse should be offered extra time, support, information and counselling before and after this examination.

Further reading

Couch-Hockedy S 1989 Women's experience of gynaecology. Professional Nurse 4(4): 173–175
Fogel C, Woods N 1995 Women's health care. Sage, London
Gould D 1990 Nursing care of women. Prentice Hall, London
Gregory S, McKie L 1990 Smear tactics. Nursing Times 86(19): 38–40
Hunter C 1985 Easing the tension. Nursing Times 81(3): 40–43
Nicholson J 1989 Smear campaign. Nursing Times 85(13): 40–42
Roper N, Logan W, Tierney A 1996 The elements of nursing, 4th edn. Churchill Livingstone, Edinburgh
Sadler C 1989 The unmet gynaecological needs of older women. Nursing 3(47): 34
Smith R, Hoppe R 1991 The patient's story: integrating the patient and physician-centred approaches to interviewing. Annals of Internal Medicine 111(6): 470–477

51 Vaginal Pessary Insertion

Learning outcomes	By the end of this section you should know how to: - prepare the patient for this nursing practice - collect and prepare the equipment - administer the prescribed pessaries to the patient.
Background knowledge required	Revision of the anatomy and physiology of the cervix and vagina.
Indications and rationale for administering medicinal vaginal pessaries	Vaginal pessaries are cones or cylinders of medication which are inserted into the vagina, where they dissolve and have their effect topically or by absorption. They are used *to administer medication*, e.g. antibiotics
Equipment	Tray Prescribed pessaries Disposable gloves Water-soluble lubricant Medical wipes/tissues Protective pad Receptacle for soiled disposables.
Guidelines and rationale for this nursing practice	- explain the nursing practice to the patient *to gain her consent and cooperation*. Ideally the woman should be taught to insert the pessary herself *and thereby increase her participation in her care* (Fig. 51.1) - collect, check and prepare the equipment *for efficiency of practice* - ensure maximum privacy and assist the patient into the position agreed by her and the nurse. *See* Vaginal examination for a description of suitable positions (p. 363) - observe the patient throughout this activity *to detect signs of discomfort or distress* - lubricate the end of the pessary *to ease the insertion into the vagina* - put on the disposable gloves - part the labia majora with the non-dominant hand and, on locating the

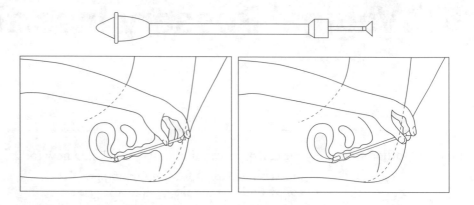

Figure 51.1 *Patient inserting vaginal pessary using applicator*

vagina, insert the pessary in an upward and backward direction with the dominant hand for the length of the index finger if possible. *This should allow the pessary to dissolve and obtain maximum absorption*
- put a protective pad over the patient's vulval area *to protect the patient's underwear from being stained by the dissolving pessary*
- ensure the patient is left feeling as comfortable as possible *with underwear adequately protected*
- dispose of the equipment safely *for the safety of others*
- document this nursing practice appropriately, monitor after-effects and report abnormal findings immediately.

Relevance to the activities of living

Maintaining a safe environment

Although this practice does not require aseptic technique, the equipment should be disposable and the nurse should wash her hands before commencing and on completion of the nursing practice.

Communicating

A clear explanation should be given to gain the patient's consent and cooperation, which should make the administering of the pessary easier. The majority of women should be able to insert the pessary themselves if adequate information and support is given.

Eliminating

The patient should be given the opportunity to empty her bowel and bladder before the pessary is administered. This gives the pessary time to dissolve and be absorbed before the patient's next visit to the toilet.

Mobilising

It should be suggested to the patient that she move around as little as possible for half an hour after the insertion of the pessary, so that it can dissolve and be absorbed.

Expressing sexuality

This can be an embarrassing practice for some patients, and maximum privacy is important. Self-administration of the pessary can help to reduce embarrassment and increase the woman's sense of control.

Further reading

Fogel C, Woods N 1995 Women's health care. Sage, London
Gould D 1990 Nursing care of women. Prentice Hall, London
Roper N, Logan W, Tierney A 1996 The elements of nursing, 4th edn. Churchill Livingstone, Edinburgh
Jones I 1995 Vaginal conditions. Skill update. Macmillan Magazines, London

52 Vaginal Ring Pessary Insertion

Learning outcomes

By the end of this section you should know how to:

- prepare the patient for this practice
- collect and prepare the equipment
- assist the qualified practitioner in the insertion of a ring.

Background knowledge required

Revision of the anatomy and physiology of vagina, cervix and uterus.

Indications and rationale for the insertion of vaginal ring pessaries

Ring pessaries are made of a PVC type of material which is flexible and compressible by hand but springs back into shape when in situ (Fig. 52.1). The pessaries are supplied sterile and individually wrapped. There is a range of sizes; the experienced practitioner will select the most appropriate size for the patient.

They are used to relieve symptoms caused by a degree of uterine prolapse when:

- *the patient is unfit for a surgical repair of her prolapse*
- *the patient does not wish to undergo surgery*

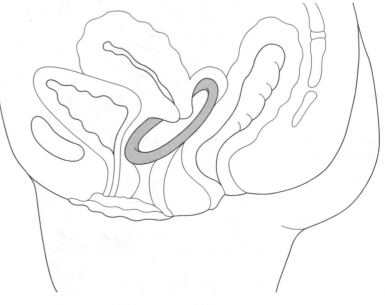

Figure 52.1 *Vaginal ring pessary in position*

Ring pessary *in situ*

- *the patient requires a temporary treatment to alleviate problems while waiting to undergo surgery.*

Equipment

Selected pessary

Disposable gloves

Water-soluble lubricant

Protective pad

Receptacle for soiled disposables.

Guidelines and rationale for this nursing practice

- explain the nursing practice to the patient *to gain her consent and cooperation*
- collect, check and prepare the equipment
- ensure maximum privacy for the patient and assist her into the position agreed by her and the person inserting the pessary. *See* Vaginal examination for a list of appropriate positions (p. 363)
- observe the patient throughout this activity *to detect any signs of discomfort or distress*
- put on the disposable gloves *for protection*
- lubricate the pessary and, using the thumb and forefinger of the dominant hand, squeeze the pessary into an oval shape *for ease of insertion*
- with the non-dominant hand part the labia *to expose the entrance to the vagina*
- the pessary is slid into the posterior part of the vagina and gently pushed downwards and backwards until it settles in the posterior fornix
- once it is in this position it will spring into its normal shape and the person inserting it requires to hook the front portion of the pessary into the anterior fornix behind the symphysis pubis
- ensure that the patient is left feeling comfortable
- dispose of the equipment safely
- document this nursing practice appropriately, monitor after-effects and report abnormal findings immediately.

Relevance to the activities of living

Maintaining a safe environment

Although this practice does not require an aseptic technique, the equipment used should be sterile and the nurse should wash her hands before commencing and on completion of the nursing practice. Gloves should be worn for protection.

The importance of good personal hygiene practices to avoid the risk of infection should be explained to the patient: the pessary is a foreign body in the vagina and therefore a possible focus for infection.

Communicating

If a clear explanation is given and the woman understands the reasons for the insertion of the pessary and has sufficient knowledge of her anatomy to know exactly where it will be positioned, the insertion should be made easier.

Eliminating

Micturition and bowel movements should not be interfered with by the presence of the pessary. It may improve any micturition and bowel problems that the patient was experiencing.

Mobilising

It should be suggested to the patient that she move around as much as possible after the pessary has been inserted to ensure that it is correctly fitted. The patient should be unaware of its presence.

Expressing sexuality

The presence of the pessary will not interfere with sexual intercourse. Personal hygiene is important to prevent infection developing. In older women the lining of the vagina may be dry so oestrogen cream may be prescribed to help avoid any irritation of the mucosal lining.

A slight watery discharge from the vagina is common but patients should be advised to seek help if the discharge becomes purulent, bloodstained, or of an offensive smell.

Patient education: key points

An explanation of the reasons for the insertion of the pessary will help gain the patient's cooperation.

Teaching about the importance of good personal hygiene habits to reduce the risk of infection is essential.

Assurance about the normal activities of micturition, bowel movements and sexual activity should be given.

Advice, and a contact name and telephone number, should be given in case the patient experiences problems related to the pessary.

Further reading

Alexander M, Fawcett J, Runciman P 1994 Nursing care — hospital and home: the adult. Churchill Livingstone, Edinburgh
Fogel C, Woods N 1995 Women's health care. Sage, London
Gould D 1990 Nursing care of women. Bailliere Tindall, London
Jones I 1995 Skills update. Macmillan Magazines, London
Lawler J 1991 Behind the screens. Churchill Livingstone, Edinburgh

53 Venepuncture

Learning outcomes

By the end of this section you should know how to:
- prepare the patient for this procedure
- collect and prepare the equipment
- obtain a sample of blood from a patient
- educate the patient on self-care following this procedure.

Background knowledge required

Anatomy and physiology of the venous blood system.

Principles of infection control in respect of blood-borne infection.

Different devices used in venepuncture.

UKCC 1992 *The Scope of Professional Practice*.

Health authority policy for this procedure.

Indications and rationale for venepuncture

Venepuncture is carried out in order to:
- *obtain a specimen of blood for clinical analysis*. This may include measurement of electrolyte, haemoglobin, or antibody levels within the blood
- *cross-match blood for transfusion*.

Outline of the procedure

Venepuncture is performed by the medical practitioner or phlebotomist, or by a qualified nurse who has undertaken specialised education and is competent in this practice.

Blood may be withdrawn from the vein using the traditional method of a needle and syringe. More recently vacuum container systems have been introduced in some health authorities.

Hoeltke (1995) advises that the syringe method be used when the veins are fragile or when the superficial veins in the back of the hand are used. The value of the vacuum system is that several different samples may be taken as only the tubes require to be changed (not the syringe, as is necessary in the traditional method), thus protecting the nurse from blood spillage. If the veins are too small or fragile to tolerate these techniques Hoeltke (1995) advises that a 'butterfly infusion device' be used to gain venous access. The vacuum system is not described here as the technique may differ slightly depending on the type of device. Nurses using the vacuum system must undertake additional training and follow the manufacturer's instructions.

Equipment

Clean tray for equipment

Disposable gloves

Alcohol-impregnated cleansing swab

Sterile needle(s) or infusion device (20–21 gauge)*

Sterile syringe(s)*

Disposable drape

Sterile adhesive plaster

Sterile gauze swab or cotton wool balls

Tourniquet

Sharpsbox

Receptacle for soiled material

Appropriate specimen containers*

Venepuncture vacuum container system (if used in health authority)

Completed laboratory form(s)

Plastic envelope for transferring specimen.

If a vacuum container system is used the items marked* are not required. Special needles are available for use with this system. Alternatively normal needles can be used with an adaptor produced by the manufacturer.

Guidelines and rationale for this nursing practice

- discuss the procedure with the patient and ascertain if he has an allergy to adhesive plaster *to inform the patient about the procedure, discuss any concerns or queries and identify any previous difficulties experienced with venepuncture*
- obtain consent from the patient to undertake the procedure *to ensure that the patient is aware of his rights as a patient*
- select a suitable clean surface and lay out equipment. If the procedure is being undertaken in the patient's own home protect the surface with a waterproof cover *to provide a suitable protected work surface*
- check that the laboratory forms have been completed and select the appropriate specimen containers *to ensure that the documentation is correct and that the samples are put into the correct specimen containers*
- cleanse hands using a bactericidal solution *to reduce risk of cross-infection* (Gould 1995)
- open sterile packs and attach a needle to the syringe *to ensure that equipment is ready for patient use*
- position the patient in a supine position on a bed/trolley/couch (if these are not available then patient should be seated) *to ensure patient comfort and prevent injury if patient feels faint during the procedure*
- observe and palpate the veins on both arms. The blood vessels most commonly used are the cephalic, basilic or the median cubital (in the forearm— Fig. 53.1) followed by the superficial veins on the dorsal aspect of the hand (Fig. 53.2). The nurse should be aware of the location of the brachial

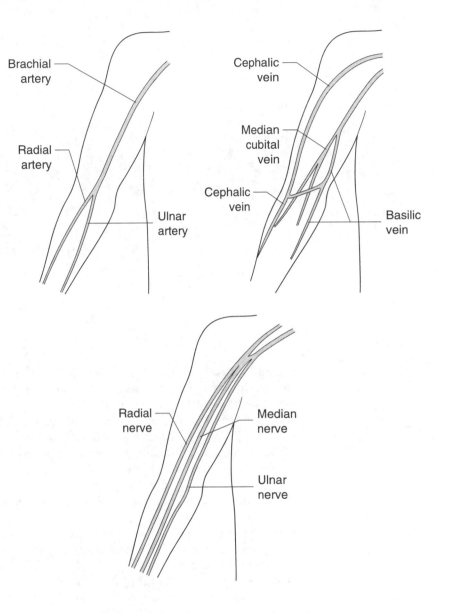

Figure 53.1
Anatomical features of forearm
A Arteries
B Veins
C Nerves

artery and median nerve (Fig. 53.1) *as injury to either will cause pain and may cause temporary or permanent damage*

- select a vein which is visible and firm to touch. If there is lymphatic impairment or the patient has had an illness/disease or surgery affecting the limb then an alternative site should be selected. Take into account the patient's own past experience of venepuncture in helping to identify the best vein *to identify the vein most likely to provide best venous access*

- place the tourniquet or sphygmomanometer cuff approximately 2–5 inches (5–12 cm) above the proposed puncture site *to promote vasodilation*. This should not remain in situ for any longer than 2 minutes

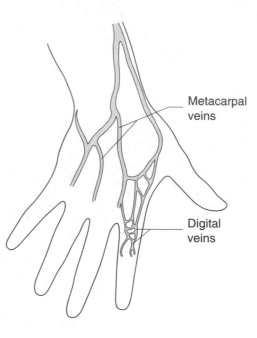

Metacarpal veins

Digital veins

Figure 53.2 *Superficial veins on dorsal aspect of hand*

- ask patient to clench his fist *to promote vasodilation*
- put on gloves *to protect patient and nurse from potential blood-borne infection* (Pollard 1990, Clulow 1994)
- select a firm visible vein and cleanse with an alcohol-impregnated cleansing swab for 5 seconds, *reducing skin flora by 97%* (Lawrence et al 1994)
- place the thumb or index finger below the proposed puncture site and pull the skin in a downward direction *to stabilise the vein*
- with the bevel facing upwards, gently and slowly insert the needle at an angle of 15° into the vein (Hoeltke 1995) *to ensure correct angle of entry into the vein*
- when the vessel wall has been punctured and blood appears in the barrel of the syringe then level off the needle and advance it slightly further into the vein *to ensure that the opposite side of the vessel is not punctured*
- gently pull back the plunger of the syringe and collect the required amount of blood *to prevent collapse of the vein and to obtain a specimen of blood*
- release the tourniquet *to prevent further compression of the blood supply and excessive bleeding at the puncture site on removal of the needle*
- if blood does not appear the needle should be removed and, adhering to health authority policy, the nurse should either undertake the procedure using another vessel or seek assistance from another practitioner *to prevent undue distress to the patient or trauma to the vein*
- remove the needle (keeping it straight), covering the puncture site with cotton wool or gauze swab *to prevent leakage of blood from the puncture site*
- apply pressure directly over the puncture site for 2–3 minutes (3–5 minutes if the patient has a clotting defect). The patient may be able to undertake this activity. The patient should not bend his arm as this may enlarge the puncture

wound, causing more bleeding (Campbell 1995) *to reduce trauma to the vein and discomfort for the patient, and to stop bleeding from vein and thus reduce the risk of formation of a haematoma*

- as soon as possible following collection, transfer the blood to the appropriate specimen container(s). If additives are present in the container then rotate it gently several times *to prevent clotting of blood*
- complete the label on the specimen container(s) *to ensure that correct investigations are carried out and that the results are returned to the correct patient*
- place the specimen container and laboratory form in the plastic bag (or follow health authority policy) *to ensure that the laboratory receives the correct specimen*
- inspect the puncture site for bleeding and/or haematoma formation and apply adhesive plaster over the site (if the patient has an allergy to the plaster apply a gauze swab and secure it firmly with hypoallergenic tape) *to ensure that clotting has occurred and that the puncture site is protected from infection/trauma*
- dispose of contaminated equipment according to health authority policy *to prevent transmission of infection*
- remove gloves and treat as above. Wash hands or cleanse with bactericidal solution *to prevent cross-infection*
- ensure that the patient is feeling well following the procedure (this is especially important if the procedure is carried out in the patient's own home) *to ensure that the patient does not feel unwell as a result of the procedure*
- discuss the points raised under Patient education: key points. If the patient is unable to participate in this stage of the procedure then the monitoring should be undertaken by the nurse or an appropriate adult carer *to ensure that the patient/carer/nurse is aware of, and understands, follow-up self-care.*

Relevance to the activities of living

Maintaining a safe environment

All precautions to prevent potential complications such as damage to nerves or other blood vessels during venepuncture should be maintained. The puncture site and surrounding area should be observed for signs of infection such as inflammation or pain. Any of these symptoms, including swelling, pain, tingling in the arm and excessive bruising/bleeding at or around the puncture site, should be reported to a medical practitioner. The nurse should adhere to health authority policy on the safe preparation, use and disposal of all equipment.

Communicating

The nurse should be aware of the information the patient needs about the practice of venepuncture, encouraging the patient to discuss her understanding of why the blood specimen is being obtained.

The nurse should also respond to the patient's need for information regarding the reason for venepuncture (this should be carried out in consultation with the medical practitioner who authorised the investigation).

Selective health education may be carried out in relation to any underlying disease, for example a diabetic patient attending for blood glucose monitoring.

Counselling may be required following diagnosis of any disease as a result of the blood test.

Personal cleansing and dressing

There has been some debate over the cleansing of puncture sites. A study carried out by Lawrence et al (1994) found that cleansing the skin for 5 seconds with a swab impregnated with 70% isopropanol reduced skin flora by 97%. Venepuncture provides an entry point for organisms directly into the vascular system; this skin cleansing regime is therefore essential prior to puncturing the skin.

Patient education: key points

- Aftercare of the puncture site:
  — report any bleeding oozing from under the adhesive plaster
  — if itching or a rash occurs at the plaster site, remove the plaster and apply a gauze swab secured with hypoallergenic tape
  — remove the adhesive plaster 24–48 hours after venepuncture
- Potential complications following venepuncture:
  — the patient should report excessive bruising radiating from the puncture site (this could relate to haematoma formation)
  — the patient should report any tingling sensation, pain or swelling in the arm (this may indicate pressure on a nerve)
- Blood sample results: inform the patient of when results will be available, and of the process for obtaining the results.

References

Campbell J 1995 Making sense of venepuncture. Nursing Times 91(31): 29–31
Clulow M 1994 A closer look at disposable gloves. An assessment of the value of vinyl, latex and plastic gloves. Professional Nurse 9(5): 324, 326–329
Gould D 1995 Now please wash your hands. Practice Nurse 10(3): 188–190
Hoeltke LB 1995 Phlebotomy: the clinical manual series. Delmar, New York
Lawrence JC, Lilly HA, Kidson A, Davies J 1994 The use of alcoholic wipes for disinfectant of injection sites. Journal of Wound Care 3(1): 11–14
Pollard C 1990 How to take blood. Practice Nurse (Sept): 215–216
UKCC 1992 The scope of professional practice. UKCC, London

Further reading

Choudhury RP, Cleator SJ 1992 An examination of needlestick injury rates, hepatitis B vaccination uptake and instruction on 'sharps' technique among medical students. Journal of Hospital Infection 22(2): 143–148

54 Wound Care

There are four parts to this section:

1 **Wound assessment**
2 **Aseptic technique**
3 **Wound drain care**
4 **Removal of stitches, clips or staples**

The concluding subsections; 'Patient education: key points' and 'Relevance to the activities of living' refer to the four practices collectively.

Learning outcomes

By the end of this section you should know how to:

- prepare the patient for these four nursing practices
- collect and prepare the equipment
- carry out these nursing practices.

Background knowledge required

Revision of wound assessment.

Revision of the physiology of wound healing and the factors which affect wound healing.

Review of the health authority policies regarding all four parts of wound care technique.

Review of the common classification of wound dressing materials and their individual properties.

1 Wound assessment

Indications and rationale for wound assessment

Wound assessment is the process the nurse uses to plan the appropriate management of individual patients who have a wound (Bale 1994). Dealey (1994) suggests two clear aims of wound assessment:

- *to provide baseline information about the state of the wound, allowing the monitoring of progress*
- *to ensure that the appropriate wound management product has been chosen.*

The assessment process should assess the following:

- the patient
- the wound
- the environment of the patient
- the appropriateness of the wound dressing materials.

Equipment	Material to record assessment details, e.g. wound assessment chart (Morison 1992)
	Clean ruler to measure wound size
	Grid to record shape of wound
	Vascular flow detector, e.g. Doppler ultrasound — commonly used with leg ulcers by skilled personnel.

Guidelines and rationale for this nursing practice	This full assessment of the patient and his wound will not be required every time the wound is dressed:

- explain the nursing practice to the patient *to gain consent and cooperation*
- collect and prepare the equipment required *to ensure that it is available and ready for use*
- ensure the patient's privacy *to reduce anxiety*
- wash hands *to reduce cross-infection* (Horton 1995)
- help the patient into a comfortable position *to create a sense of well-being*
- using an appropriate nursing model assess the patient *to identify any factors which may interfere with wound healing such as poor nutritional status, underlying disease, prescribed medications or amount of pain experienced by the patient*
- classify the wound as chronic, acute or postoperative *as each classification will determine the subsequent management* (Dealey 1994)
- assess the wound dimensions using the ruler, which should come in direct contact with the wound. *This provides baseline data which can be used to monitor the progress of wound healing* (Plassmann 1995)
- assess and record the shape of the wound using a measured grid tracing *to permit changes to the wound shape to be noted* (Benbow & Dealey 1995)
- note the amount of wound exudate *as this may determine the choice of dressing*
- assess the wound condition and appearance, which may be epithelialising, granulating, sloughy, infected or necrotic (Thomas et al 1994) *to provide information regarding the stage of healing*
- note the position of the wound on the patient's body *as this may guide the choice of dressing*
- record where the patient is being cared for, i.e. in hospital, at home or in a long-term care institution *as this may alter the initial wound management regime* (Bale 1994)
- for leg ulcers, assist a skilled practitioner in the assessment of the venous flow of the limb *as this will assist in identifying the underlying cause of the ulcer which will then determine the management of the wound* (Morison & Moffatt 1994)
- following the initial assessment evaluate the wound at regular intervals *to monitor the overall progress of the wound*
- re-assess the appropriateness of the choice of wound dressing at regular intervals, *as one wound may require different dressing materials at the various stages of healing*

- ensure that the patient is left feeling as comfortable as possible *maintaining the quality of this nursing practice*
- dispose of the equipment safely *to reduce any health hazard*
- document the nursing practice appropriately, monitor after-effects and report abnormal findings. *This provides a written record and assists in the implementation of any action should an abnormality or adverse reaction to the practice be noted.*

2 Aseptic technique

Indications and rationale for aseptic technique

This is the technique used to reduce the potential problem of introducing pathogenic microorganisms into the body when the integrity and/or effectiveness of the natural body defences has been reduced. The details of the technique may be modified according to the particular dressings pack used, but the principles are the same. The equipment, lotions and dressings used are sterile and the risk of contamination by airborne pathogenic microorganisms is kept to a minimum. Aseptic wound dressing can be indicated:

- *to remove wound discharge*
- *to apply special treatments to a wound,* e.g. venous leg ulcer
- *where signs of wound infection are present*
- *following trauma to the skin tissue,* e.g. pressure sore
- *during an invasive procedure such as catheterisation or introduction of an intravenous cannula.*

Equipment

Dressings trolley or appropriate clean surface in patient's home

Sterile dressings pack containing a gallipot or similar container, swabs, disposable forceps and drape

Sterile wound-cleansing lotion, e.g. normal saline, *or* sterile irrigating solution

Additional sterile dressing material, usually packed separately

Sterile disposable gloves

Hypoallergenic tape

Clean pair of scissors for cutting tape

Clean disposable plastic apron

Alcohol-based hand preparation lotion

Receptacle for soiled disposables.

Characteristics of an ideal dressing

Morison (1992) identified the characteristics of an ideal dressing which the nurse should be aware of when choosing the most appropriate dressing for the patient's wound. The ideal dressing should be:

- non-adherent

- impermeable to bacteria
- capable of maintaining a high humidity while removing excess exudate
- thermally insulating
- non-toxic and non-allergenic
- comfortable and conformable
- protective of the wound from further trauma
- requiring infrequent dressing changes
- cost effective
- long in shelf life
- available in hospital and community settings.

Continuity of wound care from hospital to home can present a problem for the community nurse due to the constraints of the Drug Tariff. As a result the community nurse may require to review the wound management strategy with reference to the dressing materials available (Dealey 1994).

| **Guidelines and rationale for this nursing practice** | ***Institutional*** |

- explain the nursing practice to the patient *to gain consent and cooperation*
- use a treatment room for wound dressing technique *as this reduces the incidence of cross-infection*; if this is not available prepare the environment around the patient's bed
- wash the hands *to reduce the risk of cross-infection* (Ayliffe et al 1993, Horton 1995)
- wash the dressings trolley thoroughly with detergent and water and then dry *to provide a socially clean surface*
- disinfect the dressings trolley with 70% ethyl alcohol immediately prior to every dressing technique *to reduce the number of microorganisms on the trolley surface*
- collect and prepare the equipment, check all packaging for damage such as tears or leakage and check the expiry dates of all the equipment *to ensure the equipment has not been contaminated*
- place all the equipment on the bottom shelf of the trolley, preferably in order of use, *to leave the top shelf free and clean during the practice and to permit easy access to the equipment*
- attach the receptacle for soiled disposables to the side of the trolley below the level of the top shelf. *This assists in reducing contamination from the soiled disposables to the top shelf of the dressing trolley during the dressing*
- ensure the patient's privacy *to reduce anxiety*
- observe the patient throughout this activity, *noting any signs of distress*
- help the patient into a comfortable position *to allow him to maintain the position during the practice*
- adjust the patient's clothing to expose the wound area *to give easy access to the wound for the nurse*
- wash the hands *to reduce cross-infection* (Horton 1995)
- apply the plastic disposable apron *to reduce the adherence of microorganisms to the nurse's uniform which could be a source of cross-infection* (Ayliffe et al 1993)

- open the outer packaging of the dressings pack and slip onto the top shelf of the dressings trolley *allowing the inner cover of the dressings pack to contact a clean surface*
- loosen the outer dressing covering the patient's wound *to ease removal after the nurse has commenced the dressing*
- wash the hands using the alcohol-based hand lotion *to reduce cross-infection* (Horton 1995)
- open the dressings pack, touching the sterile covering as little as possible *to reduce contamination by the dresser's hands*
- if using forceps from the contents of the dressings pack arrange the equipment on the sterile field *to maintain asepsis*
- if using sterile gloves, apply and arrange equipment on the sterile field *to maintain asepsis*
- open additional equipment and drop onto the sterile field. If using a sachet of skin cleansing lotion pour into the gallipot *thereby preparing all equipment ready for use*
- using forceps or a gloved hand remove the soiled dressing and discard both the dressing and forceps *to remove all contaminated material from the wound site*
- drape the wound with the sterile drape if used *to act as an extra surface to work from*
- note the condition of the wound and surrounding tissue *to assess and evaluate the wound's progress*
- use the irrigating solution *to remove any visible debris and cleanse the wound*
- apply the fresh dressing which is part of the wound management strategy *to create the optimum wound healing environment*
- discard gloves or forceps *to remove contaminated materials*
- *to maintain the position of the dressing* secure by the chosen method
- apply any secondary material such as compression bandaging for a patient with a venous leg ulcer, *to assist in the overall healing environment of the wound* (Morison 1994)
- ensure that the patient is left feeling as comfortable as possible *maintaining the quality of this nursing practice*
- dispose of all equipment safely *to reduce any health hazard*
- document this nursing practice appropriately, monitor after-effects and report abnormal findings immediately *providing a written record and assisting in the implementation of any action should an abnormality or adverse reaction to the practice be noted.*

Community

- explain the nursing practice to the patient *to gain consent and cooperation*
- identify an adequate surface within the patient's home *to provide a working environment which is as clean and dry as possible*
- wash the hands *to reduce the risk of cross-infection* (Ayliffe et al 1993, Horton 1995)
- collect and prepare the equipment, check all packaging for damage such as

tears or leakage and check the expiry dates of all the equipment *to ensure the equipment has not been contaminated*

- attach the receptacle for soiled disposables to a nearby surface. *This provides a collection point for all used materials*
- ensure the patient's privacy *to reduce anxiety*
- observe the patient throughout this activity *noting any signs of distress*
- help the patient into a comfortable position *to allow him to maintain the position during the practice*
- adjust the patient's clothing to expose the wound area *to give easy access to the wound for the nurse*
- wash the hands *to reduce cross-infection* (Horton 1995)
- apply the plastic disposable apron *to reduce the adherence of microorganisms to the nurse's uniform which could be a source of cross-infection* (Ayliffe et al 1993)
- open the outer packaging of the dressings pack and slip onto the surface *allowing the inner cover of the dressings pack to contact a clean surface*
- loosen the outer dressing covering the patients wound *to ease removal after the nurse has commenced the dressing*
- wash the hands using the alcohol-based hand lotion *to reduce cross-infection* (Horton 1995)
- open the dressings pack, touching the sterile covering as little as possible, *to reduce contamination by the dresser's hands*
- if using forceps from the contents of the dressings pack arrange the equipment on the sterile field *to maintain asepsis*
- if using sterile gloves, apply and arrange equipment on the sterile field *to maintain asepsis*
- open additional equipment and drop onto the sterile field. If using a sachet of skin cleansing lotion pour into the gallipot *thereby preparing all equipment ready for use*
- using forceps or a gloved hand remove the soiled dressing and discard both the dressing and forceps *to remove all contaminated material from the wound site*
- drape the wound with the sterile drape if used *to act as an extra surface to work from or a barrier for spillages*
- note the condition of the wound and surrounding tissue *to assess and evaluate the wound's progress*
- use the irrigating solution *to remove any visible debris and cleanse the wound*
- apply the fresh dressing which is part of the wound management strategy *to create the optimum wound healing environment*
- discard gloves or forceps *to remove contaminated materials*
- *to maintain the position of the dressing* secure by the chosen method
- apply any secondary material such as compression bandaging for a patient with a venous leg ulcer *to assist in the overall healing environment of the wound* (Morison & Moffat 1994)
- ensure that the patient is left feeling as comfortable as possible *maintaining the quality of this nursing practice*
- dispose of all equipment safely *to reduce any health hazard*
- document this nursing practice appropriately, monitor after-effects and report

abnormal findings immediately *providing a written record and assisting in the implementation of any action should an abnormality or adverse reaction to the practice be noted.*

3   Wound drain care

Indications and rationale for wound drain care

Wound drains are inserted at the time of surgical intervention by the medical practitioner *to prevent fluid collecting at the operation or wound site, a factor which may retard tissue healing.* The extent and site of the surgery will influence the type and number of drains used. Drains may be inserted away from the original incision to be dressed and heal independently. *This will help prevent transmission of infection between the incision/operation site and the exit site for the wound drain.* Drains are frequently stitched in position and attached to a closed circuit drainage bag, or portable suction if required (Nightingale 1989).

Some types of wound drains

Figure 54.1   *Wound care: a portable vacuum drain*

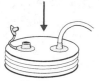

Use hand pressure to expel air

Replace stopper while maintaining pressure to create vacuum

Hollow plastic tube   This is a deep drain with drainage holes at the proximal (drainage site) end. It is usually stitched in position and attached to a closed circuit drainage bag. It may be used following major abdominal surgery to drain any collection of fluid.

Corrugated rubber drain   This is a superficial drain which usually drains directly into the dressing. It may be used to drain an incision site.

T-tube   This is a specialised tube inserted into the common bile duct following a cholecystectomy. It allows bile to drain into a closed circuit bag for 6–10 days postoperatively, until normal drainage is re-established.

Portable vacuum suction drain   This is a perforated plastic catheter attached to a specialised sterile vacuum suction bag (Fig. 54.1). Two or more may be attached to the same vacuum bag with a Y connection. *This system is used to prevent a haematoma forming by maintaining gentle suction. It may be used following joint replacement surgery or surgery in the face or neck area where fluid may collect rapidly due to the efficient blood supply in the area.*

Equipment

As for Aseptic technique, p. 383.

Additional equipment as required

- Sterile gloves
- Sterile scissors
- Sterile stitch cutters
- Sterile drainage bag
- Portable wound suction equipment
- Sterile specialised keyhole dressing
- Extra sterile dressings material (Thomas et al 1993)
- Sterile safety pin

- Sterile wound pads
- Measuring jug
- Sterile specimen container.

Sterile gloves should be used when dressing wound drains to help maintain asepsis and to protect nursing staff from infected body fluids.

Guidelines and rationale for this nursing practice

- explain the nursing practice to the patient *to gain consent and cooperation and encourage participation in care*
- ensure the patient's privacy *to respect his individuality*
- help the patient into a comfortable position depending on the area of the wound drain *so that the area for dressing is easily accessible and the patient is able to maintain his position with minimum distress.* In some instances carefully timed prescribed analgesia may be given *to ensure maximum effect during the wound care*
- observe the patient throughout this activity *to monitor any adverse effect.* This continual evaluation ensures that nursing or medical intervention can be altered as necessary
- collect and prepare the equipment *to ensure efficient use of time and resources*
- remove clothes and covers from the area of the wound, ensuring that with the exception of that area the patient remains covered *to expose only the site for wound care and respect the patient's dignity*
- perform the dressing for the surgical incision line first if necessary, maintaining asepsis. Normally dressings will be removed from the incision line after 24 hours and the wound covered by plastic spray dressing *to encourage healing by first intention.* After this only the drainage tube sites need to be dressed *to promote healing and prevent infection* (Guilding 1993)
- prepare the sterile field for dressing the drainage tube site *as an essential component of aseptic technique*
- don sterile gloves after efficient hand washing *to prevent any contamination with body fluids*
- proceed as for Aseptic technique until the drainage tube is exposed
- cleanse the skin round the wound drain with wound cleansing lotion if there is any exudate *to prevent any spread of infection occurring* (Young 1995) (Fig. 54.2)
- dry the skin round the wound drain *to reduce any infection*
- prepare a 'keyhole dressing'. *This allows the dressing to fit snugly round the drain* (Fig. 54.3)
- shorten the drain as ordered by the medical practitioner. This will depend on the healing process of the individual wound
- apply the keyhole dressing or other as required *to maintain asepsis and promote healing*
- secure the dressing *to prevent it slipping*
- change the drainage bag and secure it in such a position *that gravity will help the fluid drain away from the wound efficiently*
- measure the drainage fluid and note its colour, consistency and smell *so that the process of healing can be monitored and any adverse condition reported*

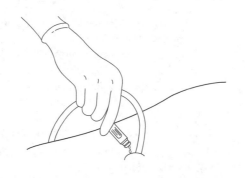

Figure 54.2 *Cleansing the skin round the wound drain*

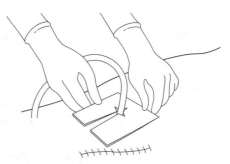

Figure 54.3 *Applying a keyhole dressing*

- ensure that the patient is left as comfortable as possible *to create an environment which will promote healing*
- dispose of the equipment safely *to maintain a safe environment*
- document this nursing practice appropriately, monitor after-effects and report abnormal findings immediately *so that any nursing or medical intervention can be evaluated and altered as required.*

Shortening wound drains

Deep wound drains may be shortened once or twice during the postoperative period as healing proceeds, as ordered by the medical practitioner.

- expose the drain site, maintaining asepsis and cleansing the skin as before. Sterile gloves should be worn after effective hand washing *to prevent contamination with body fluids*
- remove any stitches holding the drain in position (*see* Removal of stitches, p. 391) *to release the drain*
- support the skin round the drain site with one hand using a sterile swab and gently withdraw the drain as far as ordered by the medical practitioner, e.g.

3–5 cm; *supporting the surrounding area reduces discomfort and prevents damage to healthy tissue*
- insert a sterile safety pin through the drain near the entry sites. *This prevents the drain falling back into the wound*
- cut off the extra length of drain if necessary *so that it lies neatly at the drain site and causes no discomfort.* Drains attached to drainage bags will not need to be cut
- apply a sterile keyhole dressing under the safety pin, and another over the safety pin. *This helps to maintain the drain in position and prevents the safety pin from damaging the skin*
- secure the dressing in position *to prevent any drag on the drain or contamination of the wound* (Pagget 1992)
- proceed as for Guidelines and rationale for this nursing practice.

Removing wound drains

This will be ordered by the medical practitioner when there is no longer any significant drainage from the wound.

- expose the drain site and cleanse the skin as before, maintaining asepsis. Sterile gloves should be worn *to prevent contamination with body fluids*
- remove any stitches holding the drain in position
- support the skin round the drain site with one hand, using a sterile swab, and gently withdraw the drain using either a sterile gloved hand or sterile forceps held in the other hand. *This prevents damage to surrounding tissues and helps to reduce discomfort as well as maintaining asepsis.* The tip of the drain should be cut off with sterile scissors and placed in a sterile specimen container, maintaining asepsis, *if it is required for microbiological investigation*
- cleanse and dry the wound site again if necessary (Young 1995)
- apply and secure an appropriate sterile dressing *to maintain asepsis and promote healing*
- proceed as for Guidelines and rationale for this nursing practice
- dispatch the labelled specimen to the laboratory immediately with the completed form *so that investigative procedures may be completed as soon as possible.*

Emptying the portable wound suction container

The containers should be emptied as soon as they are no longer maintaining a vacuum suction, or every 12 hours as required *to measure drainage and prevent ascending infection.*

- clamp the drainage tubing above the level of the wound drainage container *to prevent backflow*
- remove the stopper or bung from the container, maintaining asepsis, *to release the vacuum*
- obtain a specimen of drainage fluid *for microbiological investigation if required*
- pour the remaining contents into a measuring jug *avoiding contamination*
- wipe the outside of the entry channel with alcohol solution, e.g. Mediswab, *to remove any drainage fluid which might cause infection*

- press the two rigid surfaces of the container together and maintain the pressure until the stopper is firmly in position. Once the pressure is removed a gentle vacuum suction is created
- secure the drainage bag in postion as before
- document the amount and details of the drainage fluid in the patient's records *so that accurate monitoring of the healing process and evaluation of treatment can continue.*

4   Removal of stitches, clips or staples

Indications and rationale for removal of stitches, clips or staples

Following surgery, stitches, clips or staples are used to place the skin edges in apposition and promote rapid healing. These are removed when there is:
- *evidence of the wound having healed*
- *infection in part of the wound.*

Equipment

Sterile dressings pack

Sterile normal saline

Sterile stitch cutter or scissors, clip or staple remover

Receptacle for soiled disposables.

Guidelines and rationale for this nursing practice

- explain the procedure to the patient *to gain consent and cooperation*
- ensure the patient's privacy *to maintain dignity and sense of 'self'*
- collect the equipment *to help the efficiency of the practice*
- observe the patient throughout this activity *to detect any signs of discomfort or distress*
- clean the wound with solution only if it is necessary to get access to stitches, clips or staples *as studies have shown that unnecessary washing increases the risk of infection being introduced* (Leaper 1986, Harding 1992).

Removing sutures

- hold the stitch cutter or scissors in the dominant hand and the dissecting forceps in the other hand to gently lift the knot of the stitch (Fig. 54.4)
- cut between the knot and the skin, so that no part of the stitch above the skin surface is pulled under the tissues, then gently pull out the cut stitch. *This helps reduce the risk of introducing infection*
- ensure that no piece of the stitch is left in the wound, *as this could eventually form a wound sinus.*

Removing clips or staples

- hold the remover in the dominant hand and the dissecting forceps in the other hand when removing clips or staples (Fig. 54.4)

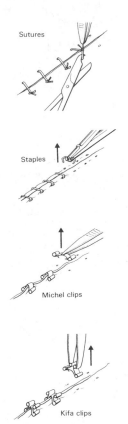

Figure 54.4   *Removal of sutures, clips and staples*

- steady the clips or staples with the dissecting forceps. Depending on the type of clip or staple, either insert one blade of the remover under the centre of the clip or staple and the other blade over, then gently squeeze the blades together *or* place a blade of the remover on the outside of each wing on top of the clip and squeeze the blades together. Depending on the clip or staple type, one or other of these actions should lift the clip from the skin on either side of the wound
- follow health authority policy for the aftercare of a wound. The wound may be cleaned if necessary then left exposed or covered with a semipermeable membrane
- ensure the patient is left as comfortable as possible
- dispose of all equipment safely *for the protection of others*
- document the nursing practice appropriately, monitor after-effects and report abnormal findings immediately.

Relevance to the activities of living	***Maintaining a safe environment***

In a healthy individual the skin and mucous membranes act as a natural defence against the entry of pathogenic microorganisms. When continuity of these tissues is lost even temporarily, there is the potential for creating infection (Ayliffe et al 1993). Infection of any kind is an extremely debilitating process. It can cause a great deal of discomfort and inconvenience to the patient, as well as increasing the length of stay in hospital, with its alteration of lifestyle and huge health costs (Morison & Moffatt 1994).

In an institutional environment airborne pathogenic microorganisms can be reduced by utilising a well ventilated room used solely for procedures involving aseptic technique, or by performing procedures at least 30 minutes after completion of ward cleaning and bedmaking (Ayliffe et al 1993). This may not always be possible in the home setting where the community nurse has little control over the environment (Bale 1994).

There is no need for the nurse to wear a disposable cap or face mask but verbal communication should be kept to a minimum during aseptic technique, to reduce droplet contamination (Ayliffe et al 1993). When a number of aseptic wound dressings are to be performed, a known contaminated and/or infected wound should be treated last to reduce the environmental contamination.

In an institutional setting careful preparation of the equipment to be used can further reduce environmental contamination. The dressings trolley should be washed daily using detergent and water then dried, and immediately prior to preparation for aseptic technique it should be disinfected with 70% ethyl alcohol. It is preferable that the dressings trolley be solely used for that purpose. All equipment packaging should be checked for damage and date of expiry which would render the equipment non-sterile.

At home the nurse should assess each situation on an individual basis and, where possible, create a clean environment; the nurse may therefore have to adopt an educative role (Bale 1994).

The member of staff who performs aseptic technique also requires specific preparation. Due to the nature of the nurse's work her uniform and hands can be a catchment area for pathogenic microorganisms. A disposable plastic apron should be worn to provide a barrier to transmission of microorganisms. Thorough hand washing *prior to* the dressing must be performed while further hand preparation should be performed *during* the aseptic technique as stated in the Guidelines, and when the nurse accidentally contaminates her hands (Ayliffe et al 1993). Alcohol-based hand rub is used for the subsequent hand preparation; it has the benefit that the nurse does not have to leave the patient during the practice.

It is preferable that the skin cleansing lotion be supplied as an individual single-use sterile sachet or bottle. Once a bottle has been opened environmental contamination can occur, so any residual lotion should be discarded. If an aerosol can of irrigating fluid is used, the nurse should ensure that the dispensing nozzle does not become contaminated to act as a source of infection.

Continual use of aseptic skin cleansing lotion may have a detrimental effect on granulation tissue (Cameron & Leiper 1988). Adequate cleansing of an open granulating wound can be achieved with the use of sterile normal saline.

Thomlinson (1987) noted that during the cleansing of a chronic wound the microorganisms were redistributed throughout the tissue rather than being removed from the wound bed.

A non-touch technique reduces the potential problem of contamination from the nurse's hands to the wound. Sterile forceps or gloves can be used, the latter having the benefit of easing manipulative skills and promoting comfort for the patient. As the soiled dressing and equipment used during removal may be contaminated, all items must be discarded before continuing with the aseptic technique. The wound should be cleansed and dried thoroughly, using each swab once only, working from the centre of the wound outwards and from the cleanest part first. These measures may reduce cross-infection from one part of the wound to another. The use of cotton wool balls has been found to be detrimental to the wound healing process as cotton fibres can be left within the wound surface (Johnson 1988).

On completion of the aseptic technique discard all equipment in the appropriate receptacles and seal them, before leaving the patient, to reduce environmental contamination from the soiled equipment. In an institutional setting the trolley should be washed, dried and returned to its place of storage; at home the surface should be cleared of any visible contaminating materials. The nurse should thoroughly wash her hands using soap and water only.

Wound care is a dynamic and evolving process, especially where wound dressing materials are concerned. The nurse has a legal, moral and professional responsibility to ensure that her knowledge and practice of wound care is based on recent research findings (Bennett & Moody 1995).

As a wound drain is in direct contact with the underlying tissues, pathogenic microorganisms could gain entry to a wound through the drain site (Dealey 1994). Maintenance of a closed drainage system and aseptic technique may help to reduce the chance of wound infection.

A wound drain site should be dressed after the incision site to minimise the risk of cross-infection. Gauze swabs should not be cut for keyhole dressings as small pieces of cut gauze may remain within the wound. Commercial keyhole dressings with sealed edges are available. If these are unavailable any suitable sterile dressing may be placed around the drain and secured in position to cover the drain site.

During suture, clip or staple removal, care must be taken to prevent the sharp equipment causing accidental injury to the patient.

Communicating

The nursing practice should be explained simply to the patient. Any discomfort or pain should be anticipated by the nurse and the appropriate analgesic offered, as prescribed by a medical practitioner. At home the nurse should confirm with the patient the date and time of the next dressing change; this will allow the patient to administer a painkiller to reduce the potential discomfort.

The nurse should inform the patient of her intended actions during the nursing practice as this may help to reduce his anxiety.

An explanation for reduced verbal communication during aseptic technique should be given. The nurse must be alert to the fact that her non-verbal communication can often be interpreted by a patient, e.g. when faced with a malodorous or unsightly wound a reaction of disgust must not be evident. The patient's non-verbal communication may be an indicator of his acceptance of a change in his body image if the wound is defacing.

The nurse should observe and note any sign of inflammation such as increased heat, redness or swelling around the wound as this may indicate the presence of infection.

Breathing

The patient's respiration and pulse rates may increase due to anxiety.

Eliminating

The patient should empty his bladder prior to these nursing interventions to facilitate his comfort.

Personal cleansing and dressing

Care must be taken during the performance of this activity of living that the wound dressing or drain comes to no harm.

In some hospital departments, surgical wounds are left exposed to the environment within the first few days of surgery. If this is practised the dried blood along the suture line should not be removed because it acts as a protective barrier.

When securing a dressing with tape, allow for body movement when applying the tape, i.e. stretch out any natural skin creases during the application. Wet wound dressings should be changed immediately except during the first 24 hours following surgery, when the dressing is used as an estimation of approximate fluid loss.

Even before the removal of sutures, clips or staples, an immersion bath or shower can usually be performed by the patient with assistance from the nurse or carer, but this will vary in different health care settings.

Following removal of sutures, clips and staples, advice may have to be given to the patient about aftercare of a healing wound and the most appropriate clothing to wear. The area should be washed and dried carefully each day. The clothing worn on top of the wound should not be tight but may be gently supportive if desired.

Wound dressing deodorants may be found to be useful in concealing the smell from a malodorous wound.

A patient with a chronic wound should be given advice regarding the appropriate care for this Activity of living. For example, the patient with a venous leg ulcer who also has compression bandages in situ will require advice about the most suitable method of personal cleansing and the most appropriate form of hosiery to wear.

Controlling body temperature

A patient with an infected wound may develop pyrexia. The nurse should implement the appropriate nursing intervention to assist the patient if this complication occurs.

Mobilising

A wound dressing should not impede mobilising, but discomfort caused by the presence of a wound drain or awkwardness of the site of the wound may interfere with the patient's normal form of mobilising.

A patient may fear that the sutures, clips or staples holding the wound may give way when mobilising. The nurse should allay his fears and explain the importance and benefit of adequate mobilisation.

The patient may fear that the wound will open up following removal of the wound closures. Some education and guidance may be necessary — many surgical units have printed leaflets with advice and information which can be given to the patient to read at leisure.

Expressing sexuality

Adequate provision of privacy is essential in reducing patient anxiety during these interventions. The nurse should assist the patient in adjusting to his altered body image whether the disfigurement is temporary or permanent.

Sleeping

The patient's normal sleep pattern may be altered due to the discomfort caused by the wound and/or drain. The most appropriate nursing intervention may be to help the patient to find a more comfortable position, or to listen to his concerns and help to allay anxiety, or to administer a prescribed analgesic to reduce discomfort and pain.

Patient education: key points

The nurse should discuss the identified factors which may interfere with wound healing for each patient and, where possible, agree realistic goals for these factors with the patient.

The nurse should provide information and education for the patient and/or carer in the care of the wound between each dressing change.

The community nurse should agree and confirm the place, date and time of the next dressing change with the patient.

At home the patient or carer may assume some or all of the responsibilty for wound care; the nurse therefore has an important role in the education of all concerned.

Some education and guidance may have to be given to allay patients' fears that the wound may open up once the clips or sutures have been removed.

Advice and guidance should be given on any lifestyle restrictions.

References

Wound assessment and aseptic technique

Ayliffe G, Lowbury E, Geddes A, Williams J 1993 Control of hospital infection. Chapman & Hall, London

Bale S 1994 Wound healing. In: Alexander M, Fawcett J, Runciman P (eds) Nursing practice — hospital and home: the adult. Churchill Livingstone, Edinburgh

Benbow M, Dealey C 1995 Parameters of wound assessment. British Journal of Nursing 4(11): 647–651

Bennett G, Moody M 1995 Wound care for health professionals. Chapman & Hall, London

Cameron S, Leiper D 1988 Antiseptic toxicity in open wounds. Nursing Times 84(25): 77–79

Dealey C 1994 The care of wounds. Blackwell Scientific, London

Horton R 1995 Handwashing: the fundamental infection control principle. British Journal of Nursing 4(16): 926–933

Johnson A 1988 Wound care. Community Outlook, February

Morison M 1992 A colour guide to the nursing management of wounds. Wolfe, London

Morison M, Moffat C 1994 A colour guide to the assessment and management of leg ulcers (2nd edn). Mosby-Times Mirror International Publishers, London

Plassmann P 1995 Measuring wounds. Journal of Wound Care 4(6): 269–272

Thomas S, Fear M, Humphreys J 1994 Assessment of patients with chronic wounds. Journal of Wound Care 3(3): 151–154

Thomlinson D 1987 To clean or not to clean. Nursing Times March 4: 71–75

Further reading

Wound assessment and aseptic technique

Alexander J, O'Connor H 1982 The Hampshire dressing aid. Nursing 2(8) (suppl): 6–7

Benbow M 1994 Hydrocolloid dressings. Community Outlook 4(7): 25–30

Benbow M 1995 Intrinsic factors affecting the management of chronic wounds. British Journal of Nursing 4(7): 407–410

Benbow M 1995 Extrinsic factors affecting the management of chronic wounds. British Journal of Nursing 4(9): 534–538

Brunner L, Suddarth D 1992 The textbook of adult nursing. Chapman & Hall, London, ch 2

Charles H 1995 Living with a leg ulcer. Journal of Community Nursing 9(7): 22–24

Fincham Gee C 1990 Nutrition and wound healing. Nursing 4(18): 26–28

Gilchrist B 1990 Washing and dressings after surgery. Nursing Times 86(50): 71

Grocott P 1995 The palliative management of fungating malignant wounds. Journal of Wound Care 4(5): 240–242

Irvine A, Black C 1990 Pressure sore practices (discusses wound dressings). Nursing Times 86(38): 74–78

Kelso H 1989 Alternative technique. Nursing Times 85(23): 40–42

Lawrence J, Lilly H, Kidson A 1994 A novel presentation of saline for wound irrigation. Journal of Wound Care 3(7): 334–337

Roper N, Logan W, Tierney A 1996 The elements of nursing, 4th edn. Churchill Livingstone, Edinburgh, pp 68–70, 81–84, 93–96, 251–253

Sutton J 1989 Accurate wound assessment. Nursing Times 85(38): 68–71

Thomas S 1990 Making sense of hydrocolloid dressings. Nursing Times 86(4): 36–38

Vowden K 1995 Common problems in wound care: wound and ulcer measurement. British Journal of nursing 4(13): 775–779

Walsh M, Ford P 1989 Nursing rituals — research and rational actions. Heinemann Nursing, Oxford, ch 2

Young T 1995 Common problems in wound care: overgranulation. British Journal of Nursing 4(3): 169–171

References

Wound drain care

Guilding 1993 Dimensions of nursing knowledge in wound care. British Journal of Nursing 2(14): 712–716

Nightingale K 1989 Making sense of wound drainage. Nursing Times 85(27): 40–42

Pagget L 1992 Wound dressing packs, a simpler alternative. Journal of Tissue Viability 2(1): 18–21

Thomas S, Loveless P, May N, Toyick N 1993 Comparing non-woven, filmated and woven gauze swabs. Journal of Wound Care 2(1): 35–41

Young T 1995 Common problems in wound care: wound cleansing. British Journal of Nursing 4(5): 286–289

Further reading

Wound drain care

Morison M 1992 A colour guide to the nursing management of wounds. Wolfe, London

Walsh M, Ford P 1989. Nursing rituals, research and rational actions. Heinemann Nursing, Oxford, pp 22–27

References

Removal of stitches, clips or staples

Harding K 1992 The wound programme. Centre for Medical Education, University of Dundee

Leaper D 1986 Antiseptics and their effect on healing tissue. Nursing Times 82(23): 45–47

Further reading

Wound sutures, clips and staples

Jones I 1994 Removal of sutures and staples. Skills update, book 3. McMillan Magazines, London

Nightingale K 1990 Making sense of wound closure. Nursing Times 86(14): 35–37

Index